Women in Engineering and Science

Series Editor
Jill S. Tietjen, Greenwood Village, CO, USA

The Springer Women in Engineering and Science series highlights women's accomplishments in these critical fields. The foundational volume in the series provides a broad overview of women's multi-faceted contributions to engineering over the last century. Each subsequent volume is dedicated to illuminating women's research and achievements in key, targeted areas of contemporary engineering and science endeavors.The goal for the series is to raise awareness of the pivotal work women are undertaking in areas of keen importance to our global community.

More information about this series at https://link.springer.com/bookseries/15424

Florence D. Hudson

Editor

Women Securing the Future with TIPPSS for Connected Healthcare

Trust, Identity, Privacy, Protection, Safety, Security

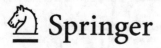 Springer

Editor
Florence D. Hudson
FDHint, LLC
Purchase
NY, USA

ISSN 2509-6427 ISSN 2509-6435 (electronic)
Women in Engineering and Science
ISBN 978-3-030-93594-8 ISBN 978-3-030-93592-4 (eBook)
https://doi.org/10.1007/978-3-030-93592-4

This Springer imprint is published by the registered company Springer Nature Switzerland AG
The registered company address is: Gewerbestrasse 11, 6330 Cham, Switzerland

This book is dedicated to my family who supports me and loves me through my weekend and vacation book writing and editing time, especially my husband George, and children Kristen and Ryan Hudson.

This book is in loving memory of my dear brother Charlie DiStefano, who passed away in May 2021 after a long and brave battle with cancer.

Preface

Welcome to the TIPPSS community. In reading this book, you are joining us on a journey that will last a lifetime. Together we are on a mission to increase awareness of the security, privacy, and safety considerations in connected healthcare and provide recommendations and approaches to improve Trust, Identity, Privacy, Protection, Safety, and Security for humans, devices, and data.

This is the second book on *Women Securing the Future with TIPPSS* in the Springer Women in Engineering and Science series. The first book, *Women Securing the Future with TIPPSS for IoT—Trust, Identity, Privacy, Protection, Safety, Security for the Internet of Things* was published in 2019 [1]. I must thank Jill Tietjan, a former President of the Society of Women Engineers (SWE) with whom I have collaborated over the years including when I was an SWE Director and Trustee, for inviting me to write and edit a few books in *the Springer Women in Engineering and Science* series. It has been a pleasure creating the vision for these books and bringing along with me dozens of women who have penned chapters to address the TIPPSS issues we have in our increasingly connected world. Having been trained as an aerospace and mechanical engineer and enjoying a series of leadership roles in engineering and technology including at NASA, Grumman, IBM, Indiana University, my FDHint consulting firm, and now Columbia University, my passions run deep to make the world a better place.

In this book, *Women Securing the Future with TIPPSS for Connected Healthcare—Trust, Identity, Privacy, Protection, Safety, Security*, you will enter a world of expertise and mission-based focus led by deep thinking and clear communications from 17 women who will increase your awareness of the challenges in connected healthcare security and privacy. We will share our thoughts on how to address these challenges with new perspectives and approaches to improve TIPPSS, with the goal to protect the patients, secure the devices and data, and enable a safer future of connected healthcare across the world. The authors of this book have written excellent perspectives on the concerns about the level of TIPPSS—Trust, Identity, Privacy, Protection, Safety, Security—that exists today in connected healthcare systems and medical devices, and the improvements which need to be made today and into the future. These women are engineers, technologists, medical professionals, neuroscientists, psychologists, ethicists, academics, educators, researchers, data scientists, lawyers, architects, business leaders, standard leaders, and patient advocates. Our expertise spans advanced technologies, medicine, healthcare, medical device security, cybersecurity, threat intelligence, counterintelligence, artificial intelligence, machine learning, privacy, trust, equity, health informatics, telehealth, standards, policy, law, ethics, inclusion, equity, accessibility, sustainability, interoperability, wireless networks, mobile medicine, industrial control systems, and rocket science.

The current reality is that all the connected medical devices and systems we know and use today are hackable. The U.S. Department of Homeland Security [2] and Food and Drug Administration [3] have issued alerts regarding cybersecurity vulnerabilities from medical devices to ransomware. We must work as a team across many disciplines in the connected healthcare ecosystem to ensure the "things" that make up the Internet of Medical Things (IoMT) and the systems they connect with are secure. This includes ensuring that the devices or services connecting to a device can be trusted, that the identity of the incoming service request or person can be validated by a trusted authority, that the privacy of the data and the individual is maintained, that the humans and the infrastructure using the device are protected, and that we maintain safety and security. This is called TIPPSS. The TIPPSS elements are as follows:

- Trust: allow only designated people or services to have device or data access
- Identity: validate the identity of people, services, and "things"
- Privacy: ensure device, personal, and sensitive data are kept private
- Protection: protect devices and users from physical, financial, and reputational harm
- Safety: provide safety for devices, infrastructure, and people
- Security: maintain security of data, devices, institutions, systems, and people

We thank the Institute of Electrical and Electronics Engineers (IEEE) and the United States National Science Foundation (NSF) for supporting the development of the TIPPSS framework, beginning with a workshop they sponsored to discuss the challenges in end-to-end trust and security technology and policy for the Internet of Things in 2016 [4]. IEEE has further developed awareness of the TIPPSS framework through articles in IEEE IT Professional Magazine [5] and Computer Magazine [6] in 2018, and through a pre-standards workstream which resulted in a paper published in 2019 on Clinical IoT Data Validation and Interoperability with Blockchain [7]. IEEE continues its commitment to connected healthcare cybersecurity and TIPPSS through the support of IEEE/UL working group P2933 which has 250 people working together from around the world to develop a standard for "Clinical Internet of Things (IoT) Data and Device Interoperability with TIPPSS—Trust, Identity, Privacy, Protection, Safety, Security." You are welcome to join us by visiting the website for the IEEE/UL working group [8]. The Global

Connected Healthcare Cybersecurity Workshop series [9], sponsored by the IEEE Standards Association and the NSF-funded Northeast Big Data Innovation Hub headquartered at Columbia University [10], is another vehicle used to engage the broader community in this endeavor.

TIPPSS is a journey. We need it in our connected healthcare [6], smart cities [11], and across all IoT-enabled systems. If it is connected, it needs to be protected. We are honored to have the women securing the future with TIPPSS for connected healthcare sharing their thoughts and insights in this book, and we look forward to continuing in this important journey together.

References

1. Hudson F.D. (Ed.) (2019) Women Securing the Future with TIPPSS for IoT - Trust, Identity, Privacy, Protection, Safety, Security for the Internet of Things. DOI https://doi.org/10.1007/978-3-030-15705-0
2. U.S. Department of Homeland Security. Cybersecurity & Infrastructure Security Agency. https://us-cert.cisa.gov/
3. U.S. Food & Drug Administration. Medical Device Safety. https://www.fda.gov/medical-devices/medical-device-safety
4. IEEE Standards Association. (2016). IEEE Trust and Security Workshop for the Internet of Things. https://internetinitiative.ieee.org/images/files/events/ieee_end_to_end_trust_meeting_recap_feb17.pdf
5. IEEE Computer Society. IT Professional Magazine. Technology Solutions for the Enterprise. "Enabling Trust and Security: TIPPSS for IoT". March/April 2018
6. IEEE Computer Society. Computer Magazine. "Wearables and Medical Interoperability: The Evolving Frontier". September 2018
7. IEEE. Pre-Standards Workstream Report: Clinical IoT Data Validation and Interoperability with Blockchain. https://ieeexplore.ieee.org/document/8764088
8. IEEE Standards Association. P2933 - Clinical Internet of Things (IoT) Data and Device Interoperability with TIPPSS Working Group. https://sagroups.ieee.org/2933/
9. IEEE Global Connected Healthcare Cybersecurity Workshop Series https://standards.ieee.org/practices/healthcare-life-sciences/gchc.html
10. Northeast Big Data Innovation Hub headquartered at Columbia University https://nebigdatahub.org/about/
11. Hudson F. Cather M. "Creating, Analysing and Sustaining Smarter Cities: A Systems Perspective". Chapter 6 "TIPPSS - Trust, Identity, Privacy, Protection, Safety and Security For Smart Cities". (2017) ISBN-10: 1848902093, ISBN-13: 978-1848902091

Other Springer Books by Florence D. Hudson

Women Securing the Future with TIPPSS for IoT—Trust, Identity, Privacy, Protection, Safety and Security for the Internet of Things—2019

ISBN 978-3-030-15704-3
ISBN 978-3-030-15707-4 (softcover)
ISBN 978-3-030-15705-0 (eBook)

Purchase, NY, USA   Florence D. Hudson

Contents

Editor and Contributors

About the Editor

Florence D. Hudson is Editor in Chief for this book *Women Securing the Future with TIPPSS for Connected Healthcare*. This is the second book in the TIPPSS series, as part of the *Springer Women in Engineering and Science* series. The first was *Women Securing the Future with TIPPSS for IoT—Trust, Identity, Privacy, Protection, Safety, Security for the Internet of Things* published by Springer Nature Switzerland in 2019.

The book title including TIPPSS is meant to have two meanings. TIPPSS is the basis for a standard Florence is leading the development of globally with IEEE and Underwriters Laboratories (UL) to improve Trust, Identity, Privacy, Protection, Safety, and Security for Clinical IoT devices and connected healthcare solutions. The other meaning is that women can provide tips on how to create a safer connected healthcare environment.

Florence is currently Executive Director of the Northeast Big Data Innovation Hub at Columbia University and Founder and CEO of FDHint, LLC, a global advanced technology and diversity and inclusion consulting firm (www.fdhint.com). She leads the COVID Information Commons (https://covidinfocommons.net) funded by the U.S. National Science Foundation (NSF), providing an open resource to explore research and enable global collaboration for COVID-19 pandemic recovery. She is a former IBM Vice President and Chief Technology Officer, Internet2 Senior Vice President and Chief Innovation Officer, Special Advisor for the NSF Cybersecurity Center of Excellence at Indiana University, and aerospace engineer at NASA and Grumman. She Chairs the global IEEE/UL P2933 Working Group on Clinical IoT Data and Device Interoperability with TIPPSS—Trust, Identity, Privacy, Protection, Safety, Security and has published books on TIPPSS. She serves on Boards for Princeton University, California Polytechnic State University San Luis Obispo, Stony Brook University, Blockchain in Healthcare Today, the IEEE Engineering in Medicine and Biology Society and the Neuroscience Outreach Network. She has a BSE in Mechanical and Aerospace Engineering from Princeton University and executive business education from Harvard and Columbia Universities.

About the Authors

Katherine Grace August, PhD is a Research Guest at Stevens Institute of Technology—ECE Intelligent Networks. Her current research projects involve humanitarian activities, Health and Justice for All, following the United Nations Sustainable Development Goals (UN SDGs) 3, 4, 10 including focus on innovating inclusion, equity, accessibility, sustainability, interoperability, and scalability in communication technologies and solutions, and employing sustainable low-cost mainstream technology to connect the unconnected with culturally and linguistically appropriate solutions (U.S. Department of Health & Human Services CLAS). Dr. August focuses on SDGs to promote health and well-being, promote gender equality, and reduce inequity, for example, to improve ease of use, curate and reduce bias in data, algorithms, processes, and in solutions. These projects promote improved opportunity for underrepresented minorities, women, and girls, with an emphasis on inventing. Dr. August has research experience in neurorehabilitation with robots, haptics, augmented and virtual reality, functional brain imaging, biological, analog and digital signal processing, wireless, systems engineering, communications, steganography, intelligent systems, search, AIML, speech processing, and the like. Dr. August is formerly a Bell Labs Member of the Technical Staff for New Service Concepts Systems Engineering 1991–2002. Eighteen US patents; 50 international patents; Citations: 3234, h index 22, i10 index 25; IEEE Dignity, Inclusion, Identity, Trust and Agency (DIITA) Workflow—Transparent Design for Wellbeing, IEEE NJ Coast Section PACE SIGHT Group Chair, AP-VT-EMC Chapter Vice Chair, Computers Chapter Vice Chair, IEEE ComSoc History Committee; Whitaker Scholar 2009–2012 at ETH Zurich, Brooklyn Academy of Music (BAM) Arts in Technology Award Virtual Actor with John Jesurun and Daniel Lee, PhD. Kit received the PhD in Biomedical Engineering, Newark College of Engineering NJIT, the MSCS-MIS, Marist College, and BFA Communications Design, Parsons the New School for Design.

Cory Brennan, JD is an attorney at Hall Render and a security advisor. As an experienced information security leader in healthcare as well as a health law attorney, she has focused her practice on developing practical, operationally focused cybersecurity, privacy, and compliance recommendations. Her healthcare operations background and qualification as a Certified Information Systems Security Professional (CISSP) allow her to bring a functional perspective to complex privacy, security, and research issues with a focus on solutions that work in the real world. She has significant experience with clinical device cybersecurity and health system compliance audits and has regularly assisted with and conducted risk assessments, incident and breach response, and information governance development, as well as compliance issues, developing enterprise governance, risk, and compliance programs. She has extensive practical knowledge of healthcare information security and compliance standards, including HIPAA/HITECH, NIST, and ISO. She is a member of the Healthcare Technology Leadership Council for the Association for the Advancement of Medical Instrumentation (AAMI), the American College of Clinical Engineering (ACCE), and the American Health Law Association. Additionally, she sits on the Board of The Next IT Girl, which aims to help young women of color discover, pursue, and succeed in technology-related careers. She received a Master of Science in Cybersecurity Risk Management and a JD from Indiana University.

Zulema Belyeu Caldwell, PhD graduated with a BS in Electrical Engineering from Texas A&M University and an MS in Electrical Engineering from the University of Maryland at College Park. She completed her PhD in Information Technology with a specialization in Computer Information Security at Capella University. Zulema has a wealth of experience as a researcher, engineer, and software developer. She was the former owner and lead technical partner for a defense contracting company, which served multiple Department of Defense (DoD) agencies. Zulema has served as a technical director for several organizations within the Department of Defense, and she has also served as a program manager responsible for the budget and resources of multi-tiered national security projects. She is currently a technical director specializing in cybersecurity solutions for critical infrastructure, industrial control systems, and Industrial Internet of Things (IIoT) devices. Zulema has performed research for several projects focused on energy disaggregation, machine learning anomaly detection, and security event management for industrial control systems. She is a certified computer information security specialist (CISSP), and she has served as an instructor at several higher learning institutions. She taught computer science courses at Anne Arundel Community College, and she is currently an adjunct faculty member teaching graduate level information assurance and cybersecurity courses at the University of Maryland Global Campus, where she focuses on research for understanding the threat landscape, conducting security assessments, and identifying control measures or mitigations for a variety of information systems, including financial information systems, electronic health records management systems, telecommunications, and industrial control systems. Zulema is also a founding member of the University of Maryland Clark School Women in Engineering Advisory Board, and she devotes a significant amount of time supporting STEM programs at local elementary schools and serving as a mentor for high school and college students.

Jenny Colgate is a partner at Rothwell, Figg, Ernst & Manbeck PC, in Washington, DC. She is an experienced litigator, creative strategist, trusted advisor, and thought leader. She typically handles technology-related cases involving all areas of intellectual property including patents, trade secrets, trademarks, copyright, unfair competition, unfair trade practices, data protection, and privacy. She provides counsel on complex issues including developing and updating compliance strategies, litigation threat letters, negotiating and drafting agreements, and evaluating the legal risks of pursuing various business actions. She is also a mom, an accomplished equestrian, a former marathoner, and an animal lover. Jenny received her JD from the University of New Hampshire School of Law (formerly Franklin Pierce Law Center) and her Bachelor of Arts from the University of Pennsylvania.

Alexis Diamond is an associate with Vantage Technology Consulting Group. Alexis holds a bachelor's degree in Architecture from the University of Southern California and is an Associate AIA member. Alexis uses her background in architecture to ensure that technology is incorporated into a healthcare facility effectively. As a member of the Healthcare Information and Management Systems Society (HIMSS), Alexis promotes technology integration in major acute care and outpatient medical facilities to improve communication, workflow efficiencies, and the healing environment.

Emily Dillon is a security program manager at Indiana Health Information Exchange. She is a knowledgeable security analyst with a background in regulatory and quality compliance when related to the healthcare industry, providing subject-matter expertise for cybersecurity and risk management with proficiency in technology assessments, risk management, industry regulations and standards, and data analysis.

Sherri Douville is CEO and Board Member at Medigram and is a sought-after speaker and author in mobile medical technology, other healthcare-related industries, leadership, risk management, mobile security, and governance. Ms. Douville is honored to strategically build, grow, and lead multidisciplinary, multi-industry teams at Medigram and in the market to solve the leading cause of preventable death—a delay in information. Ms. Douville is co-chair of the technical trust and identity standard subgroup for the healthcare industry for clinical IoT through IEEE and UL and has been published and quoted in both mainstream and industry media such as CIO.com, the San Jose Mercury News, NBC, Becker's Hospital Review, ThisWeekinHealthIT.com, and HITInfrastructure.com. Other industry leadership has included serving on the board of the NorCal HIMSS and teaching continuing education credit in mobile security for CISSP, the information security certification. She is co-author for a number of technical articles and papers, a forthcoming Springer book chapter on Trust in Clinical IoT and is the lead author and editor for *Mobile Medicine: Overcoming People, Culture, and Governance* (Taylor & Francis). Ms. Douville led the development of this industry guide to mobile computing in medicine and built the international, multi-industry, and multidisciplinary team behind it. Prior to her current work in the mobile medicine, privacy, security, health IT, and AI industries, Sherri worked in the medical device space consulting in the areas of physician acceptance and economic feasibility for medical devices. Prior to that, she worked for over a decade with products addressing over a dozen disease states at Johnson & Johnson and was recognized for industry thought leadership there by McGraw-Hill and won a number of awards. Ms. Douville has a Bachelor of Combined Sciences degree from Santa Clara University and has completed certificates in electrical engineering, computer science, AI, and ML through MIT. She advises and serves startups, boards, and organizations including as a member of the Board of Fellows for Santa Clara University and an advisor to the Santa Clara University Leavey School of Business Corporate Board Education initiatives, the Black Corporate Board Readiness, and Women's Corporate Board Readiness programs.

Joanna Lyn Grama is an associate vice president with Vantage Technology Consulting Group. Joanna has more than 20 years of experience with a strong focus in law, higher education, information security, and data privacy. A former member of the U.S. Department of Homeland Security's Data Privacy and Integrity Advisory Committee, Joanna is a frequent author and regular speaker on information security and privacy topics. Joanna received her JD from the University of Illinois College of Law with honors, her BA in International Relations from the University of Minnesota, and holds a number of security and privacy industry certifications.

Gabrielle E. Hempel is a system engineer at RSA Security. She is a graduate of the University of Cincinnati, where she studied Neuroscience and Psychology. She started her career in pharmaceutical/medical device regulation, where she led specialized committees targeting Phase I and emergency use research. She still serves on a board as a regulatory/genetic science consultant and moved to cybersecurity in 2018, working as a Cloud Security Engineer in healthcare. She also serves as a member of the Marine Corps Cyber Auxiliary and a consultant for the National Security Innovation Network (NSIN). She continues to pursue education through a master's program in Global Security, Conflict, and Cybercrime at New York University and has obtained certifications in threat intelligence, counterintelligence, and human trafficking investigation through the McAfee Institute. She collaborates with a variety of law enforcement entities and task forces to assist in and educate on use of digital forensics and information security to combat trafficking. She has spoken at numerous national conferences and guest lectured on medical device security and trafficking. Her continued areas of research include embedded/vehicle security, IoT vulnerabilities, and medical device/healthcare security.

Jennifer Maisel is a partner at Rothwell, Figg, Ernst & Manbeck PC in Washington, DC, where she focuses on intellectual property and privacy law matters involving cutting-edge technology. Her practice encompasses all aspects of intellectual property law including litigation, post-grant review proceedings before the Patent Trial and Appeal Board, patent prosecution, transactions, opinions, and counselling. She is also a Certified Information Privacy Professional in the United States (CIPP/US) and counsels clients on privacy and data security matters. She is selected to the Washington, DC Super Lawyers "Rising Star" list (2018–2021) and is included in Best Lawyers: Ones to Watch (2021–2022), which recognizes extraordinary lawyers who have been in private practice for less than 10 years.

Melissa Markey is a shareholder with Hall, Render, Killian, Heath & Lyman, one of the nation's top health law firms, in the Denver, Colorado office, and is licensed to practice as an attorney in Texas, Michigan, Utah, and Colorado. Melissa's practice focuses on cybersecurity, privacy, and life sciences issues, particularly research misconduct and grant compliance, mobile medical applications, and innovations in health technology. She leads the Life Sciences team at Hall Render and has a particular interest in cybersecurity and legal issues at the developing edge of technology. Ms. Markey is a Certified Information Systems Security Professional (CISSP), a paramedic, was on the Board of Directors and is now a Fellow of the

American Health Lawyers Association, is a member of the Healthcare Information and Management Systems Society (HIMSS) and the computer law sections of the American Bar Association as well as the State Bars of Texas, Utah, and Michigan. She is a nationally recognized author and presenter on data privacy and security, clinical research and human subject protection, the clinical-technology interface, research misconduct, and emergency preparedness and response law.

Ann Mongoven, PhD, MPH is a healthcare ethicist with a focus on public health. Currently working in Covid-response for Heluna Health under contract to Santa Clara County, she previously held academic positions in healthcare ethics at Indiana University, Michigan State University, and Santa Clara University. Her training includes a BA in Science Policy from Princeton University, an MPH from Johns Hopkins University and a PhD in Religious Studies and Ethics from the University of Virginia. In addition to teaching healthcare ethics to undergraduate, graduate, nursing, and medical students, she served on several hospital and medical association ethics committees, and on a state institutional review board. Mongoven facilitated community-engaged and policy-engaged research on transplantation ethics and biobanking ethics. She has special interest in ethical challenges of developing trustworthy complex health systems to serve diverse patients.

Paula Muller, PhD Founder of Sociavi, has a lifelong passion for technology applied to healthcare beginning with her MS in Biomedical Engineering in Chile working with the blind, then her work in Switzerland analyzing EEGs to prevent epileptic seizures, followed by her PhD and Post-doc work at Rutgers with Parkinson patients, and later at Authentidate with Telehealth products and services. Paula is a Certified Alzheimer's Disease and Dementia Care Training (CADDCT) and Certified Dementia Practitioner (CDP) and volunteers as a bilingual Community Educator for the Alzheimer's Association. The concept of Sociavi evolved from her professional background as well as her strong commitment to family relations and lifetime connections. Thus, SOCIAVI was born, meaning in Latin to "share" and "unite," with the goal of keeping those aging in place and their families connected and closer together. Their specifically designed, touch screen communication device, the Sociavi C2M (Connect To Me), provides the users with a "small appliance," that is simple to operate and easily integrates into their daily life. Simplicity is the Cornerstone of Sociavi: No Login, No Password, No Username, No Account Setup. Just a 13-in. screen hands-free device simple to navigate along with an array of brain fitness activities that stimulate and soothe the mind. Paula and her company were awarded two patents from the USPTO in 2020 on the methods and devices for a Communication System for Use with Protected Persons. At Sociavi, they are proud to give Peace of Mind to families and caregivers through their Sociavi C2M that allows families to connect with their Loved Ones Far, Near, Simply, and Globally.

Tanja Pavleska is a researcher at the Laboratory for Open Systems and Networks at Jozef Stefan Institute. She graduated from the Faculty of Electrical Engineering in Skopje, Macedonia. She obtained her PhD from the Jozef Stefan International

Postgraduate School in the area of Computational Trust and Reputation Systems. Her main interests are trust and reputation management, user behavior in digital platforms, critical infrastructure security, cybernetics and complexity in online systems, Internet governance, digital policies and regulatory frameworks, and IoT in Healthcare. She coordinates and performs research for both national and EU projects in her area of interests. She coordinated the development of the cybersecurity evaluation methodology for large-scale pilots (e-Justice, e-Health, e-Agriculture, e-Business, e-Procurement, etc.) in the EU FP7 e-SENS (Electronic Simple European Networked Services) project, as well as the development of the policies and regulatory frameworks for online misinformation in the H2020 EU project COMPACT. Currently, she is leading the work on EU governance landscape in the H2020 project DE4A (Digital Europe for All) and has developed the methodology for assessment of the architecture building block in the same project. Tanja is also the Chair of the Slovenian Internet Society (ISOC) chapter.

Jodyn Platt, PhD, MPH is an Assistant Professor of Learning Health Sciences trained in Medical Sociology and Health Policy. She is widely published in trust in informatics and information systems with more than 30 peer-reviewed papers. She has been the Principal Investigator on grants >$3.3 million funded by the National Institutes of Health and foundations. She regularly speaks at national conferences and invited presentations on trust, equity, and ethics as they relate to emerging health information technologies. She is also a mentor and teacher and has designed and taught graduate-level courses in policy and ethics of health IT for students studying health informatics, implementation science, and other interdisciplinary health sciences. Her research focuses on and addresses ethical and policy issues raised by using the health information of individuals in "Big Data" and data analytics. She is passionate about and expert in understanding what makes health information systems trusted by diverse stakeholders and interdisciplinary teams. She is motivated by the goal of serving people and institutions in their mission to become sustainable partners in the care ecosystem.

Mathini Sellathurai, PhD is Dean Science and Engineering at Heriot Watt University, Edinburgh, UK and Full Professor of Signal Processing and Intelligent Systems. She was previously at Bell Laboratories, New Jersey, USA, as a visiting researcher and at the Communications Research Centre, Ottawa, Canada, as a senior research scientist. She holds an honorary Professorship at McMaster University, Ontario, Canada. She is leading research (over 215 IEEE papers) in signal processing and machine learning for wireless communications and radar. She has won the IEEE Communication Society Fred W. Ellersick Best Paper Award 2005, Industry Canada Public Service Awards for contributions in science and technology, 2005, and the Best PhD Thesis Award/Medal from NSERC Canada, 2002. She is a member of the IEEE SPCOM Technical Strategy Committee, an Editor of IEEE TSP and was the General Chair of IEEE SPAWC 2016 in Edinburgh. She is also a fellow of Higher Education Academy, UK. Presently funded by EPSRC and DSTL. The research group is also involved in European Union FrameWork 7 projects cognitive radio-oriented wireless networks and interference alignment.

Oshani Seneviratne is the Director of Health Data Research at the Institute for Data Exploration and Applications at the Rensselaer Polytechnic Institute. Oshani obtained her SM and PhD degrees in Computer Science from MIT in 2009 and 2014, respectively, under the supervision of Sir Tim Berners-Lee, the inventor of the World Wide Web. Oshani's current research interests span knowledge representation and decentralized systems. Oshani leads the Smart Contracts Augmented with Analytics Learning and Semantics (SCALeS) project at Rensselaer and is also involved in the Health Empowerment by Analytics, Learning, and Semantics (HEALS) project. Before Rensselaer, Oshani worked at Oracle, specializing in distributed systems, provenance, and healthcare-related research. Oshani has published over 50 research articles. She has co-organized many technical events, including the Personal Health Knowledge Graph Workshops at the Knowledge Graph Conference (2020–2021), IEEE AIChain workshop series (2019–2021), AAAI Fall Symposium on AI for Social Good (2019–2020), Developers Day at the Web Conference (2016), and the AAAI Symposium on Structured Data for Humanitarian Technologies (2015). Oshani is a co-editor of Semantic Technologies for Data and Algorithmic Governance, and actively reviews for the Journals of Web Semantics, Medical Internet Research, Biomedical and Health Informatics, and many conferences.

Abbreviations

AAL	Ambient Assisted Living
AAMI	Association for the Advancement of Medical Instrumentation
ACCE	American College of Clinical Engineering
ADA	Americans with Disabilities Act
AES	Advanced Encryption Standard
AI	Artificial Intelligence
AIDS	Acquired Immunodeficiency Syndrome
AMI	Acute Myocardial Infarction
APPE	Association of Practical and Professional Ethics
APHA	American Public Health Association
ASBH	American Society for Bioethics and Humanities
BIPA	Biometric Information Privacy Act
BLE	Bluetooth Low Energy
BMI	Body Mass Index
BSC	Balanced scorecard
CAGR	Compound Annual Growth Rate
CARE	Collective benefit, Authority, Responsibility, Ethics
CCPA	California Consumer Privacy Act
CDC	Centers for Disease Control and Prevention
CEES	Center for Engineering Ethics and Society
CFR	Code of Federal Regulations
CIA	Confidentiality, Integrity, Availability
CIO	Chief Information Officers
CIS	Center for Internet Security
CISA	Cybersecurity and Infrastructure Security Agency
CL	Connected Lifestyles
CLAS	Culturally and Linguistically Appropriate Services
CMS	Centers for Medicare and Medicaid Services
CNL	Cannot Locate
COPD	Chronic Obstructive Pulmonary Disease

COPPA	Children's Online Privacy Protection Act
CPAP	Continuous Positive Airway Pressure Machine
CPU	Central Processing Unit
CRT-D	Cardiac Resynchronization Therapy Defibrillator
CT	Computed Tomography
CSC	Crisis Standards of Care
CVSS	Common Vulnerability Scoring System
dB	Decibel
DBIR	Data Breach Investigation Report
DBS	Deep Brain Stimulation
DDoS	Distributed Denial of Service
DHS	U.S. Department of Homeland Security
DKA	Diabetic Ketoacidosis
DNA	Deoxyribonucleic Acid
EA	Enterprise Architecture
EC	European Commission
ECG	Electrocardiogram
EEG	Electroencephalograph
EHR	Electronic Health Record
EIRA	European Interoperability Reference Architecture
eMBB	Enhanced Mobile Broadband
EMF	Electromagnetic Field
EMR	Electronic Medical Record
EMS	Emergency Medical Services
ENISA	European Union Agency for Cybersecurity
eSENS	Electronic Simple European Networked Services
EU	European Union
FAA	Federal Aviation Administration
FAIR	Findability, Accessibility, Interoperability, and Reusability
FCC	Federal Communications Commission
FDA	Food and Drug Administration
FHIR	Fast Healthcare Interoperability Resources
FHS	Framingham Heart Study
FIPPs	Fair Information Practice Principles
FTC	Federal Trade Commission
FUD	Fear, Uncertainty and Doubt
GA	Genetic Alliance
GARB	Genetic Alliance Registry and Biobank
GB	Gigabyte
GDPR	General Data Protection Regulation
GHz	Gigahertz
GINA	Genetic Information Nondiscrimination Act
GPS	Global Positioning Systems
GQM	Goal-Question Metrics
HDO	Health Delivery Organization

HHNS	Hyperosmolar Hyperglycemic Nonketotic Syndrome
HHS	U.S. Department of Health & Human Services
HIPAA	Health Insurance Portability and Accountability Act
HITECH	Health Information Technology for Economic and Clinical Health
HIV	Human Immunodeficiency Virus
HL7	Health Level Seven, Inc.
HotF	Hospital of the Future
HPH	Healthcare and Public Health
HSCC	Healthcare Sector Coordinating Council
HVAC	Heating, Ventilation, and Air Conditioning
H2H	Human to Human
ICD	Implantable Cardioverter Defibrillators
ICS	Industrial Control Systems
ICU	Intensive Care Unit
IDC	International Data Corporation
IEC	International Electrotechnical Commission
IEEE	Institute of Electrical and Electronics Engineers
IEM	Ingestible Event Marker
IHE	Integrating the Health Enterprise
IIC	Industrial Internet Consortium
IIHS	Insurance Institute for Highway Safety
IIRA	Industrial Internet Reference Architecture
IIS	Industrial Internet Systems
IMDRF	International Medical Device Regulators Forum
IoMT	Internet of Medical Things
IoT	Internet of Things
IP address	Internet Protocol address
IPFS	Inter Planetary File System
IPNet	Internet Protocol Network
IPSec	Internet Protocol Security
IRB	Institutional Review Board
ISO	International Organization for Standardization
ISO/IEC JTC 1/SC 27	Standardization subcommittee of the Joint Technical Committee ISO/IEC JTC 1 of the International Organization for Standardization and the International Electrotechnical Commission
ISO IoT RA	The ISO Reference Architecture for IoT
ISP	Internet Service Provider
IST	Institute for Security and Technology
IT	Information Technology
ITU	International Telecommunications Union
JAMA	Journal of the American Medical Association
JSP	Joint Security Plan
Kbps	Kilobits per second

LoRaWAN	Long Range Wide-Area Network
LPWAN	Low-Power Wide-Area Network
MAC address	Media Access Control address
MAUDE	Manufacturer and User Facility Device Experience
MCAE	Markkula Center for Applied Ethics at Santa Clara University
MDCG	Medical Device Coordination Group
MDDT	Medical Device Development Tool
MDISS	Medical Device Innovation, Safety, and Security Consortium
MDS	Movement Disorder Society
MDSAP	Medical Device Single Audit Program
MIMO	Massive Multi-Input Multi-Output
MIT	Massachusetts Institute of Technology
ML	Machine Learning
m:m	many to many
mMTC	massive Machine-Type Communication
MOSA2	MOdular Security Aware Architecture
MQTT	Message Queuing Telemetry Transport
MRI	Magnetic Resonance Imaging
ms	Millisecond
MTTD	Mean Time To Detection
MTTF	Mean Time To Fix or Failure
MTTR	Mean Time To Repair or Recovery
NCCoE	National Cybersecurity Center of Excellence
NEST	National Evaluation System for Health Technology
NFC	Near Field Communication
NHS	National Health Service in the UK
NHTSA	National Highway Traffic Safety Administration
NIS Directive	Network and Information Systems Directive
NIST	National Institute of Standards and Technology
NOMA	Non-Orthogonal Multiple Access
NP	Non-deterministic Polynomial acceptable problems
NSA	National Security Agency
NSIN	National Security Innovation Network
NSPE	National Society of Professional Engineers
NYU	New York University
OCTA	Organised Crime Threat Assessment
OFAC	Office of Foreign Assets Control
ONC	Office of the National Coordinator for Health IT
OR	Oregon
OSE	Operating System Embedded
OTS	Off-The-Shelf
PAR	Periodic Automatic Replenishment
PC	Personal Computer

PET	Positron Emission Tomography
PHT	Personal Health Train
PI	Personal Information
PII	Personally Identifiable Information
PKG	Parkinson's KinetiGraph
PLC	Programmable Logic Controllers
POC	Proof Of Concept
PPACA	Patient Protection and Affordable Care Act
PPE	Personal Protective Equipment
PrEP	Pre-Exposure Prophylaxis
QS	Quality System (QS) Regulation
RAMI	Reference Architecture Model for Industry
RDP	Remote Desktop Protocol
RF	Radio Frequency
RMIAS	Reference Model for Information And Security
RTF	Ransomware Task Force
RTLS	Real Time Location System
SaMD	Software as a Medical Device
SBOM	Software Bill Of Materials
SCADA	Supervisory Control And Data Acquisition
SDLC	Security Development Life Cycle
SDN	Specially Designated Nationals and Blocked Persons List
SLA	Service Level Agreement
SMB	Server Message Block
SMS	Short Message Service
SON	Self-Organizing Network
SPM	Security Process Management
SUPPORT	Surfactant, Positive Pressure, and Oxygenation Randomized Trial
TAP	Trust, Accessibility, and Privacy
TIPPSS	Trust, Identity, Privacy, Protection, Safety, Security
TIR	Technical Information Report
TJC	The Joint Commission
TKIP	Temporal Key Integrity Protocol
TLP	Traffic Light Protocol
TOGAF	The Open Group Architecture Framework
TRUST	Transparency, Responsibility, User focus, Sustainability, and Technology
TTPs	Tactics, Techniques, and Procedures
UAV	Unmanned Aerial Vehicles
UDAP	Unfair and Deceptive Acts and Practices
UE	User Equipment
UIX	User Interaction and Experience
UL	Underwriters Laboratories
UN	United Nations

UNCTAD	United Nations Conference on Trade and Development
UNDP	United Nations Development Programme
URL	Uniform Resource Locator
URLLC	Ultra- Reliable Low- Latency Communication
US	United States of America
USD	United States Dollars
WEP	Wired Equivalent Privacy
WHO	World Health Organization
WiFi	Wireless Fidelity
WPA	WiFi Protected Access
WPA2	WiFi Protected Access II
ZB	Zettabyte
3G	Third-generation wireless communication technology
5G	Fifth-generation wireless communication technology

Chapter 1
Health Data Management for Internet of Medical Things

Oshani Seneviratne

Contents

1.1 Introduction

The explosion of big data and advances in information technology has profoundly changed how information is stored, exchanged, managed, and analyzed in healthcare. Electronic Health Records (EHR) have enabled the digitization of patient records and substantially transformed the healthcare delivery system. At the same time, the emergence of IoMT devices has been increasingly applied in remote patient health monitoring, healthcare decision-making, and medical research by offering various physiological data to a broad group of health data stakeholders. In

O. Seneviratne (✉)
Rensselaer Polytechnic Institute, Troy, NY, USA
e-mail: senevo@rpi.edu

© Springer Nature Switzerland AG 2022
F. D. Hudson (eds.), *Women Securing the Future with TIPPSS for Connected Healthcare*, Women in Engineering and Science,
https://doi.org/10.1007/978-3-030-93592-4_1

some estimates, the IoMT device data market will be worth over half a trillion USD by 2027 [1]. According to Justin Fanelli, Chief Architect of Defense Medical Intelligence Data and the Technical Director at the Naval Information Warfare Center, "before 1950, healthcare data doubled every 50 years, now it is doubling about every 50 days, and over 30% of the world's data are healthcare data" [2]. Therefore, it is fair to say that a reasonable percentage of the healthcare data can be attributed to data generated by IoMT devices. The International Data Corporation predicted that the wearable market would continue to grow and have a compound annual growth rate of 18.4% with 222.3 million shipments in 2021 [3]. Therefore, there is a need to organize and utilize the massive amount of data generated from IoMT devices in a scalable way.

The data collected from IoMT devices have received the most attention because those can be used to monitor patients outside of healthcare settings (i.e., in their homes), register fine motor body movements, and be cheaper and easier to set up. Such personal health data may be gleaned from various data sources such as EHR from health care providers, personal genome sequences, imaging data, and increasingly continuous data coming from personal IoMT devices such as fitness trackers and other wearable medical devices. As technology-supported disease monitoring works are objective, more concise, and more precise than traditional methods, they can utilize a variety of sensory inputs, including ambient-based (sensors installed in a room), video-based (cameras recording patients), and wearable-based (people porting the devices) in recommending an actionable insight to a healthcare provider. Therefore, patient-generated physiological and behavioral measures collected via IoMT devices can be used to explain, influence, or predict many health outcomes, if the data is utilized and combined with the appropriate data streams.

One of the biggest challenges of healthcare data is organizing and making sense of it. This challenge is directly correlated with the need to develop the proper infrastructure to pipe data in and out of the healthcare settings in the appropriate manner that fuels analytics that would better inform the healthcare providers in treating their patients. For example, many valuable insights can be gained from combining genomic data with personal wearable devices to provide comprehensive genomic and environmental metrics of a person's well-being from their activity as determined by their IoMT devices. Coupled with authoritative and up-to-date medical guidelines, an intelligent agent could predict the early detection of coronary artery disease and proactively suggest preventative action to the individual. For example, the agent could suggest that if they were to move $x\%$ (as determined by their IoMT wearable devices), they would be $y\%$ less susceptible to heart disease coupled with explanations for that prediction based on aggregated population-level data as well as scientific literature on pre-dispositions of individuals with the given genetic makeup to heart disease as an example. Furthermore, by having longitudinal records of individuals collected over a while, life-saving medical research can be accelerated beyond what was even imaginable even a decade ago.

The large volume of data offered through IoMT creates opportunities for new models of care and supports the delivery of predictive, preventive, personalized, and participatory medicine. For instance, healthcare providers can use algorithms and templates that model health guidelines to understand IoMT device data and determine whether the patient's health is within normal limits or requires medical attention. As a result, it allows for quicker healthcare interventions, which prevent unnecessary and costly visits to the emergency room and allow patients' symptoms to be resolved at a much faster pace than in current healthcare workflows. Moreover, studies have shown that simple reminders or alerts in the form of text messages or emails can change patients' behavior and improve their health [4–6]. However, such interventions from providers are not readily available due to the lack of personal health data management infrastructures, and thus, patients have to undertake most of the responsibility to stay compliant and follow the proper treatment regimen. Therefore, this chapter highlights that the need for robust, interoperable, standards-based data management infrastructures is as vital as the innovations in IoMT device technology to reap the benefits of the wealth of the data collected through the IoMT devices.

1.2 Motivating Use Cases

This section illustrates several exemplary IoMT use cases that motivate the need to have a robust data collection and management infrastructure for personal health data. Although we have only selected two use cases, we posit that the IoMT wearable health devices could assist in many diseases with the right kind of data architectures supplementing it. Undoubtedly, the rich data collected with the built-in sensors and processing units of our smartphones and IoMT devices have already shown much promise for different types of passive and continuous measurement of various health biomarkers. These, in turn, can be used to develop all sorts of new health sensing apps and interventions.

1.2.1 Remote Monitoring Comorbid Chronic Conditions

IoMT can improve access to and speed of diagnosis with advanced point of care diagnostics and deliver more targeted precision treatments. For example, a patient with several chronic comorbid conditions, such as diabetes and hypertension, might want an easy way to monitor their progress between visits to a clinic, which may span 3–6 months. The patient and their healthcare provider may rely on several IoMT devices for this purpose. Specifically:

- An insulin pump may deliver life-saving medication to the patient.
- Skin patches and continuous blood sugar monitors may be used in measuring blood glucose levels automatically.
- Blood pressure cuffs measure the blood pressure and record any irregularities.
- Smart pill bottles are used for tracking medication intake and adherence.

- Smartwatches and activity trackers are used to assess the patient's activity levels and food intake, two factors that are equally important as the medication prescribed to the patient.

The patient and their healthcare provider must decide what kinds of data and information should be collected from the wearable IoMT devices at their disposal (some of which are described above), what kinds and aspects of the data should be stored, and ultimately brought together to monitor their disease(s). Through the data collected by the IoMT devices, the healthcare provider can gauge how the patient's health has either improved, declined, or remained the same in-between the health visits and can corroborate these insights with lab reports such as the Hemoglobin A1C and other pertinent parameters. If the patient has not been taking their medication (as determined by the data relayed through the smart pillbox), the healthcare provider could provide suggestions for a behavioral change instead of prescribing another medication.

In all such cases, the healthcare provider treating this patient needs to ascertain if the data received and the combinations of the various data streams are trustworthy, usable in the provider's clinical setting, and valuable to the patient's unique circumstances. Determining trust in these kinds of settings requires robust infrastructures that are standards-compliant, interoperable with the various data streams integrated, reactive, efficient in day-to-day use, and intelligent enough to alert the healthcare provider in case of an emergency.

1.2.2 Monitoring Elderly Patients for Fall Detection and Prevention

A report by Deloitte estimates that the percentage of people aged 65 and over is expected to double by 2050 [7], and the United Nations estimates the worldwide prevalence of older adults ($\geq$65 years old) will increase from nearly 10% to 18% in the next 40 years, corresponding to over 1.8 billion in 2060 [8]. Therefore, as more people are living longer, there is a rise in the need for constant monitoring and care for the aging population in Ambient Assisted Living (AAL) environments [9]. The advances in remote patient monitoring with advanced sensing capabilities in AAL environments include sensors placed under the patient's mattress [10] or within a wheelchair [11] that continuously measure vital signs to provide precious information with a fraction of the cost. They also provide the much-needed autonomy for the elderly patient to live their lives with dignity. As falls are one of the main concerns for the elderly population, in recent years, many technologies for fall detection have emerged [12–14]. Furthermore, for detecting complications arising from a disease such as Parkinson's, most wearable-based approaches focus on motor symptoms like tremor [15], bradykinesia (i.e., slowness of movement) [16, 17], gait disturbances [18–20], voice alterations [21, 22], or motor fluctuations determined through a wrist-worn sensor [23]. Among these approaches, accelerometer data has wide popularity, sometimes complemented by gyroscope data, audio recordings, or video recordings depending on the monitored feature. IoMT devices, including wearable sensors, passive in-house monitors, and combinations thereof, promise to alert caregivers or emergency personnel once a fall is detected.

However, most current technology and care solutions are based on a one-dimensional approach, i.e., detect the fall and send help. For many individuals, detecting a fall once it has occurred is already too late as the damage has been done, outcomes are typically poor, and the cost is always high. Therefore, there is a need for a robust architecture to keep all the IoMT sensorimeter data in place and apply learning algorithms to detect if a fall is about to happen and take any precautionary action, if possible. However, the causes leading up to a fall are varied and are better understood by assessing information at different scales and even across different populations under varying circumstances. Therefore, a data integration architecture that ingests IoMT device data obtained from AAL settings would be the ideal solution for this problem. The collected data can be analyzed, and making sense of the various multi-modal data is highly important. Furthermore, this would give an opportunity to analyze and characterize how biomechanical and physiological parameters associated with fall risk have been established by testing/collecting relevant cohort data at the population levels. Then these features can be used for personalized assessments in diverse AAL environments for health assessments utilizing multi-modal, time-varying physiological, and biomechanical fall risk characteristics utilizing a variety of subjective and objective techniques.

1.3 Capabilities of IoMT Data Infrastructures

This section discusses the requisite capabilities of IoMT data infrastructures, including regulatory, technical, and social. There are serious questions about where and how the data streams collected from IoMT devices are stored, collected, and utilized. A connected health application may involve mobile application development, data services, visualization, machine learning, and sensor signal processing, needing multidisciplinary teams, including professional software engineers gathering requirements for data collection [24]. Therefore, the data infrastructure developed must cater to a broad group of stakeholders and must be versatile while honoring the applicable rules and regulations.

1.3.1 Regulation

First and foremost, IoMT data architectures would be subjected to broad healthcare privacy regulations, as such architectures would be storing personally identifiable health data information in them.

The EU General Data Protection Regulation (GDPR) [25] is intended to strengthen and unify data protection for all individuals within the EU. GDPR has imposed strict restrictions regarding data sharing and has set three specific requirements that need to be met. (1) *Data concerning health* containing any data related to a person's physical or mental health, including the type of care they have received, as the latter type of data could be used to infer the patient's health status. (2) *Genetic data* that includes data on an individual's genetic makeup and biological sample analysis. (3) *Biometric data* containing information related to a patient's physical or behavioral characteristics, including facial images, fingerprints, gait traits, and any such personal characteristics.

Similarly, the Health Insurance Portability & Accountability Act (HIPAA) [26] is intended to protect patient privacy in the USA. HIPAA deals with protected health information of the patient, which includes diagnoses, treatment information, medical test results, prescription information, genetic data, and biometrics.

As biometrics are key pieces protected by both the GDPR and HIPAA regulations, the IoMT data architectures must have sufficient safeguards to protect the personal information collected and managed in these systems and must be auditable if the regulatory bodies need to assess the compliance to the stated rules. Furthermore, both the GDPR and HIPAA require informed consent from the patient when sharing the data with third parties. These informed consent declarations, once received, must be stored and available for later use for things such as compliance checking. Therefore there is a need for an innovative, scalable, transparent solution that could ease the consent implementation process and its comprehension by individuals.

1.3.2   Interoperability

Interoperability describes the extent to which systems and devices can exchange and interpret shared data. Interoperability in healthcare is highly complex and relies on establishing connectivity and communication between IoMT devices and EHR systems and between data and workflows while enabling secure and transparent data exchange through standards and protocols. Unfortunately, there is a significant lack of interoperability between the current clinical data infrastructures [27, 28]. When it comes to clinical data, they are still primarily stored and managed in a fragmented manner, which creates friction in information exchange at the point of care and hinders effective decision-making on patient data. Unsurprisingly, these drawbacks translate to IoMT data integration as well.

Fast Healthcare Interoperability of Resources (FHIR) Standard [29] is a system of requirements and guidelines on EHR system development created by the standards organization HL7. The FHIR system is developed based on resources, which are fundamental building blocks representing different types of interchangeable content. As per the FHIR documentation, a resource consists of the following: "A common way to define and represent them [resources], building them from data types that define common reusable patterns of elements, a common set of metadata, and a human-readable part." As a result, one primary implementation point for an IoMT data architecture is determining if a patient's health data can be represented as a resource that can be transferred and used by a standard EHR system. That way, FHIR resources can be easily queried by third parties through a set of REST APIs defined by the FHIR standard. Furthermore, as more and more IoMT device manufacturers adopt the FHIR resources such as specification in representing the data output from the devices, using FHIR resources such as Device, and Observation, the IoMT data architectures would be able to integrate the device data seamlessly. Providing interoperability in such a ground-up manner would lead to interoperability all around, as the applications that consume the data would understand and emit the data in the standards-based schema, further propagating interoperability throughout the entire healthcare ecosystem.

1.3.3 Connectivity

Connectivity technologies are the backbone of the IoMT ecosystem. These technologies include wireless technologies such as Wi-Fi, Bluetooth Low Energy (BLE), Near Field Communication (NFC), Zigbee, and cellular and satellite technologies. Personal health devices such as fitness bands, pedometers, heart rate sensors in smartwatches, among others, require a functional architecture for data collection. The M2M communications standard developed by the European Telecommunication Standards Institute [30] and its extension on the OneM2M standard defined the main functionalities of this type of architecture [31].

Factors that facilitate seamless wireless connections are interoperability between wireless standards, low energy consumption, and range extension. In some instances, more than one peripheral or sensor is simultaneously needed to gather quality data. Therefore, connectivity is a significant factor for collecting high-quality data in data management infrastructures for IoMT devices as many external sensors rely on the standards mentioned above for communication, and these protocols should be able to send/receive data in different formats, from lower-level communication to files (text, images, sound). Many IoMT device manufacturers provide higher-level software development kits and application programming interfaces that make the integration tighter. SMS communication is another method for data gathering, but it is primarily used in no or unreliable Internet access settings. The data management infrastructure would then rely on these endpoints to gather the data via a push or a pull model.

1.3.4   Security and Privacy

The increasing interconnectivity of IoMT enabled devices to collect and share personal health data significantly increases the number of potential vulnerabilities within a system. In terms of the connectivity layer, as medical devices are connected to home networks, public Wi-Fi, or cellular networks to transmit information back to the hospital's network, if the data is unencrypted, the sensitive information could be exploited, and the privacy of the individuals concerned will be at risk.

Ownership of the data as to who controls or who processes these private health data collections is a significant concern for many stakeholders involved, as the more centralized the data silos are, the more vulnerable the data will be, especially if there are no adequate security measures such as encryption and digital signatures. The data stored in centralized systems increases the risk of a significant data breach, which is evident by the recent uptick in healthcare data breaches. From August 2020 to the end of July 2021 alone, more than 44 million patient medical records have been leaked or compromised [32]. Therefore, while current data security methods are in place, more work is necessary to enhance patient security while allowing healthcare systems to be interoperable.

Another worrying trend in the healthcare space is the increase in ransomware attacks [33]. Many of these attacks lock up the EHRs preventing healthcare providers from accessing valuable information in their patients' EHRs. One possible method to mitigate this risk is through the decentralization of medical data. By decentralizing data, information is instead shared as a peer-to-peer network that removes the need for trusting a specific third party to secure crucial medical information. Secondly, if a malicious actor manages to access some information through a peer, the entire system of data is still not compromised, and even if the data is locked up in one system, the critical information could still be accessed as there would be a failsafe provided through the peer-to-peer architecture of the decentralized system.

1.3.5   Machine Learning Readiness

A system that integrates personal health data could have more far-reaching impacts by facilitating the application of Artificial Intelligence (AI)/Machine Learning (ML) technology. With AI/ML techniques, we can correlate background, actions, and outcomes to find paths to optimal health for patients in personalized ways. Data from such an integrated system is more likely to form a complete and accurate health profile of patients, which is critical to ML algorithm training. Otherwise, these algorithms would be trained on mostly biased, truncated, or even distorted data. Therefore, training AI/ML models on "wholesome" data available in robust data architectures can potentially enhance the value of ML in evidence-based medicine [34].

Keeping the privacy of the individuals as a priority and ensuring that the data privacy regulations have been met, population-level health data could be filtered from the data collected in the personal health data management infrastructures by employing differential privacy [35]. Such filtered population-level health information can potentially be incorporated into the federated machine learning algorithms [36, 37]. The findings from these federated learning systems may assist healthcare providers in making more viable treatment plans for complicated patients, any underrepresented populations, and even help reduce health disparity between groups. In particular, completeness and accuracy in training data are crucial for successful machine learning. However, a lot of development of algorithms is currently based on limited datasets due to failure in interoperability, as noted earlier, but may be alleviated as more and more data providers will start adopting interoperable data standards such as FHIR. Mobile devices present new opportunities for health monitoring outside the clinic, especially in technology-enabled interventions such as Digital Therapeutics [38], which can provide feedback to the patient about their lifestyle choices, drive behavioral change, and supplement conventional treatment determined through an AI/ML algorithm. In summary IoMT based data architectures would need to cater to tried and tested clinical decision support systems [39] as well as emerging AI/ML paradigms such as federated learning [40], privacy-preserving deep learning [41], and swarm learning [42]. The latter architectures ensure that data does not leave the patient's end, thus assuring the patient's privacy.

1.3.6   Distributed Ledger Technology

Blockchain is a distributed system to store a series of time-stamped records in a decentralized network, and the use of blockchain in healthcare would primarily rely on "established cryptographic techniques to allow each participant in a network to interact without pre-existing trust between these parties" [43]. Blockchain can address many of the IoMT issues by maintaining flexibility, interoperability through common protocol usage, and enforcing data sovereignty. A blockchain-based architecture's decentralized and distributed features reduce the risk of a cyber-attack, which has plagued many centralized patient data management systems. Moreover, the interaction associated with data transfer can be managed through smart contracts [44], specifying under what conditions and to which extent the receiver can access and manipulate the data. These smart contracts can manage patient alerts and interventions as well.

Blockchain is also featured with a clear definition of data ownership, which has started to focus on healthcare data management. As centralized solutions are administered and regulated by third parties and are often opaque to the data subjects, there has been an emerging trend with decentralized data storage mechanisms. In the context of blockchain-based storage solutions, Inter-Planetary File System (IPFS) [45] provides a content-based addressing mechanism to store data. However, since health data is protected by HIPAA and GDPR, the IPFS storage needs several augmentations if the data were to live in a decentralized system. Even encrypted data is considered under the umbrella of GDPR since the data subject can be indirectly identified [46]. The combination of blockchain and off-chain storage is becoming a standard answer to address privacy concerns of storing data on-chain [47].

Data could be stored locally at the patient's end in devices owned and administered by themselves and retrieved through federated data access mechanisms as demonstrated by a system that connects Blockchain and IoMT devices called BlockIoT [48]. BlockIoT is still a research prototype. Therefore, more robust enterprise-ready systems that bring out similar features to integrate EHR systems with IoMT devices utilizing blockchain and interoperable standards are needed in the healthcare ecosystem. Furthermore, given the many benefits of utilizing a blockchain to record transactions on data access and usage, IoMT data infrastructure developers need to consider whether a blockchain-based mechanism makes sense for their particular use case, especially for enabling trust between two or more mutually distrusting parties.

1.4 Existing Frameworks for Managing IoMT Data

The myriad of connected devices and data points will have little value unless the millions of data points generated through them are managed in a privacy-aware data management framework and turned into actionable insights. So far, we have briefly introduced several prototypes, mostly still available in research labs, which implement the technical features described in the previous section. This section outlines the existing frameworks for managing personal health data collected through IoMT devices with a particular emphasis on community-based open-source solutions vs. proprietary solutions.

1.4.1 Community-Based Open-Source Solutions

National biomedical research initiatives are emerging, such as the All of Us Research Program [49] and the Million Veteran Program [50], which invite persons to share their digital health data and biospecimens with researchers. There are also collaborative initiatives such as Patients Like Me [51] that enable contributing personal health data for citizen science projects. Whether a person wants to participate in one of these research initiatives or play an active role in staying healthy, they face a challenge in deciding what personal health information is important enough to collect, store, manage, and share. Such challenges further necessitate the need to have a transparent and accountable data sharing ecosystem between patients and providers. To that end, there are several existing personal health data management infrastructures to supplement initiatives such as those mentioned above and any other data integration efforts described below.

A survey on IoMT architectures observed that two to five layers were commonly used in many such IoMT architectures, with three-layered architectures (with things, intermediate, and integrated application layers that store vast amounts of data and processes them through several applications) being the most common [52]. One of the more successful community-based methods for health data collection from a patient's end, in addition to the data available in the traditional EHR systems, is OpenEHR [53]. OpenEHR enables the separation of medical semantics from data representation of electronic health records. However, OpenEHR does not address the question of interoperability between various personal IoMT device-based data collection. In order to address this problem, IoMT-focused OpenM2M-based OpenEHR architecture with support for FHIR APIs, as well as data analytics techniques and online analytic processing through Hadoop, is discussed in [54]. Furthermore, Verma and Sood proposed a cloud-centric IoT-based framework for monitoring disease diagnosing, which automatically predicts potential diseases and their level of severity [55]. There also exist several platforms developed to empower practitioners to design and deploy interventions, such as the *LifeGuide* [56] that applies a "person-based approach" for weight management, or a framework that uses contextual data, such as location and weather, added to interaction patterns with the device, to monitor behavior variables that can be mapped to the progression of Parkinson's disease [57].

A platform that integrates different IoMT solutions through connectors, which are specific programs for a systematic extraction of data from each vendor, is described in [58]. The data are then changed to a particular format, stored in a non-standardized EHR, and re-transformed to resources in FHIR and other open data formats. However, the platform does neither integrate IoMT device data nor provide a data management infrastructure for effective analysis. The Open Humans project aims at providing a path to share data, such as genetic, activity, or social media data, with researchers [59], where the data is ingested using connectors to different external sources, and users can store data privately to archive and analyze data or opt to contribute data to projects proposed by the community. The Hypercore protocol (previously known as the Dat protocol) is a data sharing protocol supported by a decentralized architecture [60]. Its goal was to archive and share scientific data with a secure signed append-only log with efficient replication and a filesystem called *Hyperdrive*. A similar architecture powered by the hypercore protocol could be used in powering IoMT based data architectures.

The Personal Health Train (PHT) initiative promotes the use of FAIR principles and citizen-controlled privacy-by-design infrastructure health data lockers [61]. The PHT architecture contains three components: (1) healthcare sites (i.e., "stations") containing FAIR data, (2) technical network connections and legal frameworks (i.e., "tracks"), and (3) statistical learning applications (i.e., "trains"). The PHT project has demonstrated distributed machine learning on over 20,000 lung cancer patients quickly and at scale by connecting eight oncology institutes from 5 countries (Amsterdam, Cardiff, Maastricht, Manchester, Nijmegen, Rome, Rotterdam, Shanghai) in 4 months using the PHT [62], and this infrastructure has demonstrated how it can overcome patient privacy barriers to healthcare data sharing. One could imagine one of the "stations" to be IoMT data endpoints in an IoMT data management infrastructure.

The Solid project [63] spearheaded by the inventor of the world wide web, Sir Tim Berners-Lee, champions the idea of *data pods*, which an individual could use to manage all their data either by themselves or through trusted delegated data providers. Instead of centralized silos keeping various pieces of our health data, including IoMT data, this provides an attractive alternative solution in which our data remains with us, and the applications that operate on the data are delivered to us, primarily through existing web and mobile technologies, i.e., through browser or mobile apps. The solid architecture is currently being piloted by the National Health Service in the UK in the Greater Manchester area, focusing on treating dementia patients using data gleaned from third-party applications. Such data sources include music preferences of the patient or any movement/activity preferences learned by the data collected through an IoMT device. Such data are not typically included in the patient's medical record, and might have a calming effect on a given patient and could be considered in their dementia treatment regimen [64].

Other community-based projects include the Open Health Archive, which is a proposal put forward to creating a shared forum for maintaining and archiving personal health records [65], and the MIDATA.coop initiative in Switzerland pushing for the democratization of personal data with different national cooperatives and nonprofit organizations [66]. However, there are no technical implementations with the requisite capabilities identified in the previous section backing their proposal as of current writing.

1.4.2   Proprietary Solutions

Given that data integration is the bread and butter of many commercial entities, it is no surprise that healthcare products promise to perform data integration seamlessly. Many players have already ventured into providing HIPAA compliance on their existing cloud infrastructure, and the description below is by no means comprehensive. We have selected a platform that connects to several EHR systems in a standards compatible manner and an IoMT vendor that provides a data integration architecture, as examples.

Microsoft Azure (previously Microsoft Health Vault) FHIR Connector can be used to store health data oriented to businesses (including hospitals, pharmacies, and lab testing companies) and consumers. For example, consumers can use the service to gather, store, use, and share data of themselves, children, and other family members. In their Microsoft Azure project's GitHub repository [67], they provide device connector templates and FHIR mapping files to manage the configuration and connection to the personal health device data, which is a great direction. The bridge to community and the use of standards will pave the way for more interoperable solutions to be made available on the Microsoft Azure platform.

Similarly, the Medtronic CareLink network service [68] can be used to transmit data from various implantable cardiac IoMT devices to be remotely monitored through a network accessible to a clinician on demand. Evidence from the operation of CareLink for patients with heart failure suggests that the system results in a decrease in the time from the detection of a clinical event to a clinical decision and decreases the number of emergency visits and overall health care use in people with heart failure compared to standard face-to-face follow-up [68]. Therefore, data integration solutions with IoMT have already shown success in improving patient outcomes.

1.5   Future Directions

This section outlines the future directions for more robust architectures for personal health data management.

One of the most exciting directions in IoMT is the range of sensory inputs that data would be collected from. Since many medical-grade sensors can be invasive and cumbersome to wear in everyday use, researchers are innovating on wearable health sensing with everyday clothing in textile sensors. These wearable clothing would collect physiological data from everyday clothing items, just like with pervasive wearable devices such as Fitbit and Apple watches. As an example, the fiber-enhanced pyjama called "Phyjama" [69] can be used to measure heartbeats, respiration, and joint movements, and a specially designed eyewear called the "Phymask" can be used to acquire all signals of interest to sleep solely using comfortable textile sensors placed on the patient's eyes or the head [70]. With the explosion of such wearable IoMT devices, including clothing, we must carefully investigate the effective means by which we can manage the large volumes of data from a diverse range of inputs that will be available in our data management infrastructure.

Another critical aspect for IoMT device development as well as data integration is to consider healthcare equity. As an example, pulse oxygen meters have been used to monitor patients with COVID-19 remotely, but it was revealed that these devices are less accurate on dark-skinned people compared to light-skinned people [71]. Therefore, different IoMT devices will need to be calibrated for different genders, races, and age groups. Such calibrations may need to be done at the data infrastructure level to adjust to various parameters collected from various other data sources.

On the regulatory front, the next-generation IoMT data integration technologies must cater to existing data protection regulations such as GDPR and HIPPA. They must also be agile to cater to any new regulation because IoMT devices have become ever more sophisticated and innovative with the increasing use of a growing number of technologies. Although traditionally, regulations in most countries have failed to keep pace with scientific and technical developments, once a change has been instituted, failing to adhere to regulation can be disastrous for all the stakeholders involved. IoMT devices are evaluated through a cycle of development, proof-of-concept tests, quality improvement, and trials. For both, continuous surveillance is required to detect unexpected safety issues [72, 73]. With the rise in AI/ML systems that operate on the sea of data that is available in healthcare systems, the approval of medical AI products is on the upswing at the US Food and Drug Administration (FDA), with some estimates saying that it could reach 600 products annually by 2025 [74]. Most of these IoMT based AI products are currently approved under a standard that requires demonstrating "substantial equivalence" in safety and efficacy to similar already-approved systems [75]. This standard was established in 1976 without medical AI or IoMT devices in mind [76]. Also, unlike drugs, there is a dearth of publicly available information about how well they work because the FDA does not need systematic documentation of the development and validation processes for the *AI products*, which includes the composition of training and test datasets and the populations involved [77]. Only very few manufacturers had disclosed the number of patients in the test dataset, which ranged from about 100 to 15,000 patients [74]. Even fewer manufacturers revealed whether the data they used for training and testing had come from more than one facility, which is an essential factor in proving the product's general utility. While a recent FDA action plan for regulating AI aims to compel manufacturers to evaluate their IoMT based AI products more rigorously [78], it may be the responsibility of the data management infrastructure to manage the data to provide the explainability aspects for the regulation and audit-tracing purposes. Such enhanced data-driven architectures would ensure to the FDA that AI systems will render accurate diagnoses, recommend appropriate treatments, and treat minority populations fairly with equitable healthcare decisions.

Finally, data integration data architectures supplemented by IoMT can greatly assist clinical research. Clinical studies of drugs and devices are highly resource-intensive and often require multiple sites, where dedicated personnel must gather data efficiently and track subjects reliably. Robust IoMT data architectures could provide an excellent solution for running the clinical trials of tomorrow in a privacy-preserving yet very scalable and flexible manner.

1.6 Conclusion

Much of the future data management architectures will be designed to provide personalized medical insights to individuals by taking observations of daily living collected through IoMT devices into account. However, integrating connected IoMT devices into established care pathways is challenging. It requires significant cooperation from multiple stakeholders, and there are complex circumstances within which lifestyle behaviors occur and the learning performed on sensor data is insufficient to capture and use pertinent knowledge about an individual. However, with the right kind of data integration and management architectures, such challenges will be lessened. These data management architectures will not only provide benefits in medical diagnosis, but they would also benefit in high-stakes, high-reward endeavors. The immense throughput of IoMT devices enables more timely interventions and allows for more focused and valuable interventions than just trivial reminders via AI/ML algorithms. As for drug development in traditional medical research, health AI research requires long-term and rigorous studies to generate scientifically valid evidence that is reproducible over time and across populations that would entail longitudinal data collected from various IoMT devices and other data sources. The next-generation data collection architectures powered by IoMT devices would provide the platform to get such intelligent health product developments off the ground and into the masses and benefit humanity with more equitable access to data in a privacy-preserving, transparent, and accountable manner.

Acknowledgments This work is partially supported by IBM Research AI through the AI Horizons Network. The author wishes to thank her various past and present collaborators, listed in alphabetical order below, for their thought-provoking discussions that shaped many of the ideas presented in this chapter: Tim Berners-Lee, Shruthi Chari, Ching-Hua Chen, Amar K. Das, Ying Ding, John S. Erickson, Daniel Gruen, James A. Hendler, Lalana Kagal, Jianjing Lin, Giuseppe Loseto, Jamie P. McCusker, Deborah L. McGuinness, Marco Monti, Thilanka Munasinghe, Evan W. Patton, Floriano Scioscia, Manan Shukla, William Van Woensel, and Mohammed J. Zaki.

References

1. Global News Wire, "Medical Devices Market Size Worth Around US\$ 671.49 Bn by 2027," https://www.globenewswire.com/news-release/2020/11/11/2124829/0/en/Medical-Devices-Market-Size-Worth-Around-US-671-49-Bn-by-2027.html, Nov. 2020, online; accessed Aug 20, 2021.
2. Harvard Data Science Review, "Healthcare Data: Who Takes Care of it and How Healthy is it?" https://hdsr.podbean.com/e/healthcare-data-who-takes-care-of-it-and-how-healthy-is-it, Aug. 2021, online; accessed Aug 26, 2021.
3. IDC, "IDC Forecasts Shipments of Wearable Devices to Nearly Double by 2021 as Smart Watches and New Product Categories Gain Traction," https://www.businesswire.com/news/home/20171220005110/en/IDC-Forecasts-Shipments-of-Wearable-Devices-to-Nearly-Double-by-2021-as-Smart-Watches-and-New-Product-Categories-Gain-Traction,   2017, online; accessed Jul 17, 2021.
4. D. L. Roter, J. A. Hall, R. Merisca, B. Nordstrom, D. Cretin, and B. Svarstad, "Effectiveness of interventions to improve patient compliance: a meta-analysis," *Medical care*, pp. 1138–1161, 1998.
5. R. Neff and J. Fry, "Periodic prompts and reminders in health promotion and health behavior interventions: systematic review," *Journal of medical Internet research*, vol. 11, no. 2, p. e16, 2009.
6. J. C. J. Vann, R. M. Jacobson, T. Coyne-Beasley, J. K. Asafu-Adjei, and P. G. Szilagyi, "Patient reminder and recall interventions to improve immunization rates," *Cochrane Database of Systematic Reviews*, 2018.
7. Deloitte Center for Health Care Solutions, "Medtech and the Internet of Medical Things: How connected medical devices are transforming health care," https://www2.deloitte.com/content/dam/Deloitte/global/Documents/Life-Sciences-Health-Care/gx-lshc-medtech-iomt-brochure.pdf, Jul. 2018, online; accessed Jul 17, 2021.

8. United Nations Department of Economic and Social Affairs, "World Population Prospects 2019," https://population.un.org/wpp/, 2019, online; accessed Aug 26, 2021.
9. M. Y. Nilsson, S. Andersson, L. Magnusson, and E. Hanson, "Ambient assisted living technology-mediated interventions for older people and their informal carers in the context of healthy ageing: A scoping review," *Health science reports*, vol. 4, no. 1, 2021.
10. V. Joshi, M. Holtzman, A. Arcelus, R. Goubran, and F. Knoefel, "Highly survivable bed pressure mat remote patient monitoring system for mhealth," in *2012 Annual International Conference of the IEEE Engineering in Medicine and Biology Society*. IEEE, 2012, pp. 268–271.
11. L. Yang, Y. Ge, W. Li, W. Rao, and W. Shen, "A home mobile healthcare system for wheelchair users," in *Proceedings of the 2014 IEEE 18th international conference on computer supported cooperative work in design (CSCWD)*. IEEE, 2014, pp. 609–614.
12. O. Ojetola, E. I. Gaura, and J. Brusey, "Fall detection with wearable sensors–safe (smart fall detection)," in *2011 Seventh International Conference on Intelligent Environments*. IEEE, 2011, pp. 318–321.
13. M. A. Habib, M. S. Mohktar, S. B. Kamaruzzaman, K. S. Lim, T. M. Pin, and F. Ibrahim, "Smartphone-based solutions for fall detection and prevention: challenges and open issues," *Sensors*, vol. 14, no. 4, pp. 7181–7208, 2014.
14. X. Yu, "Approaches and principles of fall detection for elderly and patient," in *HealthCom 2008-10th International Conference on e-health Networking, Applications and Services*. IEEE, 2008, pp. 42–47.
15. S. Patel, K. Lorincz, R. Hughes, N. Huggins, J. Growdon, D. Standaert, M. Akay, J. Dy, M. Welsh, and P. Bonato, "Monitoring motor fluctuations in patients with Parkinson's disease using wearable sensors," *IEEE transactions on information technology in biomedicine*, vol. 13, no. 6, pp. 864–873, 2009.
16. S. Patel, B.-r. Chen, C. Mancinelli, S. Paganoni, L. Shih, M. Welsh, J. Dy, and P. Bonato, "Longitudinal monitoring of patients with Parkinson's disease via wearable sensor technology in the home setting," in *2011 Annual International Conference of the IEEE Engineering in Medicine and Biology Society*. IEEE, 2011, pp. 1552–1555.
17. M. Sung, C. Marci, and A. Pentland, "Wearable feedback systems for rehabilitation," *Journal of neuroengineering and rehabilitation*, vol. 2, no. 1, pp. 1–12, 2005.
18. J. Barth, J. Klucken, P. Kugler, T. Kammerer, R. Steidl, J. Winkler, J. Hornegger, and B. Eskofier, "Biometric and mobile gait analysis for early diagnosis and therapy monitoring in Parkinson's disease," in *2011 Annual International Conference of the IEEE Engineering in Medicine and Biology Society*. IEEE, 2011, pp. 868–871.
19. M. Pansera, J. J. Estrada, L. Pastor, J. Cancela, R. Greenlaw, and M. T. Arredondo, "Multi-parametric system for the continuous assessment and monitoring of motor status in Parkinson's disease: an entropy-based gait comparison," in *2009 Annual International Conference of the IEEE Engineering in Medicine and Biology Society*. IEEE, 2009, pp. 1242–1245.
20. A. Weiss, S. Sharifi, M. Plotnik, J. P. van Vugt, N. Giladi, and J. M. Hausdorff, "Toward automated, at-home assessment of mobility among patients with Parkinson disease, using a body-worn accelerometer," *Neurorehabilitation and neural repair*, vol. 25, no. 9, pp. 810–818, 2011.
21. Ö. Eskidere, F. Ertaş, and C. Hanilçi, "A comparison of regression methods for remote tracking of Parkinson's disease progression," *Expert Systems with Applications*, vol. 39, no. 5, pp. 5523–5528, 2012.
22. A. Tsanas, M. A. Little, P. E. McSharry, and L. O. Ramig, "Nonlinear speech analysis algorithms mapped to a standard metric achieve clinically useful quantification of average Parkinson's disease symptom severity," *Journal of the royal society interface*, vol. 8, no. 59, pp. 842–855, 2011.
23. C. Pérez-López, A. Samà, D. Rodríguez-Martín, A. Català, J. Cabestany, E. De Mingo, and A. Rodríguez-Molinero, "Monitoring motor fluctuations in Parkinson's disease using a waist-worn inertial sensor," in *International Work-Conference on Artificial Neural Networks*. Springer, 2015, pp. 461–474.

24. J. J. D. Veiga and T. E. Ward, "Data collection requirements for mobile connected health: an end user development approach," in *Proceedings of the 1st International Workshop on Mobile Development*, 2016, pp. 23–30.
25. P. Voigt and A. Von dem Bussche, "The EU General Data Protection Regulation (GDPR)," *A Practical Guide, 1st Ed., Cham: Springer International Publishing*, vol. 10, p. 3152676, 2017.
26. U.S. Department of Health & Human Services, "Health Information Privacy," https://www.hhs.gov/hipaa/index.html, online; accessed Aug 20, 2021.
27. D. Kalra, "Electronic health record standards," *Yearbook of medical informatics*, vol. 15, no. 01, pp. 136–144, 2006.
28. F. Wozak, E. Ammenwerth, A. Hörbst, P. Sögner, R. Mair, and T. Schabetsberger, "Ihe based interoperability-benefits and challenges," in *MIE*, vol. 136, 2008, pp. 771–776.
29. D. Bender and K. Sartipi, "Hl7 fhir: An agile and restful approach to healthcare information exchange," in *Proceedings of the 26th IEEE international symposium on computer-based medical systems*. IEEE, 2013, pp. 326–331.
30. European Telecommunication Standards Institute – ETSI TS 102 690 V2.1.1 (2013-10), "Machine-to-Machine communications (M2M); Functional architecture," https://www.etsi.org/deliver/etsi_ts/102600_102699/102690/02.01.01_60/ts_102690v020101p.pdf, 10 2013, online; accessed Jul 17, 2021.
31. European Telecommunication Standards Institute, "One M2M – The IoT Standard," https://www.onem2m.org, 10 2013, online; accessed Jul 17, 2021.
32. HIPAA Journal, "July 2021 Healthcare Data Breach Report," https://www.hipaajournal.com/july-2021-healthcare-data-breach-report, Jul. 2021, online; accessed Aug 20, 2021.
33. Rebecca Pifer, "More than 1/3 of health organizations hit by ransomware last year, report finds," https://www.healthcaredive.com/news/more-than-13-of-health-organizations-hit-by-ransomware-last-year-report-f/602329, Jun. 2021, online; accessed Aug 20, 2021.
34. I. A. Scott, "Machine learning and evidence-based medicine," *Annals of Internal Medicine*, vol. 169, no. 1, pp. 44–46, 2018.
35. C. Dwork, A. Roth *et al.*, "The algorithmic foundations of differential privacy." *Found. Trends Theor. Comput. Sci.*, vol. 9, no. 3-4, pp. 211–407, 2014.
36. N. Rieke, J. Hancox, W. Li, F. Milletari, H. R. Roth, S. Albarqouni, S. Bakas, M. N. Galtier, B. A. Landman, K. Maier-Hein *et al.*, "The future of digital health with federated learning," *NPJ digital medicine*, vol. 3, no. 1, pp. 1–7, 2020.
37. T. S. Brisimi, R. Chen, T. Mela, A. Olshevsky, I. C. Paschalidis, and W. Shi, "Federated learning of predictive models from federated electronic health records," *International journal of medical informatics*, vol. 112, pp. 59–67, 2018.
38. N. A. Patel and A. J. Butte, "Characteristics and challenges of the clinical pipeline of digital therapeutics," *NPJ digital medicine*, vol. 3, no. 1, pp. 1–5, 2020.
39. E. S. Berner, *Clinical decision support systems*. Springer, 2007, vol. 233.
40. A. Jochems, T. M. Deist, J. Van Soest, M. Eble, P. Bulens, P. Coucke, W. Dries, P. Lambin, and A. Dekker, "Distributed learning: developing a predictive model based on data from multiple hospitals without data leaving the hospital–a real life proof of concept," *Radiotherapy and Oncology*, vol. 121, no. 3, pp. 459–467, 2016.
41. R. Shokri and V. Shmatikov, "Privacy-preserving deep learning," in *Proceedings of the 22nd ACM SIGSAC conference on computer and communications security*, 2015, pp. 1310–1321.
42. S. Warnat-Herresthal, H. Schultze, K. L. Shastry, S. Manamohan, S. Mukherjee, V. Garg, R. Sarveswara, K. Händler, P. Pickkers, N. A. Aziz *et al.*, "Swarm learning for decentralized and confidential clinical machine learning," *Nature*, vol. 594, no. 7862, pp. 265–270, 2021.
43. R. Krawiec, D. Housman, M. White, M. Filipova, F. Quarre, D. Barr, A. Nesbitt, K. Fedosova, J. Killmeyer, A. Israel *et al.*, "Blockchain: Opportunities for health care," in *Proc. NIST Workshop Blockchain Healthcare*, 2016, pp. 1–16.
44. V. Buterin *et al.*, "A next-generation smart contract and decentralized application platform," *white paper*, vol. 3, no. 37, 2014.
45. J. Benet, "Ipfs-content addressed, versioned, p2p file system," *arXiv preprint arXiv:1407.3561*, 2014.

46. M. Finck, "Blockchains and data protection in the European Union," *Eur. Data Prot. L. Rev.*, vol. 4, p. 17, 2018.
47. G. Zyskind, O. Nathan *et al.*, "Decentralizing privacy: Using blockchain to protect personal data," in *2015 IEEE Security and Privacy Workshops*. IEEE, 2015, pp. 180–184.
48. M. Shukla, J. Lin, and O. Seneviratne, "BlockIoT: Blockchain-based Health Data Integration using IoT Devices," *American Medical Informatics Association*, 2021.
49. A. of Us Research Program Investigators, "The "all of us" research program," *New England Journal of Medicine*, vol. 381, no. 7, pp. 668–676, 2019.
50. J. M. Gaziano, J. Concato, M. Brophy, L. Fiore, S. Pyarajan, J. Breeling, S. Whitbourne, J. Deen, C. Shannon, D. Humphries *et al.*, "Million veteran program: A mega-biobank to study genetic influences on health and disease," *Journal of clinical epidemiology*, vol. 70, pp. 214–223, 2016.
51. P. Wicks, M. Massagli, J. Frost, C. Brownstein, S. Okun, T. Vaughan, R. Bradley, and J. Heywood, "Sharing health data for better outcomes on PatientsLikeMe," *Journal of medical Internet research*, vol. 12, no. 2, p. e1549, 2010.
52. M. Irfan and N. Ahmad, "Internet of medical things: Architectural model, motivational factors and impediments," in *2018 15th learning and technology conference (L&T)*. IEEE, 2018, pp. 6–13.
53. D. Kalra, T. Beale, and S. Heard, "The openehr foundation," *Studies in health technology and informatics*, vol. 115, pp. 153–173, 2005.
54. J. N. S Rubí and P. R. L Gondim, "IoMT platform for pervasive healthcare data aggregation, processing, and sharing based on OneM2M and OpenEHR," *Sensors*, vol. 19, no. 19, p. 4283, 2019.
55. P. Verma and S. K. Sood, "Cloud-centric IoT based disease diagnosis healthcare framework," *Journal of Parallel and Distributed Computing*, vol. 116, pp. 27–38, 2018.
56. S. Williams, L. Yardley, M. Weal, and G. Wills, "Introduction to LifeGuide: Open-source software for creating online interventions for health care, health promotion and training," *Knowledge Resources*, vol. 187, p. 90, 2010.
57. J. Vega, "Monitoring Parkinson's disease progression using behavioural inferences, mobile devices and web technologies," in *Proceedings of the 25th International Conference Companion on World Wide Web*, 2016, pp. 323–327.
58. N. Boutros-Saikali, K. Saikali, and R. Abou Naoum, "An iomt platform to simplify the development of healthcare monitoring applications," in *2018 Third International Conference on Electrical and Biomedical Engineering, Clean Energy and Green Computing (EBECEGC)*. IEEE, 2018, pp. 6–11.
59. Open Humans, "Explore, analyze, and donate your data – doing research together!" https://www.openhumans.org, online; accessed Jul 17, 2021.
60. Hypercore Protocol, "Peer-to-peer data sharing," https://hypercore-protocol.org, online; accessed Jul 17, 2021.
61. A. Choudhury, J. van Soest, S. Nayak, and A. Dekker, "Personal health train on fhir: A privacy preserving federated approach for analyzing fair data in healthcare," in *International Conference on Machine Learning, Image Processing, Network Security and Data Sciences*. Springer, 2020, pp. 85–95.
62. T. M. Deist, F. J. Dankers, P. Ojha, M. S. Marshall, T. Janssen, C. Faivre-Finn, C. Masciocchi, V. Valentini, J. Wang, J. Chen *et al.*, "Distributed learning on 20 000+ lung cancer patients–the personal health train," *Radiotherapy and Oncology*, vol. 144, pp. 189–200, 2020.
63. E. Mansour, A. V. Sambra, S. Hawke, M. Zereba, S. Capadisli, A. Ghanem, A. Aboulnaga, and T. Berners-Lee, "A demonstration of the solid platform for social web applications," in *Proceedings of the 25th International Conference Companion on World Wide Web*, 2016, pp. 223–226.
64. Rory Cellan-Jones, "NHS data: Can web creator Sir Tim Berners-Lee fix it?" https://www.bbc.com/news/technology-54871705, Nov. 2020, online; accessed Aug 20, 2021.

65. V. Estrada-Galinanes and K. Wac, "Visions and challenges in managing and preserving data to measure quality of life," in *2018 IEEE 3rd International Workshops on Foundations and Applications of Self* Systems (FAS* W)*. IEEE, 2018, pp. 92–99.
66. MIDATA, "My Data – Our Health," https://www.midata.coop/en/home, online; accessed Jul 17, 2021.
67. Microsoft/iomt-fhir contributors, "IoMT FHIR Connector for Azure," https://github.com/microsoft/iomt-fhir, 2021, online; accessed Jul 17, 2021.
68. Medtronic, "CareLink remote monitoring network: Heart failure," https://www.medtronic.com/uk-en/patients/treatments-therapies, 2018, online; accessed Jul 17, 2021.
69. A. Kiaghadi, S. Z. Homayounfar, J. Gummeson, T. Andrew, and D. Ganesan, "Phyjama: physiological sensing via fiber-enhanced pyjamas," *Proceedings of the ACM on Interactive, Mobile, Wearable and Ubiquitous Technologies*, vol. 3, no. 3, pp. 1–29, 2019.
70. S. Rostaminia, S. Z. Homayounfar, A. Kiaghadi, T. L. Andrew, and D. Ganesan, "Phymask: Robust sensing of brain activity and physiological signals during sleep with an all-textile eye mask," *arXiv preprint arXiv:2106.07645*, 2021.
71. Laura Lovett, "FDA warns pulse oximeters less accurate for people with darker skin," https://www.mobihealthnews.com/news/fda-warns-pulse-oximeters-less-accurate-people-darker-skin, Feb. 2021, online; accessed Aug 20, 2021.
72. M. S. Lipsky and L. K. Sharp, "From idea to market: the drug approval process." *The Journal of the American Board of Family Practice*, vol. 14, no. 5, pp. 362–367, 2001.
73. O. Faris and J. Shuren, "An fda viewpoint on unique considerations for medical-device clinical trials," *New England Journal of Medicine*, vol. 376, no. 14, pp. 1350–1357, 2017.
74. Casey Ross. (2021, Feb.) Explore STAT's database of FDA-cleared AI tools. [Online]. Available: https://www.statnews.com/2021/02/03/fda-artificial-intelligence-clearance-products/
75. The US Food and Drug Administration. (2020, Mar.) What is Substantial Equivalence. [Online]. Available: https://www.fda.gov/medical-devices/premarket-submissions/premarket-notification-510k
76. The US Food and Drug Administration . (2018, Sep.) 510(k) Clearances. [Online]. Available: https://www.fda.gov/medical-devices/device-approvals-denials-and-clearances/510k-clearances
77. Casey Ross. (2021, Feb.) As the FDA clears a flood of AI tools, missing data raise troubling questions on safety and fairness. [Online]. Available: https://www.statnews.com/2021/02/03/fda-clearances-artificial-intelligence-data
78. The US Food and Drug Administration. (2021, Jan.) Artificial Intelligence and Machine Learning in Software as a Medical Device. [Online]. Available: https://www.fda.gov/medical-devices/software-medical-device-samd/artificial-intelligence-and-machine-learning-software-medical-device

Chapter 2
Architecting and Evaluating Cybersecurity in Clinical IoT

Tanja Pavleska

Contents

T. Pavleska (✉)
Laboratory for Open Systems and Networks, Jožef Stefan Institute, Ljubljana, Slovenia
e-mail: atanja@e5.ijs.si

© Springer Nature Switzerland AG 2022
F. D. Hudson (eds.), *Women Securing the Future with TIPPSS for Connected
Healthcare*, Women in Engineering and Science,
https://doi.org/10.1007/978-3-030-93592-4_2

2.1   Introduction

In Europe, the Network and Information Systems (NIS) Directive recognizes e-Health as a critical sector, enforcing security as an essential property [1]. Moreover, article 25 of the European data protection regulation is concerned with security and data protection by design, recognizing medical documents as a special category, and providing a specific definition for health data [2]. Similar security requirements are applicable in the USA as well [3, 4]. The regulatory prescriptions in terms of cybersecurity requirements are thus not separated from the technical requirements and span across all levels of the healthcare environment, from infrastructures up to doctors' workstations and medical devices.

The Internet of Things (IoT) in the healthcare industry offers benefits such as end-to-end connectivity and affordability, continuous monitoring and reporting, data processing and analysis, and remote medical assistance, facilitating patients' lives and healthcare professionals' work. In a business context, IoT serves to facilitate disease management and to reduce healthcare costs and administrative burden. The IoT healthcare market was valued at USD 28.42 Billion in 2015 and is projected to reach USD 337.41 billion by 2025, growing at a CAGR of 28.2% over the forecast period. In order to enable organizations to derive maximum value from their assets, these goals are achieved by reliance on innovative digital paradigms, enabling evidence-based treatment and providing real-time data to aid decision-making. Evidence-based treatment, however, calls for an evidence-based design. As stated in the IEEE Pre-Standards Workstream Report "Clinical IoT Data Validation and Interoperability with Blockchain" [5]: "A key component to the evidence-based design is consideration of risk as part of the overall cybersecurity equation. By understanding risk, each participant in the healthcare ecosystem can make educated decisions on current and future technology implementations."

However, evidence-based design and risk analysis require knowledge of the system's past behavior, which assumes an operational environment in place. This is often not possible, preventing a complete consideration of the desired cybersecurity goal. Therefore, accounting for the risks and the threats must be complemented with an account of the security goals, regardless of whether the architecture is yet to be established or an intervention in its functionality is to be done as part of an organization's change management. The work presented here is a direct contribution to this end, as it takes a goal-based approach to both embedding cybersecurity principles in the architecture design and evaluating the devised architecture afterwards.

The provision of IoT end-to-end connectivity does not only refer to a single implementation context. As citizens may enjoy their freedom of movement and relocate to other countries, they have the right to benefit from the healthcare systems in those countries. Therefore, technology barriers causing non-optimal mobility or patient treatment cannot be accepted. In that sense, interoperability is directly related to patient safety: failure in availability during data transfer, especially in emergency situations, may be detrimental for the patient. This also testifies to the close relationship between system design and system security, especially in contexts where connectivity is at the core of the system functionalities and the system architect is not able to manually intervene at every adaptation step. Addressing these issues only through the adoption of international standards is insufficient, as standards, like any other asset, undergo continuous evolution, re-introducing lack of interoperability. Therefore, a governance model on standards is needed in critical sectors to guarantee sustainability and long-term interoperability [6]. Thus, the main design concerns in a complex environment where a diverse set of entities exchange healthcare data are: governance, interoperability, sustainability, and automation.

In the clinical IoT domain, interoperability is addressed by several international initiatives, such as the Integrating Health Enterprise organization (IHE) and HL7/FHIR [7]. These governance models adopt modular Enterprise Architectures where standards and solutions are confined into building blocks. Modularity implies that these building blocks are then combined into complex architectures to provide the solution. However, modular architectures, coupled with long product life cycles and high heterogeneity of mobile devices pose serious challenges in the fulfillment of high cybersecurity standards for the critical sectors. Moreover, modular approaches require constant intervention by security experts, which are becoming scarce and expensive resources, urging the companies to optimize their market presence towards a solution that is not cybersecurity-optimal. To point out the gap between design and cybersecurity (TIPPSS) principles on the one hand for comprehensive Trust, Identity, Privacy, Protection, Safety and Security, and the striving for business optimization on the other, this work elicits a taxonomy of design issues, principles, requirements, and functionalities. The taxonomy is part of an integrated architecture framework that is itself based on standard methodologies and models, aiming to facilitate the dialog between technical and non-technical stakeholders and to lower the need for constant outlook by security experts.

To address the issues outlined above, the chapter is structured as follows: first, it lays the theoretical basis needed to understand the main concepts employed throughout the text. Then, it provides a detailed survey on the described issues and architecture frameworks relevant to address them in a clinical IoT context. A comparative analysis of these frameworks in view of the desired system and TIPPSS properties is also presented as part of this overview. After establishing the rationale behind the methodological choices, some background on the pillar models of the architectures is provided before finally devising the generic architecture with a goal-based security model integrated into the viewpoints. Based on the architecture, the taxonomy is also defined. Finally, a cybersecurity-based evaluation methodology for such architectures is presented to complete the whole methodology development cycle. The chapter ends with a summary and some future directions that follow as a logical outcome of this work.

2.2 Theoretical Background

The underlying terms of the TIPPSS framework already require some basic definitions:

- *Trust* in this chapter is defined as the willingness to put one's welfare into the hands of another entity to trust [8]. As such, trust incorporates risk and uncertainty, which is what makes it different from confidence [9]. However, this definition leaves the impression that trust is mainly to be seen as a social construct. Therefore, for a computational context, trust was introduced and adapted by Marsh [10], who gave a formal model for representing trust in mathematical terms.
- *Identity*, according to the National Institute of Standards and Technology (NIST), is defined as information that is unique within a security domain and which is recognized as denoting a particular entity within that domain [11]. In that sense, identity-based security is defined as a security policy based on the identities and/or attributes of the object (system policy IT-related risk resource) being accessed and of the subject (user, group of users, process, or device) requesting access.
- *Privacy* in its general meaning is understood as the right to be let alone, or freedom from interference or intrusion [12]. Information privacy is the right to have some control over how your personal information is collected and used [13].
- *Protection and Safety* are seen as the condition of the system operating without causing unacceptable risk of physical injury or damage to the health of people, either directly, or indirectly as a result of damage to property or to the environment [14].
- *Security* is the condition of the system operating without allowing unintended or unauthorized access, change, or destruction of the system or the data and information it encompasses [15].

In addition to the basic cybersecurity concept, this work employs architecture design principles, terminology, and artifacts that are compliant with The Open Group Architecture Framework—TOGAF.[1] The two ground concepts in the architecture design process are the Reference Architecture and the Solution Architecture.

- *Reference Architecture* is the generic architecture providing guidelines and options for developing specific architectures and solution implementations. In this chapter, it refers to the set of all available clinical IoT-related profiles used to build a *solution architecture*.
- *Solution Architecture* describes the specific business operations/activities and the ways in which information systems and technology support them. It typically

---

[1] TOGAF provides an approach for designing, planning, implementing, and governing an enterprise information technology architecture.

applies to a single project/organization. In this chapter, it translates to a cohesive ensemble of architectural constructs (see *profiles*) intended to solve a specific business problem or respond to a set of use-case requirements.

Aside from the general architecture terms, some concepts from a governance perspective in the specific healthcare context are also employed throughout this work. These mainly come from the Integrating the Health Enterprise (IHE) organization, i.e., from its *IT Infrastructure Technical Framework* [16] and are defined to the necessary details later in Sect. 2.4.

* **Solution architecture design** practically consists of: (a) translation of business requirements into a solution vision; and (b) derivation of a set of IT specifications. The former produces an initial subset of *profiles* that result directly from the requirements and the associated use-cases; the latter outputs a superset of the initial *profiles* by resolving all functional interdependencies (through an operation called *grouping*). Our work is a proof that the process of profiling can be formalized to enable an automated solution architecture design.

2.3 Related Work

2.3.1 TIPPSS in Healthcare

Following Marsh's work on computational trust [10], many computational trust models have been developed for calculating trust in both centralized and distributed environments [17–20]. Some were even devised for medical IoT purposes [21]. However, there is no taxonomy of trust developed for the medical/clinical IoT context. Most of the taxonomies either refer to the categorization of the healthcare system sectors in general [22], the IoT technology employed [23], or to some aspect of security and privacy [24–27].

In order to enforce governance rules and principles to guarantee interoperability, many critical sectors had already deployed mechanisms relying on Enterprise Architectures [28–30]. By treating standards as architectural constructs, a proper governance scheme enables interoperability at all levels, prevents standards' lock-in and leads to long-term sustainability of the implemented solutions. One of the most advanced governance schemes relying on architectural principles is the Integrating the Healthcare Enterprise (IHE), implemented in the healthcare sector [16]. With the support of industry and academia, and initially run by the Radiological Society of North America, IHE aimed to provide a governance model for building the infrastructure to securely share medical records.

However, in terms of system design, there are very few design approaches that try to address both cybersecurity and architecture throughout as part of a single methodological framework. Those that focus on one of the desired architectural properties (interoperability, governance, and sustainability) are still in their early research phase, with almost no practical implementation existing. This lack of a common architecture development methodology was also noted by [31].

A work that resembles the approach in this chapter is presented in [32] for the context of Active Assisted Living. It provides an architectural model for mapping use-cases to a three-dimensional model for assisted living. Unlike Muñoz et al., the framework developed here is generic and resembles an IoT use-case translated to a clinical domain. In that sense, we establish a common design language across domains, addressing a well-known problem of scarcity of security expertise. This problem has also been noticed and approached in [33], where a set of "modular security safeguards" is defined and assembled into holistic "security requirement profiles." However, Zuccato's model only serves the solution developers and is mainly concerned with the technical aspects. Moreover, although it provides some tools to be reused for other implementations, it provides no framework that would allow addressing a full set of security goals at an architectural level and by design. In that sense, our work is a contribution for the further development of IoT architecture frameworks along cybersecurity lines. It complements any security assessment framework that is based on architectural principles, such as the one presented in [34], as it is not tied to a particular model, technology, or context.

As architecture design is at the core of this work, we elaborate in greater detail in a separate subsection on the relevant architecture frameworks taken into account in devising the generic architecture in this chapter.

2.3.2   Overview of Relevant Architecture Frameworks

This section reviews the most notable reference architectures in the relevant domains that were considered for the development of the architectural approach in this chapter. It results in a comparative analysis between these frameworks from the view of a set of required architecture qualities and provides the rationale for employing one particular reference architecture as the pillar of the developed methodology.

2.3.2.1   International Standards Organization IoT Reference Architecture (ISO IoT RA)

The International Standards Organization IoT Reference Architecture covers the general context of the Internet of Things by defining system characteristics, a conceptual model, a reference model, and architecture views for the IoT [35]. It is being developed by Work Group 10 of the Joint Technical Committee 1 of the International Organization for Standardization and the International Electrotechnical Commission (ISO/IEC JTC1 WG10) with the aim to become an International Standard and an authoritative reference for terminology and concepts for the IoT. The conceptual model contains an overall IoT model based on five concepts: *Domains, Identity, Service and Communication, IoT-User*, and *IoT Device* concept.

It takes a systemic approach in that it not only defines the system entities, but it also accounts for the interrelations between them in a particular context. Thus, it has an *Entity-based Reference Model* that shows how users, systems, networks, gateways, devices, and physical entities relate to each other, and a *Domain-based Reference Model* showing the relations between the User, Operations and Management, Application Service, IoT Resource and Interchange, Sensing and Control, and Physical Entity domains.

The ISO IoT RA integrates five architectural viewpoints: Usage, Functional, Information, System, and Communication.

2.3.2.2 Industrial Internet Reference Architecture (IIRA)

The Industrial Internet Reference Architecture (IIRA) is a standards-based open architecture for Industrial Internet Systems (IIS) [36]. It documents and communicates the development of an architecture framework developed by the Industrial Internet Consortium (IIC), which describes the conventions, principles, and practices for the description of architectures established within a specific domain of application and/or community of stakeholders. It has broad industry applicability to drive interoperability, to map applicable technologies, and to guide technology and standards development. The IIRA design is independent from any technologies and is able to identify technology gaps based on the architectural requirements. The various concerns of an IIS are classified and grouped together as four viewpoints of the IIRA: Business, Usage, Functional, and Implementation. Each of the viewpoints also accounts for certain security concerns relevant for the particular viewpoint and in relation to the stakeholders' requirements. This consideration of security right from the design phase makes the IIRA a suitable starting point for our methodology. Therefore, its aforementioned properties are discussed in greater detail in Sect. 2.4 as well.

2.3.2.3 ISO/IEC 10746 Reference Architecture

The ISO/IEC 10746-3:2009 provides a coordinating framework for the standardization of open distributed processing [37]. Much like the IIRA, it aims to be independent from platform and technology. In addition, it aims to support distribution, interplay, and portability. To that end, the standard establishes an enterprise architecture framework for the specification of open distributed systems by defining the specification for an open distributed processing system from five viewpoints. The viewpoints are subdivisions of the specification of the system and serve to establish a common structure of the particular pieces of information relevant to some stakeholder or to the particular area of concern.

The overall framework consists of four building blocks that revolve around object modeling of the system specification, a specification procedure following the interrelated viewpoints, defining the infrastructure that provides distribution transparencies for the envisaged applications, and specifying a framework to assess system conformance to the standard.

In that sense, the structure of this work follows the same development procedure: we specify an architecture model, define a taxonomy of interrelations, and provide an evaluation method for conformance. However, the work presented here provides a much more granular view of the cybersecurity principles relevant at design level and in view of the TIPPSS principles for the particular context of clinical IoT. In addition, the methodology is developed in a way that enables automation of the solution architecture design, thus lowering the need for exhaustive efforts by security experts in the architecture definition.

2.3.2.4 Reference Architecture Model for Industry 4.0

The Reference Architecture Model for Industry 4.0 (RAMI 4.0) provides an architectural basis for the IoT and cyber-physical systems in the industrial manufacturing domain [38]. It mainly focuses on industrial applications and use of computerized tooling for system design. By concept, RAMI 4.0 is a three-dimensional matrix that can be used to position standards and describe use-cases. It addresses integration within and between factories, end-to-end engineering, and human value stream orchestration. To provide this functionality, it is structured along two horizontal dimensions and a vertical dimension. The horizontal dimensions are: *Life Cycle & Value Stream*; and *Hierarchy*. The vertical dimension incorporates six layers: *Business, Functional, Information, Communication, Integration*, and *Asset*. RAMI 4.0 also accounts for certain security considerations, especially in the life cycle dimension. However, not only do these considerations not cover the set of desired TIPPSS properties, but they are also constrained in the covered security aspect in that they mainly focus on the risk management side. In that sense, many of the architecture models elaborated here can benefit in a complementary manner from the work presented in this chapter.

2.3.2.5 e-Health and the Integrated Healthcare Enterprise (IHE) Technical Framework

IHE takes a market-oriented and academically supported, yet pragmatic stance in enabling: (a) vendors to design interoperable products, (b) product certification, and (c) a sustainable methodology (due to the architectural approach) [16, 39]. The IHE Technical Framework identifies a subset of the functional components of the healthcare enterprise, called IHE actors, and specifies their interactions in terms of a set of coordinated, standards-based transactions. Transactions are organized into functional units called integration profiles that highlight their capacity to address specific IT Infrastructure requirements. The interoperability approach used by IHE is largely followed in [4] by adopting the concepts of profiles, actors, and transactions as the main architectural constructs.

Our work adopts the IHE concepts of the technical framework by translating the concept of a TOGAF Architecture Building Block into a *profile* construct to enable the reuse of such building blocks. In addition, we extend the applicability of IHE profiles by providing the grounds for the development of a formal syntax to support automation mechanisms for solution architecture design and quality checking. This is supported with more arguments in Sect. 2.4.

2.3.2.6   eSENS European Interoperability Reference Architecture EIRA

Electronic Simple European Networked Services (eSENS) was a pan-European project for facilitating cross-border public services, involving 100 public and private actors from 22 countries [40]. Information Technology (IT) architecture-wise, it built upon and redefined the solutions from previous sectorial Large Scale Pilots into a set of cross-domain reusable building blocks. It produced the eSENS European Interoperability Reference Architecture (EIRA), which is compatible with the European Union interoperability architecture frameworks, based on TOGAF [41]. The e-Health pilot in eSENS employed the IHE process in the development of EIRA. Thus, the non-repudiation building block was created and successfully implemented in the e-Health and eProcurement pilots. Our methodology integrates this approach, allowing us to adopt the non-repudiation building block as part of the novel architecture development methodology. In addition, it integrates the aspect of goal-based security to develop a holistic cybersecurity architecture, as well as an evaluation methodology for the solution design.

2.3.2.7   The World Health Organization Enterprise Architecture (EA)

The World Health Organization (WHO) architecture development process consists of four steps from Architecture Vision to Architecture Change Management, divided into two phases. In the first phase, the Analysis and Design take place, and in the second phase, the Development and Deployment are realized. Unlike other enterprise architectures (EA), the division into viewpoint in the WHO EA is firstly done from a time perspective, and then each of these follows the stakeholders' concerns and iterates through an additional nine phases: Architecture Vision, Business, Information System, Technology, Opportunities and Solutions, Migration Planning, Implementation, Governance, and Architecture change management. All of the phases revolve around the constant iterative approach of requirements management.

2.3.2.8   The Open Group Architecture Framework (TOGAF)

TOGAF [42] is the most widely used framework for enterprise architecture that provides an approach for designing, planning, implementing, and governing an enterprise information technology architecture. It represents a high-level design framework consisting of four viewpoints: Business, Application, Data, and Technology. One of the most practical aspects of TOGAF is its modularity resembling a reference library of architecture building blocks that are reusable, standardized, and generic, tested with proven technologies and products. This enables backward compatibility of the architectures developed out of the TOGAF library and is also the backbone of our development methodology.

In this chapter, we aim to widen the scope of the presented architecture models to account for a wider set of architecture properties, while addressing security-by-design. One of the major contributions is a generic architecture that can be semantically formalized and that is lendable to automation, enabling provable quality attributes of the solution design. We also provide considerations and guidelines on how to automate that process, pointing to formal means for quality evaluation of the obtained solution.

Table 2.1 synthesizes the comparison among the discussed relevant frameworks/methodologies (including the new methodology introduced in the next section) in terms of the desired architecture properties. The ✓ is used to denote addressed property, whereas empty space means no account for the specific property.

2.4 Methodology Considerations for TIPPSS

This section presents the frameworks and models that the generic methodology is based upon and whose functionalities it extends by considering the entire set of desired properties outlined in Table 2.1. The aim is to explore the possibility to integrate these properties into a single architecture that is independent of context, technology, and platform, while incorporating security-by-design and allowing for evaluation at viewpoint level.

Table 2.1 Comparing architecture frameworks' properties

Architecture	ISO IoT RA	IIRA	ISO/IEC 10746	RAMI 4.0	IHE	eSENS EIRA	WHO EA	TOGAF	The proposed
Property									
Governance	✓		✓		✓		✓	✓	✓
Interoperability	✓	✓	✓	✓	✓	✓	✓	✓	✓
Variability			✓	✓	✓	✓	✓		✓
Automation		✓							✓
Trust						✓			✓
Identity				✓	✓	✓	✓		✓
Privacy	✓	✓			✓	✓	✓	✓	✓
Protection		✓							✓
Safety		✓		✓					✓
Security	✓	✓	✓	✓	✓	✓	✓	✓	✓

2.4.1 Integrating the Healthcare Enterprise (IHE) for TIPPSS

As stated in [16]: "The IHE Framework identifies a subset of the functional components of the healthcare enterprise, called IHE actors, and specifies their inter-actions in terms of a set of coordinated, standards-based transactions. Transactions are organized into functional units called integration profiles that highlight their capacity to address specific IT Infrastructure requirements."

The IHE governance model has three main traits working together to provide the IHE functionality:

- **Establishing standards**: IHE is not a standardization body; it selects existing standards using specific criteria (such as market penetration, security, and support for specific use-cases) as a cornerstone of its interoperability provisions.
- **Creating standards-based specifications**: IHE further profiles the standards to establish interoperability and security-by-design.
- **Quality assurance**. IHE organizes public events called Connect-a-thons, where products are tested for compliance with its specifications.

Figure 2.1 illustrates the governance model for each IHE domain[2] through which the above-described functionalities are established. Each clinical use-case is submitted to a dedicated group of technicians who select the relevant standards for the specific problem. These standards are then embedded into a **profile**—a specific

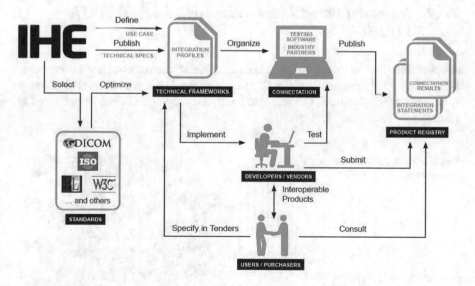

Fig. 2.1 The IHE Process. (Source: https://www.ihe.net/about_ihe/ihe_process/)

---

[2] As of 2021, IHE is composed of 11 domains: https://www.ihe.net/IHE_Domains/.

set of functionalities containing implementation details wrapped by **actors**, as well as optional **transactions**, defining in that way the **architecture variability points**. A profile's *variability* means that the diversity of the transactions impacts and determines the functionality of that profile. Vendors then test their implementation of each profile in Connect-a-thons.

Profiles are the cornerstone of the IHE methodology. They embody the governance rules for constricting standards to guarantee interoperability. Their life cycle is itself governed to guarantee overall sustainability, and they are the de facto building blocks in a Reference Architecture, containing functionalities for solving specific use-cases. IT architects design IHE-based architectures through formal procedures, by using profiles and grouping them according to specific **grouping rules**. The operation of grouping consists of merging different profile functionalities to build complex use-cases. When grouping, a new profile is created to contain the combined use-cases [16]. The final combination of profiles is the target solution architecture.

In the remainder of this work, we reuse the concepts of *domain, profile,* and *grouping* to enable an IHE-like governance model for the generic methodology. In that way, we benefit from a mature and standards-based methodology and provide backward compatibility with the frameworks that are already employed in the e-health domains.

2.4.2 Industrial Internet Reference Architecture (IIRA) for TIPPSS

As described in the overview of relevant architecture frameworks, the concerns of an Industrial Internet System (IIS) within the IIRA are integrated through four viewpoints: Business, Usage, Functional, and Implementation, as presented in Fig. 2.2.

Fig. 2.2 IIRA Architecture Viewpoints

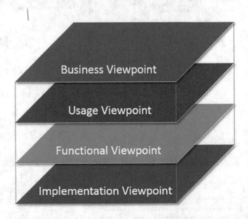

The *business viewpoint* addresses the business-oriented concerns. These include: the identification of stakeholders and their enterprise vision, the values and objectives for the context of interest, including business, ethical, legal, and regulatory context. It further identifies how these objectives are achieved by mapping them to the designed system capabilities.

The *usage viewpoint* determines the practical matching between the stakeholders' concerns and the potential system functionality. It is modeled as sequences of activities involving either human users or artificial agents that deliver the intended functionality to achieve the desired capabilities. The stakeholders at this level include: system engineers, product managers, and other individuals who are involved in the specification of the specific IIS, including end users.

The *functional viewpoint* focuses on the functional components in an IIS, accounting for their interdependencies and internal design, the nature of establishing the interactions between them, and their relation with the external environment. Through the functional viewpoint, the systems are interfaced with the outside world. Therefore, the concerns addressed at this level are of particular interest to system and component architects, developers, and integrators.

Finally, the *implementation viewpoint* deals with the concrete technologies required to realize the functional specifications, the behavioral patterns, and their life cycle considerations. All of the components at this level are coordinated by activities (through the Usage viewpoint) and facilitate the desired system capabilities (through the interface with the Business viewpoint). The concerns resolved at this level are mainly of interest to the technical personnel involved in the system design: system and component architects, developers and integrators, and system operators.

2.4.2.1 Security Concerns Across IIRA Viewpoints

Any Internet connected system calls for an integrated approach to security, spanning across the physical, the network and the business world, in order to address all cybersecurity aspects relevant for the specific enterprise/organization. At a general level, these include direct observability and monitoring of services, legal compliance in terms of consumer/patients/workers' rights, but also property rights and regulatory conformance when making contracts. This in and of itself implies that security cannot be an add-on design concern, but a property that is to be embedded from a mere design stage.

With that in mind, IIRA integrates security policies as part of the system design for the physical systems in general, including the hardware, software, and communication components. This allows security to be embedded across all architecture viewpoints:

- The business viewpoint establishes the return on investment for security, while ensuring performance and consumer satisfaction.
- The usage viewpoint makes security transparent to the user, in that way facilitating the trust establishment in an implicit way as well. In addition, it

minimizes both user involvement and the need for security expert intervention by establishing clear borders between machine-to-machine protocols and human interaction.

- The functional viewpoint defines the exact security functions that must be provided for each domain and determines the protocols for federated security management for the entire system.
- Finally, the implementation viewpoint applies the concrete security technologies and interfaces taking into account the common architecture patterns and the rest of the system components.

It is precisely due to these holistic considerations that the IIRA is chosen as the main reference architecture upon which the proposed framework in this chapter is based. In that way, we aim to both provide an enhanced view of security across all architecture viewpoints and to ensure backward compatibility with existing state of the art approaches that have proved to be practically implementable in real-world complex systems.

All elements in a clinical IoT system are subject to various threats from various types of entities, through both intentional and unintentional attacks: employees and other insiders, casual hackers, terrorists, and state-sponsored actors. Secure system design requires consideration of not only threats and the typical software issues, but also hardware design at chip and device level, physical system design, a robust personnel security program and supply chain security. The functional capabilities that address these threats manifest differently at each architecture viewpoint, as they have a business rationale and value (business viewpoint), are coordinated by specific activities and roles (usage viewpoint), have specific security functions (functional viewpoint), and dictate some architectural and deployment properties while relying on specific technologies (implementation viewpoint).

As shown in Table 2.1, IIRA addresses the biggest subset of TIPPSS principles in comparison to the other reference architectures. However, it mainly takes a threat-based approach to determining the set of security measures that are relevant for the particular context, lacking the consideration of the security goals relevant for the system in general. In addition, it provides no account on how adaptability in terms of security concerns is addressed as part of the overall organization change management. Therefore, we provide a goal-based account of security and complement the existing threat-view of IIRA in order to account for the full set of TIPPSS properties, even down to a viewpoint level. The following section presents the methodological account of this extension.

2.4.3 Reference Model for Information Assurance and Security (RMIAS) for TIPPSS

A comprehensive security model that integrates users, assets, data, and entry points must consider: the solution as a whole, the security and privacy features, the features whose failures are security relevant and the features that cross a trust boundary separating different trust levels or domains. A threat-based approach requires a history of system behavior and an operational environment to create a base to properly integrate the risk management of those threats. This is often not possible when architecting a system, preventing the designer to embed security-by-design and to devise a comprehensive security model. To address this problem, we propose to complement the existing threat-view in the IIRA with a goal-based model for security and assurance. A goal-based model allows us to first give a desired set of security goals that a system should accomplish and, by ensuring direct observability through the architecture viewpoint, to adaptively integrate the threat-view that would allow us to securely accomplish those goals. To realize this, we use the Reference Model for Information Assurance and Security (RMIAS), depicted in Fig. 2.3 [43].

With the premise that security must integrate all stages of product and system life cycles, the RMIAS accounts for the nature of information assets to protect, acknowledges the organizational risk tradeoffs in handling the assets, and develops

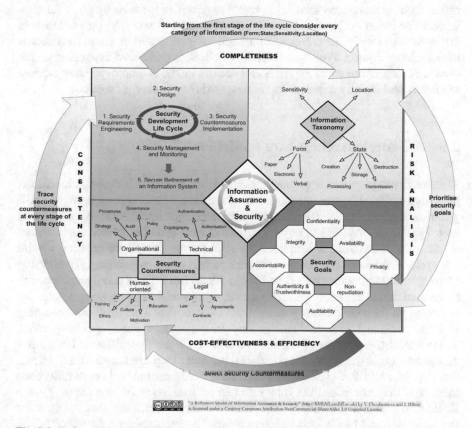

Fig. 2.3 Reference Model for Information Assurance and Security

security countermeasures to mitigate those risks and to address other vulnerabilities in the IT system. Moreover, assurance provides a means to structure the reasoning about safety, security, or resiliency in a given environment, so that architects can gain confidence that systems will work as expected. In that sense, assurance can even be a key element in the documentation of the system, as it provides a map to more detailed information regarding the security-by-design principles. The RMIAS consists of four dimensions and several steps showing their interrelationship. The security aspects (dimensions) composing the RMIAS goal-based view are: *Security Development Life Cycle (SDLC), Information Taxonomy, Security Goals,* and *Security Countermeasures.*

A preparation step is needed to adopt a security development life cycle (SDLC) and an information taxonomy suitable to the organization. RMIAS allows tailoring the SDLC to one's needs, requiring only for it to be properly embedded in the overall information system life cycle. In the first step, the information assets to protect are recognized and categorized through an information taxonomy, based on their forms, levels of sensitivity, locations, and states, producing a quadruple (Form; State; Location; Sensitivity) for each asset. When the information taxonomy is prepared, a risk analysis is performed with field experts to prioritize the security goals for each information category. Then, for each information category security countermeasures are devised to satisfy the corresponding security goal, based on cost-effectiveness and efficiency criteria. Finally, a consistency check is performed depending on the chosen SDLC. In our case, the IIRA architecture model is employed as an enabler to identify and classify the assets to protect, as shown in the next section.

2.5   A Generic Architecture Model for TIPPSS

The framework proposed here integrates standards-based methodologies to address the issues outlined in the introduction. At the core of the approach are the IHE governance principles, the IIRA architecture framework, and the RMIAS goal-based security. The methodological novelty at the technical level lies in enabling freedom of choice of the SDLC to introduce the IIRA in the overall information system life cycle. The model is envisaged to work as part of an overarching Architecture Development Methodology, as described in Algorithm 2.1 and it is generic enough to be used inside a variety of architectural frameworks. The procedure starts by operating on an initial solution in the form of a set P of IHE profiles. According to IHE, additional profiles "emerge" by following mandatory grouping rules, which establish dependencies between profiles. Each profile is dissected into IIRA viewpoints. Once the layers are populated, the outer loop implements the RMIAS, iterating over all IIRA viewpoints. After the relevant information assets have been identified, they are classified into information categories as demanded by the RMIAS information taxonomy. The desired security goals are then elicited for the categories, and finally cost-effective security countermeasures are selected. The model also checks for completeness by mapping each countermeasure to a specific transaction or actor in the IHE security profiles from P.

Algorithm 2.1 Devising a Generic Cybersecurity Architecture Model
Data: An initial set of grouped IHE profiles, P
Result: $P \cup$ {the set of additional security profiles creating a solution architecture with all the countermeasures satisfying the security goals identified by RMIAS}

    repeat
        Dissect each $p \in P$;
        Let $C = \varnothing$ be the set of security countermeasures;
        Let M be the matrix representing the i-th IIRA viewpoint;
        foreach *viewpoint in IIRA from Implementation to Business* **do**
            Let $T = \varnothing$ be the set of the RMIAS taxonomies' quadruple;
            Let $G = \varnothing$ be the set of the RMIAS security goals;
            Identify the asset m from the profile $p \in P$;
            Let $M \leftarrow m$ according to the System's security cycle;
            foreach $M \leftarrow m$ **do**
                Create a taxonomy entry t as {*Form* : *State* : *Location*: *Sensitivity* : };
                $T \leftarrow t$
            end
            foreach $T \leftarrow t$ **do**
                Outline appropriate security goals for t;
                Perform risk analysis // with field experts;
                Create a goal g and assign its priority;
                $G \leftarrow g$;
            end
            foreach $G \leftarrow g$ **do**
                Evaluate countermeasures c that satisfies g;
                $C \leftarrow c$;
            end
            if *not all countermeasures* $C \leftarrow c$ *are available in the profiles in P.*
            then
                Select or create new profile p' containing the missing counter measures;
                $P \leftarrow p'$ with its additional grouped profiles;
                dissect p';
                break – Start from Implementation layer;
            end
         end
    until *all* $C \leftarrow c$ *are available in* P;

It is important to note that the algorithm also allows for the definition of new viewpoints and concerns within each viewpoint. Moreover, it is not constrained to strictly using IIRA as the underlying architecture framework, but also supports any other architecture with well-defined viewpoints and concerns. Table 2.2 offers a

Table 2.2 Mapping between IoT reference architectures viewpoints

IoT Reference Architectures	IIRA	Draft ISO IoT RA	RAMI 4.0	TOGAF
Architecture Viewpoints	Business		Business	Business
	Usage	Usage		
	Functional	Functional	Functional	
		Information	Information	Data
				Application
		Communication	Communication	
	Implementation	System	Integration	Technology
			Asset	
			Life cycle/value chain	
			Hierarchy	

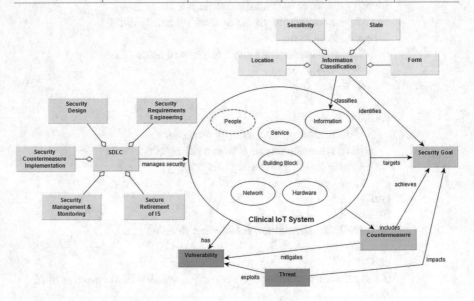

Fig. 2.4 The generic cybersecurity architecture framework

mapping between the viewpoints of the four most common reference architectures presented in the overview of relevant architecture frameworks, which can be used in adjusting Algorithm 2.1 and its application to a certain use-case and domain.

In that sense, the methodology for developing a goal-based security architecture approach is generic and applicable to contexts other than e-Health and within paradigms other than IoT. This is one of the most valuable features of the presented approach, provided by relying on general system design principles. The elements of the overall methodology are shown in Fig. 2.4.

The security aspects (i.e., dimensions) composing the RMIAS goal-based view are: Security Development Life Cycle (SDLC) (represented in green), Information

Classification (in yellow, which corresponds to the RMIAS taxonomy), Security Goals (in orange), and Countermeasures (in blue).

- SDLC illustrates how security is built up along the system development life cycle.
- Information Taxonomy characterizes the nature of information being protected.
- Security Goals contain a broadly applicable list of eight security goals: Confidentiality; Integrity; Availability; Accountability; Authentication (and Trustworthiness); Non-repudiation; Privacy and Auditability.
- Countermeasures categorize the countermeasures available for information protection.

To address the threats and vulnerabilities of the system, the goal-based model is complemented by a threat-view, which is represented by the purple blocks in Fig. 2.4.

In order to realize how the TIPPSS principles are addressed by the architecture design, the next subsection provides categorization of each aspect at a viewpoint level.

2.5.1 Architecture-Based TIPPSS Taxonomy

Based on the developed architecture model and the cybersecurity concerns outlined so far, we are now able to provide a systematized conceptual framework of TIPPSS principles in view of the individual architecture viewpoints. This is structured into a TIPPSS taxonomy, given in Table 2.3.

The taxonomy integrates design principles, methods, requirements, and system properties that are extracted from the existing taxonomies in the field and represent an intersection between the TIPPSS properties, the architecture viewpoints, and their applicability to a clinical IoT context. It is certainly not the exhaustive set of possible categorization in terms of properties, traits, and principles, but it provides a framework that is consistent with the current state of the art, while providing a common ground for reasoning on the relevant issues and allowing for extensibility.

Having such a taxonomy is useful for several reasons: for the architects, it provides direct insights into the desired system properties required to achieve TIPPSS compliance; for the decision-makers, it facilitates the definition of stakeholder concerns both in general and by architectural viewpoint; for the business owners, it creates awareness of the technical properties that should be accounted for during investment planning and supports the overall change management of the organizations as it includes the organization's dynamics in each of the security considerations; for the implementers, it provides a structured catalog of functionalities to be aware of and provides opportunities for adaptive change of those functionalities. Finally, for regulators, it gives an overview of how each aspect of the legal frameworks is transposed within the systems requirements and adapted to suit the stakeholders' needs.

Table 2.3 Architecture-based TIPPSS Taxonomy

Cybersecurity Concern	Trust	Identity	Privacy	Protection and Safety	Security
Viewpoint					
Implementation	Scoring and ranking; incentives/sanctions	Context-dependence; information sources	Information exchange; identity scheme; consent policies	Security legacy systems	End-to-end security; counter measures
Functional	Authentication; behavioral traits; preferential logic	Identity management; integrity; accountability	Data protection; personalization; user consent	Physical protection; account for human rights	Cryptographic support; ID verification in communication
Usage	Auditing; decision-making; forgiveness/forgetting (of the system)	Non-repudiation; access control; implicit knowledge	Privacy policies; transferability of data	Security monitoring; alarm systems	Security policies; cryptographic support; timestamping; auditing
Business	Business value; incentives/sanctions; reputation	Regulatory and compliance	Regulatory; auditability	Regulatory and compliance	Regulatory; auditability

In that way, the taxonomy, together with the architecture itself, facilitates the dialog between the relevant stakeholders without requiring deep technical knowledge on the one side and high-level management expertise on the other.

2.6 Evaluation of Cybersecurity Architectures

Although the IIRA integrates some security concerns introducing a threat-view across its viewpoints, it does not account for the specific threats relevant across a wider set of security domains. While such an approach suffices at the design phase, it does not offer the necessary analytics for an evaluation to be made just by considering the design principles. Therefore, we rely on an extended threat model based on the European Union Agency for Cybersecurity (ENISA) guidelines on security measures adjusted for critical sectors like the clinical IoT [44, 45] and couple them with the existing architectural goal-view on security offered by the RMIAS. In that manner, we offer an evaluation methodology for the entire architecture from both threat-based and goal-based perspectives.

We now briefly introduce the ENISA guidelines on security measures and the detailed threat-view they offer.

2.6.1 ENISA Guidelines on Security Measures and a Threat-Based View

The ENISA guidelines on security measures sublime an extensive list of national and international EU electronic communications standards into a set of security objectives divided by domain [44]. They outline 25 security objectives (as shown in Fig. 2.5), each analyzed through various security measures and supported by evidence testifying that an objective was met. The security measures are grouped in three sophistication levels, whereas the security objectives are divided into seven domains of application. This provides a suitable framework of complementary views to the goal-based security evaluation.

Clearly, all of these security assets are relevant for clinical IoT, which is why the ENISA security measures and objectives are better understood if approached by some aspect (in our case, from an architecture viewpoint) in the evaluation. To determine the relevance per viewpoint, a mapping of the contextual and security traits between the clinical IoT security needs and the ENISA provisions is performed, as presented in Fig. 2.5 showing the whole set of ENISA security objectives divided by domains. The coloring is done in relation to the relevant viewpoint (business, functional, usage, technology) and is compliant to the TOGAF architecture modeling convention: yellow is assigned to the business viewpoint; blue for the functional and purple for the usage viewpoints (in TOGAF the data and the application layers, known under the common name information system layers); and green for the technology layer.

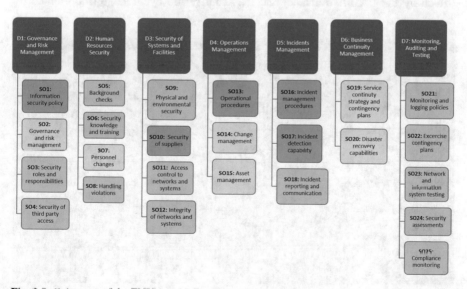

Fig. 2.5 Relevance of the ENISA guidelines by architecture viewpoint

The decision about which security objective is relevant for a particular viewpoint is highly context dependent. Therefore, the current categorization should be revised as part of a strategic dialog between the architects and the relevant stakeholders, and also in view of the precise implementation context. This in and of itself testifies that without having a set of initial security goals that correspond to the security requirements for the assets, infrastructure, and the stakeholders' needs, a threat-based view of security will be useless to provide security-by-design with no history of system behaviors. Therefore, the following section complements ENISA's threat-based framework with a goal-based view of the security measures.

2.6.2 *Complementary Goal-Based View*

Mapping the contextual and the security traits of RMIAS to the ENISA framework provides sufficient practical and scientific rigor in accomplishing the task of a holistic cybersecurity evaluation. Moreover, it enables the extraction of specific guidelines and recommendations for the security measures that must be adopted to meet the security objectives.

Next, we map each dimension of the Reference Model for Information Assurance and Security to each ENISA domain (D1 through D7) and security objective (SO 1 through SO 25). Then, we determine the relevance of that mapping for each of the architecture viewpoints and for the overall architecture. This mapping is shown in Fig. 2.6 and results in a 25 × 25 matrix as a granular representation of the context (given by the ENISA domains) and the security life cycle stage (represented by

RMIAS		ENISA guidelines	D1				D2				D3				D4			D5			D6		D7				
			SO 1	SO 2	SO 3	SO 4	SO 5	SO 6	SO 7	SO 8	SO 9	SO 10	SO 11	SO 12	SO 13	SO 14	SO 15	SO 16	SO 17	SO 18	SO 19	SO 20	SO 21	SO 22	SO 23	SO 24	SO 25
Security goals		Confidentiality																									
Security goals		Integrity																									
Security goals		Availability																									
Security goals		Privacy																									
Security goals		Authentication																									
Security goals		Non-repudiation																									
Security goals		Accountability																									
Security goals		Auditability																									
Information taxonomy	State	Creation																									
Information taxonomy	State	Processing																									
Information taxonomy	State	Storage																									
Information taxonomy	State	Transmission																									
Information taxonomy	State	Destruction																									
Information taxonomy		Form																									
Information taxonomy		Sensitivity																									
Information taxonomy		Location																									
Counter-measures		Technical																									
Counter-measures		Legal																									
Counter-measures		Organizational																									
Counter-measures		Human-oriented																									
Security System lifecycle		Design																									
Security System lifecycle		Implementation																									
Security System lifecycle		Management and monitoring																									
Security System lifecycle		Redundancy and fault-tolerance																									
Security System lifecycle		System retirement																									

Fig. 2.6 Mapping RMIAS to ENISA guidelines by relevance for each architecture viewpoint

the RMIAS dimensions), with an additional dimension for architecture viewpoint (represented by the colors that correspond to the IIRA layers).

The coloring in the figure shows a case where the highest security standards are followed throughout the entire healthcare system. It does not focus on a particular use-case, where not every security measure would be considered relevant. Thus, the same methodology can be followed at a use-case level as well, and it will most likely result in a case where not all of the matrix cells of Fig. 2.6 are colored, i.e., not all of the security measures are required to address the desired security goals throughout the architecture viewpoints. For instance, a remote sensor for home usage will not have the same requirements and security goals as a patient file within the premises of the healthcare facility. Even for a same security goal like "Privacy," the specific security measures devised by the methodology will differ. This is also one of the strengths of the mixed goal-threat-based methodology—high level of context awareness and adaptive security measures.

Finally, it is worth noting that this table can further be checked for compliance with international standards by comparing it against the mapping of ENISA domains and security objectives to international standards in Section 6 of the ENISA guidelines on security measures [44].

2.7 Summary

Clinical IoT is a data-driven critical sector where the interconnectedness of entities (people, devices, and services) create a complex system for collection, exchange, and processing of data at different system levels: from the patient's body area network to trans-continental IT infrastructure. Such settings change the classical concept of a hospital, extending the services' capabilities, but also exposing a wider attack surface to cyber threats and introducing new security challenges, as more of the entities become transparent to the outside environment.

This chapter presented a holistic architectural account of security, right from the design stage of establishing the system architecture. It enables the account of an extensive set of desired architecture properties, both from system perspective (governance, sustainability, interoperability, automation, and variability) and from cybersecurity perspective (trust, identity, privacy, protection, safety, and security). Based on the devised architecture viewpoints, it categorizes the security methods, the design principles, and systems properties into an architecture-based TIPPSS taxonomy that is meant to provide a common ground for a multi-stakeholder dialog and a starting point for defining a clinical IoT cybersecurity ontology. Finally, this work offers an evaluation framework for the development of a methodology that adds a goal-based view to the current threat aspect of security in the architecture framework in order to provide adaptive cybersecurity for the existing and future change management in healthcare organizations.

It is important to stress that the methodology outlined in this chapter is based on a well-established set of standards, enabling security-by-design at the architecture level without disrupting the existing systems in production.

2.8 Future Work

Our current work is focused on providing a complete toolchain for automation of all the steps proposed by the methodology in this chapter. In particular, we have been working on defining an Architecture Description Language named Modeling Security Architecture Aspects (MOSA2) [46], which provides a formalism for automatic consistency check (as a final step of the integration of the RMIAS into the architecture levels). Next, we will investigate the possibility to enable integration of regulatory requirements as part of the security objectives. This will be initiated through a semantic vocabulary that would allow for definition of an extensive set of security goals and offer the possibilities for formal specification that can be made testable and reusable. In addition, we will integrate it into the existing methodology to aid the cost and efficiency evaluation, which are currently done manually by the architect and also requires additional security expertise.

Acknowledgments The work presented in this chapter has been carried out in close collaboration with my dear colleagues Massimilano Masi, Giampaolo Sellitto, Helder Aranha, and Eric Grandry, to whom I owe much of the appreciation for architecture modeling and the notion of cybersecurity by design. Their support, availability, and guidance also helped me in shaping a holistic attitude towards critical infrastructures security in general, and healthcare systems in particular.

References

1. NIS. Directive (EU) 2016/1148 of the European Parliament and of the Council of 6 July 2016 concerning measures for a high common level of security of network and information systems across the Union [Internet]. 194, 32016L1148 Jul 19, 2016. Available from: http://data.europa.eu/eli/dir/2016/1148/oj/eng
2. GDPR. REGULATION (EU) 2016/679 OF THE EUROPEAN PARLIAMENT AND OF THE COUNCIL [Internet]. Official Journal of the European Union. 2016 [cited 2020 Nov 1]. Available from: https://eur-lex.europa.eu/legal-content/EN/TXT/HTML/?uri=CELEX:32016R0679&from=it
3. HIPPA. Health Insurance Portability and Accountability Act of 1996 (HIPAA) | CDC [Internet]. 2019 [cited 2020 Nov 1]. Available from: https://www.cdc.gov/phlp/publications/topic/hipaa.html
4. Scholl M, Stine K, Hash J, Bowen P, Johnson L, Smith C, et al. An Introductory Resource Guide for Implementing the Health Insurance Portability and Accountability Act (HIPAA) Security Rule [Internet]. National Institute of Standards and Technology; 2008 Oct [cited 2020 Nov 1]. Report No.: NIST Special Publication (SP) 800-66 Rev. 1. Available from: https://csrc.nist.gov/publications/detail/sp/800-66/rev-1/final

5. "Pre-Standards Workstream Report: Clinical IoT Data Validation and Interoperability with Blockchain," in *Pre-Standards Workstream Report: Clinical IoT Data Validation and Interoperability with Blockchain*, vol., no., pp. 1-29, 28 June 2019.
6. (EU) 2015/1302. Commission Decision (EU) 2015/1302 of 28 July 2015 on the identification of Integrating the Healthcare Enterprise profiles for referencing in public procurement [Internet]. 2015 [cited 2020 Nov 1]. Available from: https://eur-lex.europa.eu/legal-content/GA/TXT/?uri=CELEX%3A32015D1302
7. Continua Alliance,. CONTINUA DESIGN GUIDELINES [Internet]. 2019 [cited 2020 Nov 1]. Available from: https://www.pchalliance.org/continua-design-guidelines
8. Castelfranchi C, Falcone R. Trust Theory: A Socio-Cognitive and Computational Model. John Wiley and Sons; 2010. 388 p.
9. Luhmann N. Familiarity, Confidence, Trust: Problems and Alternatives. 2000.
10. Marsh S. Formalising trust as a computational concept. 1994 Apr;170.
11. Stoneburner G. Underlying technical models for information technology security: recommendations of the National Institute of Standards and Technology [Internet]. 0 ed. Gaithersburg, MD: National Institute of Standards and Technology; 2001 [cited 2020 Nov 17]. Report No.: NIST SP 800-33. Available from: https://nvlpubs.nist.gov/nistpubs/Legacy/SP/nistspecialpublication800-33.pdf
12. Alibeigi A, Munir AB, Karim ME. Right to Privacy, A Complicated Concept to Review [Internet]. Rochester, NY: Social Science Research Network; 2019 [cited 2020 Nov 17]. Report No.: ID 3537968. Available from: https://papers.ssrn.com/abstract=3537968
13. https://iapp.org/about/what-is-privacy/.
14. IEC. Briefing paper: Functional safety essential to overall safety – en, ru – IEC Basecamp [Internet]. 2015 [cited 2020 Oct 23]. Available from: https://basecamp.iec.ch/download/functional-safety-essential-to-overall-safety/
15. ISO/IEC JTC 1/SC 27. ISO/IEC 27000:2018 [Internet]. ISO. 2018 [cited 2020 Nov 17]. Available from: https://www.iso.org/cms/render/live/en/sites/isoorg/contents/data/standard/07/39/73906.html
16. IHE. IHE IT Infrastructure (ITI) Technical Framework [Internet]. IHE International, Inc.; 2020. Available from: https://ihe.net/uploadedFiles/Documents/ITI/IHE_ITI_TF_Vol1.pdf
17. Abdul-Rahman A, Hailes S. A distributed trust model. In: Proceedings of the 1997 workshop on New security paradigms [Internet]. New York, NY, USA: ACM; 1997 [cited 2012 Mar 16]. p. 48–60. (NSPW '97). Available from: https://doi.org/10.1145/283699.283739
18. Dellarocas C, Wood CA. The Sound of Silence in Online Feedback: Estimating Trading Risks in the Presence of Reporting Bias. Management Science. 2008 Mar 1;54(3):460–76.
19. Zhou R, Hwang K. PowerTrust: A Robust and Scalable Reputation System for Trusted Peer-to-Peer Computing. IEEE Trans Parallel Distrib Syst. 2007 Apr;18(4):460–73.
20. Wang Y, Singh MP. Evidence-based trust: A mathematical model geared for multiagent systems. ACM Transactions on Autonomous and Adaptive Systems. 2010 Nov;5(4):14:1-14:28.
21. Chakravartula RN, V NL. Trust Management Framework for IOT Based P2P Objects International Journal of Peer to Peer Networks. 2017 Aug 30;8(2/3):17–24.
22. Health Care Provider Taxonomy Codes List [Internet]. [cited 2021 Sep 17]. Available from: https://healthprovidersdata.com/hipaa/codes/taxonomycodes.aspx
23. Scarpato N, Alessandra P, Di Nunzio L, Fallucchi F. E-health-IoT universe: A review International Journal on Advanced Science, Engineering and Information Technology. 2017 Dec 30;7(6).
24. Muras J, Cahill V, Stokes E. A Taxonomy of Pervasive Healthcare Systems. 1st International Conference on Pervasive Computing Technologies for Healthcare 2006. 2007. 1 p.
25. Alsubaei F, Abuhussein A, Shiva S. Security and Privacy in the Internet of Medical Things: Taxonomy and Risk Assessment. 2017.
26. Chen K, Zhang S, Li Z, Zhang Y, Deng Q, Ray S, et al. Internet-of-Things Security and Vulnerabilities: Taxonomy, Challenges, and Practice. Journal of Hardware and Systems Security. 2018 Jun;2(2):97–110.

27. Henschke C, Panteli D, Perleth M, Busse R. TAXONOMY OF MEDICAL DEVICES IN THE LOGIC OF HEALTH TECHNOLOGY ASSESSMENT. Int J Technol Assess Health Care. 2015 Jan;31(5):324–30.
28. Gottschalk M, Uslar M, Delfs C. The Use Case and Smart Grid Architecture Model Approach: The IEC 62559-2 Use Case Template and the SGAM applied in various domains. 1st ed. 2017 edition. New York, NY: Springer; 2017. 110 p.
29. Lapalme J, Gerber A, Van der Merwe A, Zachman J, Vries MD, Hinkelmann K. Exploring the future of enterprise architecture: A Zachman perspective. Computers in Industry. 2016 Jun 1;79:103–13.
30. Franke U, Ekstedt M, Lagerström R, Saat J, Winter R. Trends in Enterprise Architecture Practice – A Survey. In: Proper E, Lankhorst MM, Schönherr M, Barjis J, Overbeek S, editors. Trends in Enterprise Architecture Research. Berlin, Heidelberg: Springer; 2010. p. 16–29. (Lecture Notes in Business Information Processing).
31. Dedic N. FEAMI: A Methodology to include and to integrate Enterprise Architecture Processes into Existing Organizational Processes. IEEE Engineering Management Review. 2020;1–1.
32. Muñoz A, Augusto JC, Villa A, Botía JA. Design and evaluation of an ambient assisted living system based on an argumentative multi-agent system. Personal and Ubiquitous Computing. 2011 Apr;15(4):377–87.
33. Zuccato A, Daniels N, Jampathom C, Nilson M. Report: Modular Safeguards to Create Holistic Security Requirement Specifications for System of Systems. In: Massacci F, Wallach D, Zannone N, editors. Engineering Secure Software and Systems. Springer Berlin Heidelberg; 2010. p. 218–30. (Lecture Notes in Computer Science).
34. Alsubaei F, Abuhussein A, Shandilya V, Shiva S. IoMT-SAF: Internet of Medical Things Security Assessment Framework. Internet of Things. 2019 Dec 1;8:100123.
35. ISO/IEC JTC 1/SC 41. ISO/IEC 30141:2018 Internet of Things (IoT)—Reference Architecture [Internet]. ISO. 2018 [cited 2020 Nov 13]. Available from: https://www.iso.org/cms/render/live/en/sites/isoorg/contents/data/standard/06/56/65695.html
36. Lin S-W, Mellor S, Miller B, Durand J, Crawford M, Lembree R. Industrial Internet Reference Architecture. 2015 Jun;(Version 1.7):100.
37. ISO/IEC JTC 1/SC 7. ISO/IEC 10746-2:2009 Information technology—Open distributed processing—Reference model: Foundations—Part 2 [Internet]. ISO. 2009 [cited 2020 Nov 13]. Available from: https://www.iso.org/cms/render/live/en/sites/isoorg/contents/data/standard/05/57/55723.html
38. Hankel M, Rexroth B. The Reference Architectural Model Industrie 4.0 (RAMI 4.0). ZVEI: Die Elektroindustrie. 2015 Apr;2.
39. IHE ITI Technical Committee. IHE IT Infrastructure Technical Framework: Mobile access to Health Documents (MHD) With XDS on FHIR [Internet]. IHE International, Inc; 2020. Available from: https://ihe.net//Documents/IuploadedFilesTI/IHE_ITI_Suppl_MHD.pdf
40. e-SENS. e-SENS White Paper Electronic Simple European Networked Services [Internet]. e-SENS Consortium; 2016. Available from: http://www.esens.eu/uploads/media/e-SENS_white_paper_general_06.pdf
41. Grandry E, e-SENS Architecture team. D6.7 e-SENS European Interoperability Reference Architecture [Internet]. European Commission; 2017. Available from: https://cordis.europa.eu/docs/projects/cnect/1/325211/080/deliverables/001-eSENSD67EuropeanInteroperabilityReferenceArchitecture.pdf
42. Harrison R. TOGAF 9 Foundation Study Guide - 3rd Edition. 3 edition. Publishing VH, editor. United Kingdom: Van Haren Publishing; 2016. 274 p. (TOGAF).
43. Cherdantseva Y, Hilton J. A Reference Model of Information Assurance & Security. In: Proceedings of the 2013 International Conference on Availability, Reliability and Security [Internet]. Washington, DC, USA: IEEE Computer Society; 2013. p. 546–55. (ARES '13). Available from: https://doi.org/10.1109/ARES.2013.72

44. ENISA. Technical Guideline on Minimum Security Measures—ENISA [Internet]. 2014 [cited 2017 Aug 31]. Available from: https://www.enisa.europa.eu/publications/technical-guideline-on-minimum-security-measures
45. ENISA. Good practices on interdependencies between OES and DSPs [Internet]. 2018 [cited 2020 Aug 11]. Available from: https://www.enisa.europa.eu/publications/good-practices-on-interdependencies-between-oes-and-dsps
46. Masi M. A Formalization of the IHE Process [Internet]. 2019 [cited 2021 Sep 17]. Available from: https://github.com/mascanc/MOSA2

Chapter 3
Do No Harm: Medical Device and Connected Hospital Security

Gabrielle E. Hempel

Contents

3.1 Hospitals: Past and Present

Tucked away near the coast of St. Augustine, Florida, lies a small, unassuming structure built in 1763 by a Scottish carpenter named William Watson. This building, among others, served as a hospital to the military during the Second Spanish Period—in which Spain reclaimed Florida. Today, it serves as a museum, a reminder of just how far medical prowess has advanced. There, visitors can immerse themselves in a world of some of the most advanced medicine of the era—early vaccinations, colonial herb gardens, a resident apothecary. Many items serve as ghosts of the technology present today—bed-wrenches for tightening ropes instead of automated-adjustment patient beds, candlesticks in lieu of surgical lights, and an

G. E. Hempel (✉)
RSA Security, New York, NY, USA

© Springer Nature Switzerland AG 2022
F. D. Hudson (eds.), *Women Securing the Future with TIPPSS for Connected Healthcare*, Women in Engineering and Science,
https://doi.org/10.1007/978-3-030-93592-4_3

isolation ward that looks eerily similar to those found today, sans the countless wires and monitors. Medical technology has grown exponentially in the centuries since the day-to-day operation of this hospital, but with growth comes growing pains. Much of the medical technology used currently has become advanced far ahead of its security measures—and technologists and attackers alike are learning of security shortcomings at a rapid pace.

Many of today's hospitals are rapidly becoming "smart" hospitals in order to apply the latest technology to patient care. To better understand the attack surface and connected medical device landscape, it is important to understand the vastness of the standard medical center.

3.2   A Typical Connected Hospital

A standard smart hospital room may look something like this: digital equipment is ubiquitous. In many medical centers, iPads and tablets display the necessary information outside the patient rooms, in the halls. These can also be helpful in terms of aiding doctors or visitors in understanding key information such as fall risks or specific safety protocols that they may need to be aware of. Once inside the room, almost all of the facility technology can be digitally controlled—the lights in the room, the media devices, the thermostat, and patient information displayed within the room. Often, the medical provider is able to pull up a patient's electronic health record and seamlessly transfer information from one platform or machine to another. Additional health-targeted devices in patient and other rooms include blood gas analyzers, diagnostic equipment like PET, MRI, and CT machines, therapeutic equipment like infusion pumps, lasers, and surgical machines, life support equipment like heart/lung machines, ventilators, extracorporeal membrane oxygen machines, and dialysis machines. The doctors and medical staff will use picture archives and communication systems that are often connected in order to communicate with patients and other staff.

Even venturing outside the room, there are many aspects of the hospital that are connected. Much of the security is managed via video surveillance, "smart" door locks and entry systems, and connected fire alarms. Building management systems will utilize connected power monitoring, power distribution, energy consumption/management monitoring, and elevators/transport. The environmental controls are also often connected and are extremely critical—these include HVAC, lighting, room control, water quality, humidity monitoring, and tissue/blood refrigeration. There will also be the standard technological infrastructure, usually including firewalls, intrusion detection and prevention systems, endpoint protection, antivirus, and encryption controls mandated by HIPAA. All of these devices and systems that could potentially be exploited make up the threat landscape (Fig. 3.1).

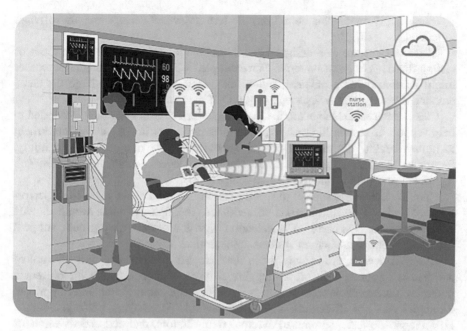

Fig. 3.1 Connected Hospital Room

3.3   Medical Devices

In order to best evaluate this vast ecosystem of medical devices, one must first understand the long history of devices in medicine. One of the first medical devices recorded dates back to 7000 BC in Balochistan, where Neolithic dentists used dental drills made of flint and bowstrings to perform procedures [1]. Archeologists have also uncovered many types of medical devices that were commonly used in ancient Rome. While it is hard to agree upon a global definition, the U.S. Food and Drug Administration (FDA) considers a medical device to be an "instrument, apparatus, implement, machine, contrivance, implant, in vitro reagent, or other similar or related article, including a component part, or accessory which is:

- Recognized in the official National Formulary, or the United States Pharmacopeia, or any supplement of those.
- Intended for use in the diagnosis of disease or other conditions, or in the cure, mitigation, treatment, or prevention of disease, in man or other animals.
- Intended to affect the structure or any function of the body of man or other animals
- Which does not achieve its primary intended purposes through chemical action within or on the body of man or other animals and which is not dependent upon being metabolized for the achievement of its primary intended purposes." [2]

Interestingly, under this definition, the term "device" doesn't include software functions.

These devices are also assigned risk classifications that dictate the amount of testing the devices must undergo. For example, a bandage or a tongue depressor might be considered a medical device but would not need to undergo the same amount of testing as, say, a pacemaker or MRI machine.

Class I devices are subject to the least regulatory control and are not intended to help support or sustain life or be substantially important in preventing impairment to human health, and may not present an unreasonable risk of illness or injury. Examples of Class I devices include elastic bandages, examination gloves, and hand-held surgical instruments (e.g., a scalpel) [2].

Class II devices are subject to special labeling requirements, mandatory performance standards, and postmarket surveillance. Examples of these would include acupuncture needles, powered wheelchairs, infusion pumps, air purifiers, surgical drapes, stereotaxic navigation systems, and surgical robots [2].

Class III devices are usually those that support or sustain human life, are of substantial importance in preventing impairment of human health, or present a potential, unreasonable risk of illness or injury and require premarket approval. Examples of Class III devices include implantable pacemakers, pulse generators, HIV diagnostic tests, automated external defibrillators, and endosseous implants [2].

The European Union has different classification standards, spanning four categories (I, IIA, IIB, III) from lowest to highest risk [3].

Clinically, there are many standards that a medical device must meet in order to be approved for use. There are ISO standards that address quality and risk management. They are applicable to all providers and manufacturers of medical devices, components, contract services, and distributors of medical devices. Additionally, they set precedence because they signify that a company engages in the creation of new products. They require that the development of manufactured products have an approval process and a set of rigorous quality standards and development records before the product is distributed. Additionally, there are standards for electrical devices (IEC 60601-1), active implantable medical devices (EN45502-1), and medical software (IEC 62304). The FDA also published a series of industry guidance regarding this topic against 21 CFR 820 Subchapter H—Medical Devices. Subpart B includes quality system requirements, an essential component of which are design controls (21 CFR 820.30) [4].

A 2011 study by Dr. Diana Zuckerman and Paul Brown of the National Center for Health Research, and Dr. Steven Nissen of the Cleveland Clinic, published in the Archives of Internal Medicine, showed that most medical devices recalled in the last 5 years for "serious health problems or death" had been previously approved by the FDA using the less stringent, and cheaper, 510(k) process. In a few cases, the devices had been deemed so low risk that they did not undergo any FDA regulatory review. Of the 113 devices recalled in the 2006–2011 timeframe by the US FDA, 35 were for cardiovascular issues [5]. This study was the topic of Congressional hearings re-evaluating FDA procedures and oversight.

A 2014 study by Dr. Diana Zuckerman, Paul Brown, and Dr. Aditi Das of the National Center for Health Research, published in JAMA Internal Medicine, examined the scientific evidence that is publicly available about medical implants that were cleared by the FDA 510(k) process from 2008 to 2012. They found that scientific evidence supporting "substantial equivalence" to other devices already on the market was required by law to be publicly available, but the information was available for only 16% of the randomly selected implants, and only 10% provided clinical data. Of the more than 1100 predicate implants that the new implants were substantially equivalent to, only 3% had any publicly available scientific evidence, and only 1% had clinical evidence of safety or effectiveness [5]. The researchers concluded that publicly available scientific evidence on implants was needed to protect the public health.

In 2014–2015 a new international agreement, the Medical Device Single Audit Program (MDSAP), was implemented with five participant countries: Australia, Brazil, Canada, Japan, and the United States. The aim of this program was to "develop a process that allows a single audit or inspection to ensure the medical device regulatory requirements for all five countries are satisfied" [6].

In 2017, a study by Dr. Jay Ronquillo and Dr. Diana Zuckerman published in the peer-reviewed policy journal Milbank Quarterly found that electronic health records and other device software were recalled due to life-threatening flaws. The article pointed out the lack of safeguards against hacking and other cybersecurity threats, stating, "current regulations are necessary but not sufficient for ensuring patient safety by identifying and eliminating dangerous defects in software currently on the market." They added that legislative changes resulting from the law entitled the twenty-first Century Cures Act "will further deregulate health IT, reducing safeguards that facilitate the reporting and timely recall of flawed medical software that could harm patients" [7].

3.4 An Intersection of Software and Medicine

While medical software has been in use since the 1960s, the FDA didn't begin to ramp up its involvement in the development of the software deployed on these devices until nearing the end of the 1980s. A new radiation therapy device (Therac-25) had incidences of overdosing patients because of software coding errors. Medical device software is considered in the United States as "any software that meets the legal definition of a [medical] device." Because this is such a broad generalization, they can be classified based on technical nature, level of safety, or on their primary function [8].

With the invasion of smartphones in the twenty-first century, the notion of software as a medical device became even more widespread. Many of these programs fell into a gray area of regulation, as hardware was covered under the regulatory standards, but software often wasn't. In July 2011, the FDA released draft guidance on mobile medical applications, which essentially lumped it in with all other software programs as far as regulatory testing went. It was implied that it should be interpreted as "as applicable to all software ... since the test for determining whether a mobile application is a regulated mobile 'medical' application is the same test one would use to determine if any software is regulated" [9].

The territory that mobile apps cover is a wide range, including installed pacemakers, image-analysis software, graphic data like EEGs/bedside monitors, urine analyzers, glucometers, stethoscopes, spirometers, BMI calculators, heart rate monitors, and body fat calculators.

Many groups struggled to grasp the ideation behind regulating medical device software, and a universal definition has yet to be established for SaMD (Software as a Medical Device).

3.5 Present Devices

For ease of reference, this text will classify medical devices into three categories: primary, secondary, and tertiary.

A primary device is one that is implanted or that provides immediate support to a person. This could include pacemakers, defibrillators, and neurostimulators.

Secondary devices will be patient-adjacent devices. These include patient monitoring (i.e., smart med, or medicine using information technologies, such as the Internet of Things, big data, cloud computing, and artificial intelligence to transform the medical system in order to make it more efficient, effective, and convenient; infusion pumps, ventilators, incubators, telemetry, smart stethoscopes, and medical imaging), and clinical monitoring (e.g., ECG, heart rate, pulse oximetry, ventilators, capnography monitors, depth of consciousness monitors, regional oximetry, biopatch technology, and respiratory rate).

Tertiary devices will be the infrastructure devices that support both primary and secondary devices. These include smart patient room devices (smart beds, hand hygiene, fall detection), virtual care (remote ICU telemetry), tele-ology (teleneurology/teledermatology), and real-time location services (asset tracking for wheelchairs, infusion pumps, smart cabinets, medication carts, par-level management, and rental management.)

3.5.1 Connection Protocols of Medical Devices

Medical devices often operate with commercial parts, including CPUs, operating systems, or off-the-shelf software that is not intended for medical use.

Though the continued tightening of standards of medical device development is good from a regulatory perspective, security can often suffer at its hands. The FDA requires that the manufacturer of record is responsible for the approved configuration of a device. Because of this, oftentimes the end-user (i.e., the hospital, medical center, etc.) is unable to access device software and cannot install security updates and patches. Many times, upgrades need to be performed by the manufacturer, which can cause a considerable delay in the remediation of vulnerabilities.

Unlike in other fields, technology is built to last a long time in the medical industry. Oftentimes, the devices built to last for a long time are kept running for a long time as part of a hospital's infrastructure due to their expensive nature. This can lead to the devices running on outdated software, many of which aren't able to be supported by their manufacturer any longer. Additionally, any updates to this outdated software are required to be approved by the manufacturer, which often leads to even longer delays for any security updates or patches.

Another thing to consider is the limited-space design of these devices. Medical devices are often manufactured to run scaled-back versions of off-the-shelf software, often with limited memory space. When security updates and patches are eventually released, sometimes they aren't compatible or are unable to be applied to the modified software.

Medical device manufacturers are also not usually focused on using the latest software platform. The technological advancements take a backseat to the medical function of the device.

3.5.2   How Do These Devices Connect?

IEEE 11073-20702, established in 2017, has begun to standardize the integration of medical devices with familiar technology. According to Amazon Web Services, the three main connectivity methods considered for the Internet of Medical Things are WiFi, Bluetooth, and LPWAN.

3.5.2.1   WiFi

As a whole, WiFi uses radio waves to transmit information at specific frequencies. It can enable high-speed and secure communication between many different types of devices, wirelessly, over many distances. Enterprise WiFi used in your typical hospital or medical center supports two communication bands—2.4 and 5 GHz. The 2.4 GHz band can quickly become congested with guest access, wireless convenience devices, etc. Many hospitals and medical centers have dedicated the 5 GHz band for critical devices and applications.

When dealing with connected devices, WiFi security is the front line in protecting data. WIFI security can be divided into two parts to be focused on: encryption and authentication. Encryption is the scrambling of data so that it cannot be intercepted, and authentication is verification that the client receiving the data and/or accessing the device is the client who *should* be receiving the data or accessing the device.

The primary security algorithms used with WiFi are Wired Equivalent Privacy (WEP), WiFi Protected Access (WPA), and WiFi Protected Access II (WPA2) [8]. WEP is the oldest and has proven to be vulnerable and exploited many times. WPA improved upon many of the security flaws but has also been proven to be vulnerable to exploitation. WPA2 is the most current, secure choice as of 2021 when this chapter is being written. Networks using WPA2 use Temporal Key Integrity Protocol (TKIP) and Advanced Encryption Standard (AES). AES is more secure.

Along with understanding these protocols and basic security controls, there are additional ways in which connected devices can be secured. Devices can be embedded with a Root of Trust, which allows only signed and trusted software images to be loaded onto the device. This means that no suspect software can be loaded or installed on the device.

Firewalls are another important barrier. It is helpful on a network, but also on a device. It can prevent intrusions into secured, sensitive, or vital information.

3.5.2.2 Bluetooth

While Bluetooth was initially scorned by healthcare organizations, it has proven in recent years to be a valuable and widely utilized tool. Many personal devices (i.e., fitness monitors, glucose monitors, and neuromodulation) use Bluetooth for connectivity. However, operating rooms, ICUs, and other locations within hospitals or medical centers are beginning to adopt Bluetooth technology as well. As a general function, Bluetooth allows mobile devices to exchange data over short distances.

BLE, or Bluetooth Low Energy, is lower power but robust and intended for situations where battery life is more important than data transfer speeds. The lower power properties of BLE make it effective for deploying environmental sensors and room monitoring, for building or patient care monitoring, or to meet compliance requirements [9].

In 2017, Bluetooth Mesh began to replace the 1:1 Bluetooth exchange with m:m (many-to-many) relationships between Bluetooth devices. A mesh network like this can meet communication and security requirements over large areas while monitoring and managing many devices. Specifically applied to Bluetooth, mesh networking accomplishes these things while also maintaining compatibility with current PCs/tablets/smartphones and will also maintain this connection with low-energy efficiency. This is excellent for use on hospital premises. This technology works due to a concept called managed flooding—a mesh node transmits (or "floods") data omnidirectionally to all nodes within its direct range. These nodes will often then do the same—flood all nodes within their direct range. This pattern continues until the published data reaches all nodes within the network. Only applicable nodes (addressed or subscribed) act on this transmitted data. The rest simply relay the messages. Because there are no single-purpose centralized routers, Bluetooth mesh networking is reliable due to its multiple paths for published messages and the ability to self-heal, all while maintaining the low-energy features.

3.5.2.3 LPWAN

LPWAN, or a low-power wide-area network, is another type of wireless communication that is designed to be longer range but communicate at a very low bit rate among connected objects. This class of wireless frequency came to exist in the early 2000s as a way for machine-to-machine communication. Often, devices using LPWAN are able to communicate for up to 10 years on a single battery charge. Because of the efficiency of the technology, speeds range from 3 to 375 Kbps. 5G is set to completely change the LPWAN environment—it will offer low latency, low power, and high speeds of data transfer [10].

3.6 Medical Device Attacks

3.6.1 Incidents

According to a recent report by Armis, 63% of healthcare organizations have experienced security incidents related to unmanaged and IoT devices between 2018 and 2020 [11]. Healthcare continues to be the top-targeted vertical in cybercrime: money earned by reselling a healthcare record is 50× the resale price of a stolen credit card. Additionally, attacks continue to be more costly due to HIPAA penalties for breached information.

3.6.2 Targeted Attacks

2019 and 2020 saw an uptick in the number of reported risks and targets on connected medical devices. In March of 2019, the FDA became aware of security vulnerabilities that were identified in a wireless telemetry technology used for communication between Medtronic's implantable cardiac devices, clinic programmers, and home monitors. Implantable cardioverter defibrillators (ICDs) and cardiac resynchronization therapy defibrillators (CRT-Ds) are devices that provide regular rhythm for slow heart rhythms and electrical shocks or pacing to stop dangerously fast heart rhythms. They are implanted under the skin in the upper chest area with connecting insulated wires called leads that go into the heart. The programmer (Medtronic CareLink Programmer model 2090) is used during this implantation and to monitor these devices periodically. These devices are used to wirelessly connect to the patient's implanted device and read the data stored on the device. The transmitter, located in-home, sends patient data to their physician using the CareLink Network on a continuous landline, cellular, or wireless Internet connection [12].

These devices use wireless radio frequency (RF) to enable communication between the devices and allow Medtronic programmers and monitoring accessories to remotely transmit data, allow clinicians to display and print information in real-time, and to program device settings. The wireless technology that these devices were using did not use encryption, authentication, or authorization, and therefore could allow unauthorized individuals to access and manipulate the implantable device, home monitor, or clinic programmer.

In June 2019, the FDA became aware of risks in Medtronic MiniMed Paradigm insulin pumps. An unauthorized person could connect wirelessly to a nearby MiniMed insulin pump and change settings to either over-or under-deliver insulin to a patient, leading to hypoglycemia or ketoacidosis. These could not be updated, and Medtronic and the FDA recommended that users of these pumps were advised to switch to a model with more security protection [13].

In October 2019, the FDA issued an urgent bulletin with 11 vulnerabilities, titled URGENT/11. The vulnerabilities detailed existed in IPnet, a third-party software component that supports network communications between computers. Though the IPnet software was no longer supported by the vendor, some manufacturers have a license that allows them to continue to use it without support. The affected operating systems were VxWorks (by Wind River), Operating System Embedded (OSE, by ENEA), INTEGRITY (by Green Hills), ThreadX (by TRON Forum), and ZebOS (by IP Infusion). The U.S. Department of Homeland Security (DHS) issued a similar bulletin with additional information, detailing stack-based buffer overflow, heap-based buffer overflow, integer underflow, improper restriction of operations within the bounds of a memory buffer, race condition, argument injection, and null pointer dereference. These are classified as requiring a low skill level to exploit, and the public exploits were available. Medical devices and systems affected by URGENT/11 were required to be reported to the Department of Homeland Security's Cybersecurity and Infrastructure Security Agency (CISA) [14].

January 2020 rang in the new year with a report of vulnerabilities in certain GE Healthcare Clinical Information Central Stations and Telemetry Servers. These devices were primarily used in healthcare facilities for displaying information, such as the physiologic parameters of a patient (i.e., temperature, heartbeat, blood pressure), and monitoring patient status from a central location in a facility, such as a nurse's workstation. GE issued an "Urgent Medical Device Correction" letter informing consumers of security vulnerabilities that would allow an attacker to remotely take control of the medical device and silence alarms, generate false alarms, and interfere with alarms of patient monitors connected to the device [15].

In March 2020, the FDA issued a statement informing patients, providers, and manufacturers of the SweynTooth family of vulnerabilities. These vulnerabilities are associated with a wireless communication technology known as Bluetooth Low Energy (BLE), which allows two devices to "pair" and exchange information to perform their intended functions while preserving battery life. An unauthorized user could wirelessly exploit these vulnerabilities to crash the device, deadlock the device, or bypass security to access device functions available only to authorized users [16].

3.7   Current Legislation

The FDA has a variety of guidance available on medical device security. One of the earliest, published in 2005, Cybersecurity for Networked Medical Devices Containing Off-the-Shelf (OTS) Software, addressed devices that are designed to be connected to computer networks and that incorporate off-the-shelf software that could be vulnerable to attacks and threats. The guidance clarifies how existing regulations, including the Quality System Regulation, apply to activities surrounding these devices [17].

Next, in October 2014, the FDA issued a Final Guidance for the Content of Premarket Submissions for Management of Cybersecurity in Medical Devices. This guide recommended that manufacturers address device security throughout the product life cycle, including during design, development, production, distribution, deployment, and maintenance of the device. This guidance also required following the Guidance for the Content of Premarket Submissions for Software Contained in Medical Devices [18].

Third, in December 2016, the FDA issued another Final Guidance for the Post-market Management of Cybersecurity in Medical Devices. This document provides recommendations to the industry for structured and comprehensive management of postmarket cybersecurity vulnerabilities for marketed and distributed medical devices throughout the product life cycle.

Finally, in October 2018, the FDA released Draft Guidance regarding the Content of Premarket Submissions for Management of Cybersecurity in Medical Devices. This guidance provides recommendations to the industry regarding cybersecurity device design, labeling, and documentation to be included in premarket submissions for devices with cybersecurity risk [18].

The FDA also collaborated with the Federal Communications Commission (FCC) and Office of the National Coordinator for Health IT (ONC) to propose a strategy on an appropriate, risk-based regulatory framework for health IT that promotes innovation, protects patient safety, and avoids unnecessary and duplicative regulation. The FCC has worked on adopting rules and policies that promote the development of wireless medical devices while implementing important technical standards. They also created the CONNECT2HEALTH Task Force to accelerate the adoption of healthcare technologies in the areas of telehealth, mobile applications, and telemedicine.

Other branches of the government began to get involved as well. The Department of Homeland Security has also created a memorandum of agreement to implement a new framework for better coordination and cooperation between the two agencies to address security in medical devices.

Most recently, in May of 2021, President Biden signed an executive order mandating an electronically readable Software Bill of Materials (SBOM) to be included with medical devices in order to provide an inventory of components used. Compared to an "ingredient label" but for devices, many industry experts hope that this requirement will provide transparency to the components of medical devices and make it easier for entities to know whether they are affected [19].

3.8 The Future of Healthcare

The primary goal of healthcare is to provide universal access to quality care. Technology will continue to be the means to achieve these goals, and securing the technology should continue to be the primary goal.

In the next decade, there will be an increased demand for more independent living wellness solutions, artificial intelligence (AI) as an integral part of the healthcare landscape, and technology that will continue to drive innovation. Human longevity has continued to increase, and the demands for services to guarantee wellness and independence will also increase. Artificial Intelligence will be an integral part of healthcare and will assist with diagnosis, treatment protocols, drug development, custom-tailored medicine, and patient monitoring. It will be imperative to secure this technology as it continues to evolve.

References

1. BBC News, "Stone age man used dentist drill," *BBC News*, 6 April 2006.
2. Food and Drug Administration, "How to Determine if Your Product is a Medical Device," 2019. [Online]. Available: https://www.fda.gov/medical-devices/classify-your-medical-device/how-determine-if-your-product-medical-device.
3. European Union, "Regulation (EU) 2017/745," in *Regulation (EU) 2017/745*, 2017.
4. Food and Drug Administration, *Code of Federal Regulations, Title 21, part 860*, 2020.
5. D. Zuckerman and P. Brown, "Lack of publicly available scientific evidence on the safety and effectiveness of implanted medical devices," *JAMA Intern Med*, vol. 174, no. 11.
6. Food and Drug Administration, "Medical Devices Single Audit Program (MDSAP)," 2017. [Online]. Available: https://www.fda.gov/medical-devices/cdrh-international-programs/medical-device-single-audit-program-mdsap.
7. Congress, "21st Century Cures Act," 2016.
8. Cisco, "What is WiFi?," Cisco, 2021.
9. Bluetooth, "Connecting Today's Hospitals Using Bluetooth Technology," Cassia Networks, 2021.
10. M. Wedd, "What is LPWAN and the LoRaWAN Open Standard?," IoT For All, 2020. [Online]. Available: https://www.iotforall.com/what-is-lpwan-lorawan.
11. Armis, "Medical and IoT Device Security for Healthcare," 2019.
12. Food and Drug Administration, "Cybersecurity Vulnerabilities Affecting Medtronic Implantable Cardiac Devices, Programmers, and Home Monitors: FDA Safety Communication," 2019. [Online]. Available: https://www.fda.gov/medical-devices/safety-communications/cybersecurity-vulnerabilities-affecting-medtronic-implantable-cardiac-devices-programmers-and-home.
13. Food and Drug Administration, "Certain Medtronic MiniMed Insulin Pumps Have Potential Cybersecurity Risks: FDA Safety Communication," 2019. [Online]. Available: https://www.fda.gov/medical-devices/safety-communications/certain-medtronic-minimed-insulin-pumps-have-potential-cybersecurity-risks-fda-safety-communication.

14. Food and Drug Administration, "URGENT/11 Cybersecurity Vulnerabilities in a Widely-Used Third-Party Software Component May Introduce Risks During Use of Certain Medical Devices: FDA Safety Communication," 2019. [Online]. Available: https://www.fda.gov/medical-devices/safety-communications/urgent11-cybersecurity-vulnerabilities-widely-used-third-party-software-component-may-introduce.

15. Food and Drug Administration, "Cybersecurity Vulnerabilities in Certain GE Healthcare Clinical Information Central Stations and Telemetry Servers: Safety Communication," 2020. [Online]. Available: https://www.fda.gov/medical-devices/safety-communications/cybersecurity-vulnerabilities-certain-ge-healthcare-clinical-information-central-stations-and.

16. Food and Drug Administration, "SweynTooth Cybersecurity Vulnerabilities May Affect Certain Medical Devices: FDA Safety Communication," 2020. [Online]. Available: https://www.fda.gov/medical-devices/safety-communications/sweyntooth-cybersecurity-vulnerabilities-may-affect-certain-medical-devices-fda-safety-communication.

17. Food and Drug Administration, "Cybersecurity for Networked Medical Devices Containing Off-the-Shelf (OTS) Software," 2005. [Online]. Available: https://www.fda.gov/regulatory-information/search-fda-guidance-documents/cybersecurity-networked-medical-devices-containing-shelf-ots-software.

18. Food and Drug Administration, "Content of Premarket Submissions for Management of Cybersecurity in Medical Devices," 2018. [Online]. Available: https://www.fda.gov/regulatory-information/search-fda-guidance-documents/content-premarket-submissions-management-cybersecurity-medical-devices.

19. G. Slabodkin, "MedTechDive," 21 May 2021. [Online]. Available: https://www.medtechdive.com/news/biden-orders-software-bill-of-materials-to-boost-cybersecurity-advamed-wan/600594/.

Chapter 4
The Case for a Security Metric Framework to Rate Cyber Security Effectiveness for Internet of Medical Things (IoMT)

Zulema Belyeu Caldwell

Contents

4.1 Introduction

Peter Drucker, the renowned management consultant, is known for the quote, "What gets measured gets managed." [1]. When a family is purchasing a vehicle, they may consider the safety rating of the car. In the United States, the National Highway Traffic Safety Administration (NHTSA) rates cars on a five-star scale based on the aggregated results from four tests—front crash test, side crash test from another car, side crash into a pole, and the vehicle's propensity to roll over [2]. The Insurance Institute for Highway Safety (IIHS) also has created an overall rating for cars based on four different crash tests and scores from defined technologies known to

Z. B. Caldwell (✉)
University of Maryland Global Campus, Adelphi, MD, USA

© Springer Nature Switzerland AG 2022
F. D. Hudson (eds.), *Women Securing the Future with TIPPSS for Connected Healthcare*, Women in Engineering and Science,
https://doi.org/10.1007/978-3-030-93592-4_4

help ensure accident avoidance, such as effective head-restraint design, headlight performance, and ease of installation for a child's seat [2].

In a 2015 *New Yorker* article entitled "The engineer's lament: two ways of thinking about automotive safety," Malcolm Gladwell discusses the challenges an engineer faces when designing and building a vehicle. One of the key points made by Gladwell is the consumer will often see things from a different perspective than the engineer [3]. The consumer is not thinking of all of the concessions made in the design process. The typical consumer just wants to ensure the car is working and is safe and free from defects. The United States was the first country in the world to make car safety ratings more accessible to consumers, and consumers often use the safety ratings to assist with their car purchasing decisions [4].

A thought-provoking concept to consider is how consumers would respond and accept a similar approach to rating the security levels of Internet of Things (IoT) devices, especially for IoT devices in the medical field where security issues could be harmful to a person's health. Several challenges and complexities make it more challenging to establish a cybersecurity metrics program for IoT. However, it is encouraging that researchers continue to focus on improving IoT security in the medical field as the growth of the number of interconnected devices continues to explode. The International Data Corporation (IDC) estimates that there will be 55.7 billion connected Internet of Things (IoT) devices generating over 73 zettabytes (ZB) of data by 2025 [5]. As the market develops and matures, IoT will play a significant role in exchanging information between machines, people, and processes.

This chapter provides an overview of IoMT technology and the attack landscape, highlighting the various levels at which hackers can exploit IoMT technologies. It also provides an overview of security metric scoring methods and offers an analytical approach for assessing the risk in IoMT technologies. It analyzes the key components of a cybersecurity metrics framework based on IoT security taxonomy, threat indicators, and the threat landscape, as well as security controls defined through the risk assessment process. This computational security metric approach can help explain impact and attack sophistication levels for various IoMT devices. The incentives and benefits for a security metric framework can help inform the security posture of IoMT technologies, help control costs, and potentially save lives.

4.2   Internet of Medical Things (IoMT): A Technology Overview

Due to pervasive connectivity, the emergence of IoT technologies in healthcare is becoming the norm to improve medical treatments, inform patient self-care, manage chronic and critical diseases, and lower overall costs. These novel technologies are driving innovation and increasing awareness among health care practitioners and health consumers. More awareness regarding customer perspective and user benefits of connected medical devices will help technologists develop better, faster, and even cheaper healthcare solutions.

IoT is providing a personalized, user-focused form of care for consumers, which will allow individuals to self-manage and self-monitor their health and give health practitioners the ability to provide and improve medical care remotely. Modern wearable devices, such as the Fitbit health monitor, Pebble smartwatch, Apple iWatch, Samsung Gear, or Garmin, help to offer self-management and self-monitoring applications. The devices allow the patient and healthcare providers to monitor vital signs such as temperature, blood pressure, heart rate, and blood oxygen levels.

There is a debate on what exactly constitutes a medical device. The World Health Organization (WHO) defines a medical device as a machine, instrument, or apparatus that provides monitoring, treatment, diagnosis, management, and prevention capabilities for a health condition [6]. Historically, the type of equipment labeled as medical devices were items found in a medical environment, such as Magnetic Resonance Imaging (MRI) devices, intravenous machines, and blood pressure machines. With the emergence of IoT, telemedicine, and advanced technological capabilities, researchers, and practitioners must consider the new class of medical devices arising to provide remote medical care and monitoring to manage and aid with controlling diseases, such as Parkinson's Disease, and to provide preventative care for conditions such as hypertension.

Elements of the IoMT ecosystem are shown in Fig. 4.1. Devices can be "On-Body" including wearables and implantables; "In-Home" for monitoring and telemedicine; "In-Clinic" for ambulatory care; and "In-Hospital" where the human ecosystem grows with not only patients and caregivers, but also the plethora of providers including doctors, nurses, radiologists, and much more medical equipment.

The architectural model for IoMT devices, as depicted in Fig. 4.2, integrates the elements of the IoMT ecosystem in Fig. 4.1, including on-body, in-home, in-clinic, and in-hospital devices and inputs and outputs, into a framework that allows us to consider the use and security of these devices and the overall connected healthcare cybersecurity framework. Looking at the IoMT architecture and elements in a holistic fashion is essential for secure and efficacious delivery of healthcare. The patients are the core of the purpose for connected healthcare and can leverage IoMT devices and the data they collect and create with their practitioners to help inform medical treatment or even alert a patient or healthcare professional to a medical issue that may require prompt attention.

The IoMT architecture depicted in Fig. 4.2 consists of four main parts that connect the patient with the doctor or other medical providers: (a) Information collection components, (b) Applications or websites, (c) Data storage, and (d) the IoT connection network. It is critical that the entire connected healthcare data stream including the IoMT data is protected and secured from tampering, unauthorized access, or destruction. The information collection components consist of sensor devices and personal wearable devices, monitoring devices, or data input devices, such as hospital patient registration systems. The doctor, patient, or other healthcare

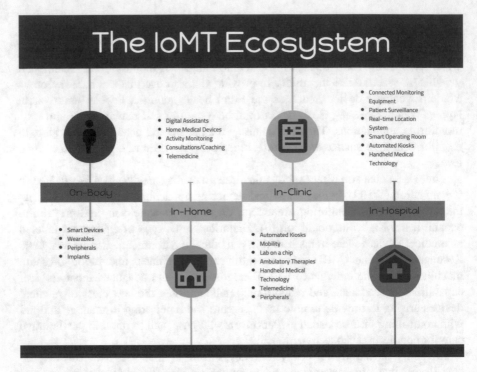

Fig. 4.1 Internet of Medical Things (IoMT) Ecosystem

providers will use an application or website to visualize and analyze the data. The data storage can either use traditional database models, but more than likely, for true IoMT solutions, the data storage will utilize a cloud-based system for storing patient data. The architecture components are connected using IoT connection infrastructure, which usually includes IoT gateways, and various IoT protocols, such as Zigbee, MQTT, or LoRaWAN.

Researchers are exploring how medical devices and wearables can help patients and health practitioners manage care before, during, and after medical procedures such as surgery. As evident with recent events such as the COVID-19 pandemic, health practitioners have turned to telemedicine to provide remote care. The healthcare crisis has been a catalyst for expanding the use of IoT technology to deliver health care. For example, to help enrich the telemedicine experience, the University of Louisville School of Medicine started a pilot program to use smart glasses for remote emergency care in rural communities and long-term care facilities. Given the risk of exposure to deadly diseases, such as COVID-19, this concept may prove to be a lifesaving measure for long-term facilities and nursing homes. For example, a physician can use smart glasses to evaluate a patient remotely and obtain vital information to provide medical care [7].

There are a host of use cases for wearables and IoT devices for the healthcare industry [8]. One such use case is highlighted with Humber River Hospital, a

IoMT Architecture

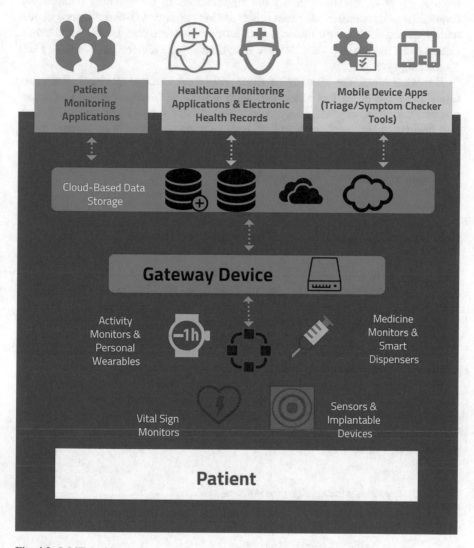

Fig. 4.2 IoMT Architecture

state-of-the-art all-digital hospital. The hospital, located in Toronto, Canada, uses IoT to provide a high level of personalized medical care. Humber River Hospital includes an online appointment scheduling and check-in process, bedside access to medical records via monitors for patients, and enhanced communication methods, such as video chat and instant messaging between patients, doctors, nurses, and family. The hospital also uses wristbands with real-time location tracking, as well as robots to prepare and mix drugs and transport goods. A 2017 literature review from Joyia et al. details over 15 IoT applications in the medical domain [9]. Example applications include smart rehabilitation systems; IoT-based kidney abnormality detection, decision-making, and home-based medical health monitoring; sleep apnea monitoring; cardiac and arrhythmia management; and remote ECG monitoring systems.

But what about the security of these IoT-based medical devices? There are numerous security vectors associated with IoMT. With the emergence of interconnected medical devices, many vulnerabilities and threats have expanded medical devices' attack surface. IoMT technologies are susceptible to various cyber threats, such as ransomware, distributed denial of service (DDoS) attacks, and data breaches. This increased attack surface can have significant ramifications for healthcare organizations and the patient.

4.3   IoMT Security Vulnerabilities and Attacks

The IoMT system includes endpoint medical devices, networking devices, gateways, back-end devices, cloud-based platforms, and mobile applications to control the endpoint medical devices, back-end management, and analytics. Just as any computer or information technology network is susceptible to cyberattacks, so are connected medical devices. Given that cyberattacks are on the rise, technologists and developers must be aware of the IoT threat landscape and how it applies to the healthcare industry and connected medical devices.

Some people may wonder if the healthcare industry is truly vulnerable and attempt to understand the attacker's motive to penetrate and attack medical devices. However, it is more than just a theoretical concept. Researchers have identified that the two main reasons attackers target the healthcare industry are for financial or political gain (Table 4.1) [10].

Table 4.1 Top Reasons for Attacking the Healthcare Industry

Top Reasons Cyberattackers Target Healthcare Industry (Coventry, 2018)	
Financial Gain	• Steal medical credentials and medical identities for health services through fraudulent claims • Steal medical identities for the sale of drug prescriptions on the dark web • Obtain personal information to open bank accounts, obtain loans or passports • Blackmail political or celebrity figures
Political Value	• Release medical information and embarrass political figures • Fuel nation-state cyberwarfare to disrupt or deny medical care and cause chaos • Blackmail political figures or release sensitive data for propaganda reasons or to impact policy decisions
Ego	• Fulfill the challenge of finding and exposing security vulnerabilities • Gain notoriety in the cybersecurity community

Healthcare software and hardware developers should understand the dataflow model, separated into four main parts—the patient, information collection, data storage, and medical devices and applications [11]. The principal vulnerabilities in this area occur during information collection from medical devices, or from data in transit between connections. Numerous threats and vulnerabilities exist, and in the healthcare domain, the consequences can pose a significant danger to patients, even potentially loss of life. To assess a technology's effectiveness and security level, we must understand the threat landscape.

As a part of information collection, IoT medical devices, such as wearables, are vulnerable to attacks that can put a patient's privacy at risk of being compromised. Practitioners and developers also must realize that the IoT medical devices and the connection used to transmit data are vulnerable to various attacks.

Examples of vulnerabilities seen in IoT devices, including medical devices, are listed below.

- Hard-coded and weak passwords—The most common vulnerabilities in IoT devices are related to password management. Some IoT devices come with passwords that are directly coded into the machine. The device may come with a default password that could grant administrative access to unauthorized users. In addition to hard-coded passwords, weak passwords are also a significant issue with IoT devices. When setting passwords, users often keep the default password or choose a common or easy-to-guess password. In some cases, the user may forgo using a password altogether.
- Command injection—Attackers use this vulnerability to access the device to execute malicious code or modify data. A familiar vector for command injection is the login field through SQL or JavaScript injections. Because IoT devices are typically running some form of the Linux operating system, they are vulnerable to command injection. This method has also been used to create botnets without the user being aware.
- Open ports—Having open ports on your devices, including ports not commonly used, can allow an attacker to access the device.
- Unencrypted services—As a part of the Confidentiality, Integrity, and Availability (CIA) triad, confidentiality is a critical part of any cybersecurity approach. When there is no encryption or weak encryption, data transmitted through connections can be intercepted or observed using packet sniffers. In some cases, the attacker may be able to manipulate the data packets.
- Insecure web interface—IoT devices may have insecure web interfaces that allow users to perform command injection, track usage, or leak data.
- Insecure network services—IoT devices that provide network services such as Telnet or Server Message Block (SMB) typically have default root logins and make the device vulnerable to ransomware attacks. Attackers may also gain access to the device using open ports and exploit certain services to elevate privilege.

Table 4.2 Common IoT Cyberattacks

Password Intrusion	*Hacking into a system with weak or default passwords*
Vulnerability Intrusion	*Exploiting identified vulnerabilities such as a weak password or privilege escalation*
Denial of Service	*Making a machine or network resource unavailable by disrupting services or flooding the resource with commands*
Elevation of Privilege	*Assuming system administration-level access to an application*
SQL Injection	*Injecting malicious statements as input into an SQL statement with the intention of the application or device executing the malicious code*
Packet Sniffing	*Intercepting and logging network traffic*
Proxy Attacks	*Intercepting and compromising network traffic by sending it to a proxy device potentially for the purposes of manipulating network communications*

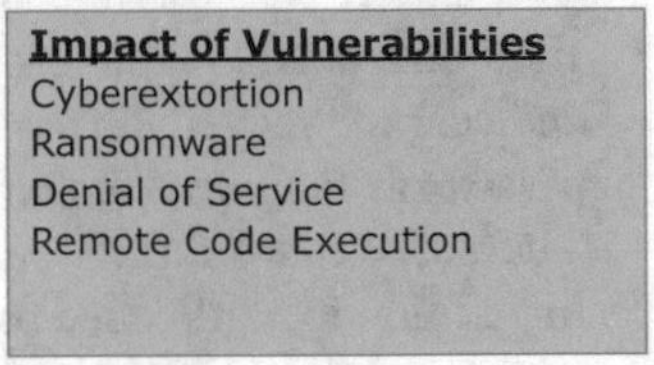

Fig. 4.3 Impact of Vulnerabilities

Impact of Vulnerabilities
Cyberextortion
Ransomware
Denial of Service
Remote Code Execution

- Account enumeration—Account enumeration occurs when a failed attempt to authenticate on a device returns a response to let the user know an incorrect username or password was used.
- Buffer overflow—Buffer overflow vulnerabilities pose a significant risk to IoT devices because of the limited amount of memory on the machines and the programming languages used. Because IoT devices are intended to conserve and use minimal power, they operate with an efficient amount of memory. The smaller the memory buffer, the easier it is to create a buffer overflow.

As a result of these vulnerabilities, IoT devices are susceptible to several attacks and threats. Table 4.2 connects some common attacks to the vulnerabilities that are being exploited in the device. Some of the common attacks for IoT devices are denial of service, botnets, ransomware, Man-in-the-Middle, Spoofing, Elevation of Privilege, Mirai, Worms, Packet Sniffing, and Proxy attacks.

The vulnerabilities can also lead to cyberextortion, as mentioned in Fig. 4.3. In the medical field, cyberextortion is becoming more prevalent. Exploiting vulnerabilities in the IoT device can allow an attacker to steal information from the system and then extort money from the system owner who wants to stop the attack and prevent the attacker from releasing the stolen data.

4.4   Security Metrics Overview

To truly understand how to apply security metrics, it is critical to define the term. Security metrics provide a way to quantify the security of systems. It is different from security monitoring, which looks for abnormal events [12]. Researchers and businesses turn their attention to security metrics to understand their security posture and quantify their systems' overall security. Based on a set of security assessment goals, metrics provide a method to assess an information system's security level.

Practitioners often use security metrics and measurements interchangeably. However, metrics allow a user to quantify data, provide awareness and critical information, and help with decision-making. On the other hand, measurement is how metrics are collected or assigned rankings/numbers to entities, similar to the car safety rating process. Researchers have applied the following definitions to metrics:

- Metrics are data used to assist with decision-making, enable accountability, and improve performance, and a measurement is a process of obtaining and analyzing the data [13].
- Metrics are a system of measurement that is based on quantifiable measures [14].
- A metric is a variable to which a measurement is assigned, consisting of two or more measures [15].
- A useful metric's characteristics are measurable, repeatable, cost-effective, contextually relevant, and represented as a cardinal number or percentage rather than a qualitative format such as low, medium, or high [16].

Quantification techniques are commonly used in other engineering areas, and they can help inform users and key stakeholders with relevant points for decision-making. Suppose we want to develop an effective system or network of IoT devices for the healthcare industry. In that case, we must quantify security effectiveness, and the understanding of security effectiveness increases with an established and dedicated set of security metrics. The main question is how to define the most useful set of security metrics for IoT medical devices, and how to leverage them to improve the cybersecurity posture of the institution, devices, and overall connected healthcare system.

The metrics should be defined as a set of measurable components that can be used to derive the device's security posture and to give the patient and end-user confidence in IoT medical devices. Prior research in the area of security metrics for IoT has ranged from using a reference architecture to providing a comprehensive view of the security elements in a network, as well as combining key elements, such as technology maturity analysis, threat analysis, threat modeling, requirements establishment, policies, mechanisms, and system behavior. Other research has used networking concepts such as Internet Protocol Security (IPSec), risk-based adaptive security frameworks, risk analysis, stochastic techniques, and attack graphs to measure the security of IoT devices [20, 21]. Ahmed et al. conducted a review of security metrics to identify a generic set of metrics that could apply to the healthcare industry [12]. The researchers divided the metrics into eight categories, as shown in Table 4.3.

Table 4.3 Categories of Cybersecurity Metrics and Recommendations

Cybersecurity Metric	Definition	Example Metrics and Recommended Actions
Indicators of Compromise (IOC)	Information to identify malicious activities occurring in a system or network [17]	• The volume of outbound traffic and any increase in the amount of outbound traffic • Volume and number of IP addresses connecting to the network from outside of the geographical area, and any significant change in the number or location • Number of simultaneous logins by the same user from different locations • Percentage of traffic from onion router not detected by network monitoring tools • Number of unknown accounts with elevated privileges found on a compromised system • *Recommendation: Develop an "IOC Real-Time Analysis System" to assess these metrics on an ongoing basis*
Indicators of Attack (IOA)	A proactive security measure could reveal an attack that is taking place before the indicators of compromise become visible [18]	• Lateral movements within the network such as moving from one vulnerable device to another • High bandwidth and increased outgoing traffic • Number of hosts communicating with external networks on non-standard ports • A high number of failed authentication attempts • Number of processes with high memory consumption • *Recommendation: Develop an ongoing "IOA Real-Time Analysis System" to avert attacks*
Resilience	The ability for a system to adapt and continue to function even when under attack [19]	• Mean Time to Repair (MTTR) • Mean Time to Failure (MTTF) • Availability of offline backups that have been fully tested • *Recommendation: Develop a "Resilience Register" with goals to monitor and improve all three metrics over time*
Vulnerability Assessment	The evaluation of weaknesses in the system which could be exploited by a threat [19]	• Mean Time to Detection (MTTD) • Percentage of critical systems with known and unpatched vulnerabilities • Exposure time • *Recommendation: Develop a "Vulnerability Register" with goals to monitor and improve all three metrics over time*

(continued)

Table 4.3 (continued)

Cybersecurity Metric	Definition	Example Metrics and Recommended Actions
Risk Assessment	The need to perform asset identification and classification to direct resources to the most critical assets [19]	• Percentage of risks with a severe or critical rating • Percentage of critical assets with no ownership assigned • Percentage of assets monitored • Number of gaps in devices and systems monitored, and as a percentage of the entire device inventory • *Recommendation: Develop a "Risk Register" with identified risks and severity and goals to improve over time*
Penetration Testing	Method for detecting security vulnerabilities in a networked environment [19]	• Percentage of penetration tests that discovered high-risk vulnerabilities • Frequency of penetration testing, especially in dynamic environments • Penetration testing coverage of critical medical systems and infrastructure • Mean Time to Fix (MTTF) • *Recommendation: Develop a "Pen Testing Register" with identified risks and severity and goals to improve over time*
Red and Blue Teaming	Red Teams attempt to penetrate the security defenses and compromise the system, Blue Teams defend the system [19]	• Resources required to breach the security defenses and compromise the systems • Required skills and knowledge of the attackers to breach the system of devices • Profiling the attackers to develop mitigation techniques • *Recommendation: Conduct Red and Blue teaming exercises to establish a baseline with annual checkups*
Intelligence-Driven Defense Metric		• Threat intelligence teams • Number of known threats groups targeting your organization or sector at any given time • Number of attacks detected and mitigated • Access to vendor threat intelligence reports • Metric from Indicators of Compromise (IOC) • Knowledge of online forums where exploits are sold or discussed • *Recommendation: Develop a "Threat Intelligence Defense Environment" leveraging internal and external intelligence*

Despite the defined categories, there are several common gaps or challenges associated with security metrics. One such gap is a lack of ability to develop a comprehensive view of the system's overall security. If an organization is not vigilant in assessing their cybersecurity posture, they may only realize how good their security is after being compromised. Organizations also must be equipped to handle the complexities associated with quantifying security metrics. In prior security surveys, practitioners and developers have identified one of the critical gaps in the security state for IoT devices as the lack of tangible metrics. In addition to quantifying the complexity of metrics, there is no established consensus on a framework most applicable for enterprise security performance measurements for IoT devices and IT networks.

4.5 Applying a Security Metric Framework Across the IoMT Architecture

Security metrics are the foundation of a security program. Organizations have also found that metrics can enable the creation of a healthy security posture. Just as with the safety ratings for automobiles, there is a certain level of trust and comfort associated with having quantifiable data to back up the product's effectiveness and quality. Metrics are increasingly more critical, which is why organizations are investing in data science and data analysis. However, the current process for metrics development is mostly manual and burdensome. Additionally, some security professionals are not sure what to measure. As a result, additional research is needed to develop a more automated process that can lead to security metric maturity, especially for the healthcare industry.

So, what should be measured to provide a confidence rating for users of IoMT devices? What metrics are quantifiable and the most efficient? If we start with the list of cybersecurity metrics identified in prior research, the type of metrics that may prove to be the most impactful at the design and development phase for IoT devices include the following:

- Percentage of code coverage analyzed from a security perspective during hardware and software testing
- Implementation of device authentication measures
- Implementation of access control measures
- Connection security
- Memory protection
- Protocol security
- Encryption techniques for data storage and devices
- Password requirements
- Input validation
- Mean Time to Fix (MTTF)

Using the IoMT Architecture in Fig. 4.2 as a reference starting at the bottom with the patient and device, metrics can be categorized based on the components within the IoMT architecture—IoMT Device, Data Storage, Internet/Network Connections, and End-User Applications. These metrics can be used to measure the categories of risk assessment, resilience, penetration testing, and vulnerability assessment for the IoMT architecture and potentially aggregate it into a rating. The metrics can be enunciated to give consumers an indicator of the level of safeguards implemented at design and production to protect the consumer's privacy and the consumer's health.

4.6 Case Study on Using Security Metrics for IoMT Devices

The following section provides an overview of three common IoMT devices—(1) cardiac implantable electronic devices; and transmitters; (2) insulin pumps and insulin pod therapy wearables; and (3) electrocardiogram (ECG or EKG) monitors—to identify potential metrics that can be used to provide a cybersecurity confidence level.

All of the IoMT devices we consider in this section will benefit from all ten of the IoMT Security Metrics suggested above.

4.6.1 Cardiac Implantable Electronic Devices

Cardiac implantable electronic devices (CIED) provide cardiac rhythm management for either a heart rate that is too slow or too fast. Pacemakers help patients manage a heart rate that is too slow, and cardioverter-defibrillators help patients manage a heart rate that is too fast. Remote monitoring of cardiac implantable electronic devices has become a routine and common practice due to increased connectivity through the Internet, advances in biomedical technology, and improvement in patient outcomes and survival. The CIED ecosystem includes the implantable device, a programmer typically in the physician's office used to query and program the implantable device, a home monitor, the cloud server, and proprietary software used by the physician's office [22]. The implantable device consists of a microprocessor, memory, telemetry circuit for transmitting and receiving data, and a timing circuit for synchronization [22]. Information flows in the system through proprietary and open-source protocols.

No cybersecurity issues have been reported to date, but researchers have proven that the risk is real in laboratory environments [22]. Multiple paths exist within the ecosystem for a hacker to exploit vulnerabilities. Areas of concern include the flow of information between the implant device and the external programmer, between the implant device and the monitor, or through the connection to the cloud server. These communication paths can be intercepted, and if not protected by encryption or authentication, an attacker can alter patient information or collect patient data [23]. An issue reported with some cardiac transmitter devices is the lack of encryption for sensitive data at rest and data in motion, such as when firmware updates are pushed to the implantable device [22].

Researchers have studied and reported multiple security vulnerabilities, which the FDA has also verified. The Muddy Water Research Report on the Abbott CIED highlighted vulnerabilities with increased radio traffic that can cause specific devices to crash [22]. The report also discussed a "battery drain" attack. Billy Rios and Jonathan Butts pointed out vulnerabilities in the wireless telemetry protocol for the Medtronic CareLink Programmer [22]. These vulnerabilities exist because of a lack of encryption or authentication with the device and a lack of digital code signing [22]. Based on the specific vulnerabilities identified with these devices, security metrics for testing with extensive code coverage, device authentication measures, access control features, connection security, protocol security, encryption techniques, password requirements, and patching programs can provide consumers with the necessary information and knowledge to respond and maintain the implantable devices.

4.6.2   Insulin Pumps and Insulin Pod Therapy Wearables

Healthcare providers prescribe insulin pumps for diabetic patients to administer insulin, usually under the skin through a thin tube. The insulin pod therapy wearable is an innovative approach for delivering insulin through a pod controlled wirelessly by a hand-held monitoring device. These diabetic devices contain patient information and allow remote commands for data delivery, treatment instructions, and insulin administration. Insulin pumps are susceptible to a host of threats and attacks that may degrade the device's functions and cause a health risk for the patient. Researchers have demonstrated the ability to attack the device, modify insulin delivery, and cause a denial of service. The attack vectors typically occur via wireless communication. IBM discovered a vulnerability that could allow a hacker to control the insulin pump, alter the patient's medication, and change the device readings [24]. The first safety notification for an insulin pump device was issued by Medtronic in June 2019 [25]. The vulnerability could allow a hacker to connect wirelessly to the Medtronic insulin pump introduced on the market before 2013, and the hacker could alter the pump's settings and take control from the patient, caregiver, or healthcare provider. The FDA announced that the vulnerability could lead to an insulin overdose or insulin stoppage. Medtronic did not classify the safety notification as a recall, but the company did offer to replace devices susceptible to the vulnerability with later generation insulin pumps [25].

Other diabetic medical products that have had cybersecurity issues include Animas One Touch Ping as well as "Do-It-Yourself" (DIY) software products to support automated insulin delivery, such as Tidepool. The FDA noted that DIY software products could be dangerous because of a security breach and are more susceptible to flawed code and malfunctioning hardware [25, 26]. Animas reported three security flaws for the One Touch Ping insulin pump—(1) communications in cleartext; (2) weak pairing between the remote and pump; and (3) lack of replay attack prevention or transmission assurance [27]. Animas made several recommendations for consumers to include disconnecting the pump's remote-control capability, limiting the amount of bolus insulin that can be delivered, enabling vibrating alarms, and checking the pump's dosing log on a regular basis [25].

The following security metrics address the vulnerabilities discovered in the described insulin pumps and could provide the consumer with relevant information to better address medical issues such as diabetes—code coverage for hardware and software testing, device authentication measures, access control features, connection security, protocol security, encryption techniques, password requirements, and patching program.

4.6.3 ECG Monitors

IoT-based electrocardiogram (ECG) monitors are cardiac event recorders. The devices record electric signals in the heart to monitor heart disease. Examples of newer and more innovative ECG monitors can work with a consumer's smartphone and communicate wirelessly with an app on the phone. The Apple Watch and the Samsung Gear are two examples of smartwatches that include a photoplethysmo-gram (PPG) sensor to measure heart rate [28]. The wearable devices include a combination of other sensors such as accelerometers and gyroscopes to estimate body movement, barometers to estimate altitude, and GPS modules for location tracking [28]. The devices usually communicate with a cloud-based application to transmit and receive data, which can be monitored by the patient and the patient's physician.

Most security issues with ECG monitors include communication issues, data protection, and device manipulation to alter readings or deny service. Researchers have identified potentially 12 security vulnerabilities, called SweynTooth, related to Bluetooth Low Energy technology commonly used on wearable ECG monitors [29]. The vulnerabilities are caused by poor implementation and can allow hackers in close proximity to the devices to remotely trigger deadlocks, crashes, and bypass security [30]. Health and Human Services (HHS) Cybersecurity Program denotes the lack of authentication, lack of access control, and leaky Bluetooth technology implementation as some weaknesses in IoT-based wearable devices such as ECG monitors [HHS]. As noted by HHS, potential mitigations for the SweynTooth vulnerabilities include asset management, endpoint protection, device maintenance, and a patching program [HHS]. These mitigations are closely linked to the security metrics identified in Sect. 4.6. With further research on measurement and consolidation, the security metrics can serve as a confidence system for manufacturers, healthcare providers, and patients.

4.7 Future Work Applying Security Measurement Methodologies

There are various measurement methodology frameworks used for security measures that can be used to evaluate the security metrics. Future work should focus on the effectiveness of the known frameworks and a need for a more tailored measurement approach for IoMT. Examples of security measurement frameworks are the Goal-Question Metrics (GQM), Security Process Management (SPM), Attack Surface Methodology, Balanced Scorecard (BSC), and Common Vulnerability Scoring System (CVSS).

4.7.1 Goal-Question Metrics (GQM)

The GQM paradigm, which applies a top-down approach for security metrics, has three levels—(1) conceptual level, which is the goal; (2) operational status, which are the questions; and (3) quantitative level, which is the metrics. It was initially designed for software development, but security practitioners use it to help businesses build measurement goals and make decisions at various stages.

4.7.2 Security Process Management (SPM)

The SPM framework is intended to capture all of the elements of the metric program. The SPM framework consists of three layers—(1) Security Metric; (2) Security Measurements Project; and (3) Security Process Improvement. The objective of SPM is to allow its users to structure the measurement activities so that security will improve over time.

4.7.3 Attack Surface Methodology

The Attack Surface methodology approach establishes metrics based on the number of paths an attacker could take to exploit the vulnerabilities in a system or device. The Attack Surface methodology uses attack graphs, which rely mostly on qualitative measures. The attack graphs are usually combined with a statistical approach such as Bayesian networks to define the probability of an attack or multiple staged attacks and help security practitioners develop a decision framework.

4.7.4 Balanced Scorecard (BSC)

The Balanced Scorecard (BSC) is mainly used for creating key business perfor-
mance indicators, but analysts have also applied it to build security metrics for
IT systems. The BSC framework addresses four main domains: (1) Financial; (2)
Internal Business Processes; (3) Learning and Growth; and (4) Customer.

4.7.5 Common Vulnerability Scoring System (CVSS)

The Common Vulnerability Scoring System (CVSS) framework assigns a numeric
value to a vulnerability, which denotes the severity of the exposure on a range of 1
to 10. CVSS has three categories—(1) base metrics; (2) temporal metrics; and (3)
environmental metrics. It includes exploitability and impact measurements to assess
the impact of the vulnerability. CVSS allocates scores to the individual exposure,
but it does not have the ability to aggregate metrics for an overall security score for
the system.

4.8 Conclusion and Next Steps

The categories of metrics identified in this chapter can be a tool to evaluate and rate
the security levels for critical IoMT devices. With the alignment of these metrics
into a tailored measurement methodology, designers and manufacturers of IoMT
devices can understand and proactively work to apply security features early in the
design life cycle and not as an afterthought.

We recommend the development of a customized "*TIDE—Threat Intelligence
Defense Environment*" that leverages the internal and external metrics as described
in Fig. 4.3, and throughout this chapter, in a tactical and strategic way to identify,
act and reduce cybersecurity risks in an IoMT environment.

This type of rating and development of a comprehensive TIDE to manage and
measure the cybersecurity risk of IoMT in the connected healthcare environment
can give consumers the safety and confidence they need for devices that may serve
a critical role in their healthcare management plan. Given the benefits, it is prudent
to continue maturing security metrics research for IoMT to help inform consumers
and vendors, to help control costs, and even to help save lives.

References

1. Prusak, L. Decision Making and Problem Solving: What Can't Be Measured. https://hbr.org/2010/10/what-cant-be-measured.
2. Evarts, E. C. What Crash Test Ratings Really Say. https://cars.usnews.com/cars-trucks/best-cars-blog/2016/09/what-crash-test-ratings-really-say. Accessed 02 January 2021.
3. Gladwell M. The engineer's lament: two ways of thinking about automotive safety. The New Yorker. 2015 May 4.
4. Mohn, T. Starflation-U.S. car safety ratings, once best in the world, now lag behind. Forbes Magazine. 2019 October 20. Accessed 26 September 2021.
5. International Data Corporation: IDC Media Center. https://www.idc.com/getdoc.jsp?containerId=prAP46737220 (2020). Accessed 26 September 2021.
6. Alsuwaidi A, Hassan A, Alkhatri F, Ali H, Mohammad QH, Alrabaee S. Security Vulnerabilities Detected in Medical Devices. In2020 12th Annual Undergraduate Research Conference on Applied Computing (URC) 2020 Apr 15 (pp. 1-6). IEEE.
7. University of Louisville Medical Xpress: Delivering health care through a new lens: smart glasses. https://louisville.edu/medicine/news/delivering-health-care-through-a-new-lens-smart-glasses. Accessed 02 January 2021.
8. Metcalf D, Milliard ST, Gomez M, Schwartz M. Wearables and the internet of things for health: Wearable, interconnected devices promise more efficient and comprehensive health care. IEEE pulse. 2016 Sep 28;7(5):35-9.
9. Joyia GJ, Liaqat RM, Farooq A, Rehman S. Internet of medical things (IoMT): Applications, benefits and future challenges in healthcare domain. Journal of Communications. 2017 Apr;12(4):240-7.
10. Coventry L, Branley D. Cybersecurity in healthcare: a narrative review of trends, threats and ways forward. Maturitas. 2018 Jul 1;113:48-52.
11. Razaque A, Amsaad F, Khan MJ, Hariri S, Chen S, Siting C, Ji X. Survey: Cybersecurity vulnerabilities, attacks and solutions in the medical domain. IEEE Access. 2019 Oct 31;7:168774-97.
12. Ahmed Y, Naqvi S, Josephs M. Aggregation of security metrics for decision making: a reference architecture. In Proceedings of the 12th European Conference on Software Architecture: Companion Proceedings 2018 Sep 24 (pp. 1-7).
13. Chew E, Clay A, Hash J, Bartol N, Brown A. Guide for Developing Performance Metrics for Information Security. National Institute of Standards and Technology; 2006 May 4.
14. Jansen WA. Directions in security metrics research. Diane Publishing; 2009.
15. Swanson MM, Bartol N, Sabato J, Hash J, Graffo L. Security metrics guide for information technology systems 2003.
16. Jaquith A. Security metrics: replacing fear, uncertainty, and doubt. Pearson Education; 2007 Mar 26.
17. Francia III GA. Automotive Vehicle Security Metrics. In Advances in Security, Networks, and Internet of Things 2021 (pp. 341-353). Springer, Cham.
18. Labuschagne WA, Veerasamy N. Metrics for smart security awareness. In European Conference on Cyber Warfare and Security 2017 Jun 1 (pp. 235-242). Academic Conferences International Limited.
19. Ahmed Y, Naqvi S, Josephs M. Cybersecurity metrics for enhanced protection of healthcare IT systems. In 2019 13th International Symposium on Medical Information and Communication Technology (ISMICT) 2019 May 8 (pp. 1-9). IEEE.
20. Savola RM, Savolainen P, Evesti A, Abie H, Sihvonen M. Risk-driven security metrics development for an e-health IoT application. In 2015 Information Security for South Africa (ISSA) 2015 Aug 12 (pp. 1-6). IEEE.
21. Yee GO. Security metrics: An introduction and literature review. Computer and Information Security Handbook. 2013 Jan 1:553-66.

22. Das S, Siroky GP, Lee S, Mehta D, Suri R. Cybersecurity: The need for data and patient safety with cardiac implantable electronic devices. Heart Rhythm. 2021 Mar 1;18(3):473-81.
23. Pycroft L, Aziz TZ. Security of implantable medical devices with wireless connections: The dangers of cyber-attacks. Expert Review of Medical Devices. 2018 Jun 3;15(6):403-6.
24. Slabodkin, G. Insulin Pumps Among Millions of Devices Facing Risk from Newly Disclosed Cyber Vulnerability, IBM Says. MedTechDie blog. 2020.
25. Klonoff D, Han J. The first recall of a diabetes device because of cybersecurity risks. Journal of Diabetes Science and Technology. 2019 Sep;13(5):817-20.
26. Klonoff DC. Cybersecurity for connected diabetes devices. Journal of diabetes science and technology. 2015 Apr 16;9(5):1143-7.
27. Beardsley T. R7-2016-07: Multiple Vulnerabilities in Animas OneTouch Ping Insulin Pump. Rapid7 blog. 2016.
28. McCaldin D, Wang K, Schreier G, Lovell NH, Marschollek M, Redmond SJ, Schukat M. Unintended Consequences of Wearable Sensor Use in Healthcare. Yearbook of Medical Informatics. 2016;25(01):73-86.
29. Garbelini ME, Wang C, Chattopadhyay S, Sumei S, Kurniawan E. {SweynTooth}: Unleashing Mayhem over Bluetooth Low Energy. In2020 USENIX Annual Technical Conference (USENIX ATC 20) 2020 (pp. 911-925).
30. Office of Information Security. [Internet]. Mar, 2020. Available from: https://www.hhs.gov/sites/default/files/hc3-intelligence-briefing-wearable-device-security.pdf

Chapter 5
How Can We Trust in IoT? The Role of Engineers in Ensuring Trust in the Clinical IoT Ecosystem

Jodyn Platt, Sherri Douville, and Ann Mongoven

Contents

5.1   Introduction 84
5.2   What Is Trust? 85
    5.2.1   Dimensions and Definitions of Trust 86
    5.2.2   Why Does Trust Matter to Engineers and Developers? 87
5.3   What Are Key Ethical Frameworks that Engineers and Developers of Trustworthy
    Clinical IoT Can Use to Evaluate Their Own Work and Professional Development? 87
    5.3.1   Engineering Codes of Ethics 88
    5.3.2   Markkula Center for Applied Ethics Framework for Ethical Decision-Making ... 90
    5.3.3   Business Ethics: Duties to Stakeholders Amidst Pressure from Shareholders 91
    5.3.4   Bioethics: From Patient Rights to Bioethics Beyond Individualism 92
        5.3.4.1   Principles of Bioethics 92
        5.3.4.2   Research Ethics 95
        5.3.4.3   Public Health Ethics 95
        5.3.4.4   Data Ethics 96
5.4   How Can High-Profile Cases from Other Areas of Engineering, Business,
    and Healthcare Inform Efforts to Build Trustworthy IoT Ecosystems? 97
    5.4.1   The Boeing 737 Max Catastrophes 97
    5.4.2   Self-Driving Cars: A New Trolley Problem? 99
    5.4.3   The SUPPORT Study 100
    5.4.4   The Havasupai Case: Genetic Alliance (GA) and Genetic Alliance
        Registry and Biobank (GARB) 102
    5.4.5   Algorithmic Bias Against African-Americans in US Healthcare................... 103
    5.4.6   Health Hacking: Kidnapping Hospitals for Ransom 104

J. Platt
Department of Learning Health Sciences, University of Michigan Medical School, Ann Arbor, MI, USA
e-mail: jeplatt@umich.edu

S. Douville (✉)
Medigram, Inc., Los Gatos, CA, USA
e-mail: sherri@medigram.com

A. Mongoven
Heluna Health, Santa Clara, CA, USA
e-mail: amongoven@pgm.helunahealth.org

© Springer Nature Switzerland AG 2022
F. D. Hudson (eds.), *Women Securing the Future with TIPPSS for Connected Healthcare*, Women in Engineering and Science,
https://doi.org/10.1007/978-3-030-93592-4_5

5.1   Introduction

Medical devices and applications are increasingly leveraging the technology of
the "Internet of Things" which connects objects via the Internet and enables
them to send and receive data. This interconnectivity may be very powerful
in healthcare—allowing providers and patients to monitor biometrics and health
status in near real-time. IoT-enabled insulin pumps can support diabetes care [1];
heart rate monitors can track data that is best collected continuously over time
[2], and medication adherence can be more easily observed when caring for the
elderly or those with chronic, complex conditions [3]. These examples indicate
how clinical IoT technologies can be embedded in implanted medical devices,
wearable technology, or smartphones with consumers either actively or passively
passing along information about their bodies and behaviors to inform their health
and healthcare. The term clinical IoT refers to data and use of data that comes
from devices and wearables being used in care settings supervised by a prescribing
clinician such as a physician or nurse practitioner.

Clinical IoT represents a subset of health-related IoT devices on the market contributing to considerable confusion and skepticism from consumers—both patients
and providers—about what clinical IoT is and what it has to offer. Within the flood
of products available, only a select few are actively approved and monitored by
the FDA for safety and efficacy. The volume of direct-to-consumer applications
is highly variable with respect to clinical utility and validity. With an estimated
300,000 health apps on the market, only a small percentage of these have been
shown to be clinically relevant by demonstrating that they meet stated claims or
otherwise show evidence of efficacy [4, 5]. Ironically, these health apps nonetheless
may influence clinical decision-making. This may cause harm from IoT devices'
generating bad data upon which decisions are made (e.g., regarding dosing) [6], or
by contributing to an excess of data which patients and providers must filter to exact
a course of best treatment [7]. From a technical perspective, the industry has yet to
agree on universal standards for privacy, security, or quality.

At risk in this laxly regulated deluge of devices is the consumer's trust. Who is
responsible for ensuring trust in clinical IoT? At present, policies which would regu-

late and enforce accountability lag behind innovations in the marketplace. Moreover, clinical IoT emerges from a complex ecosystem of (potentially) responsible parties. This clinical IoT ecosystem connects engineers and developers to health system administrators, payers, providers, policy-makers, patients and others—all involved in the development, deployment, and scalability of clinical IoT. Trustworthiness, then is distributed across this ecosystem of clinical IoT.

In this chapter, we consider the role of the engineer in ensuring this trust across the ecosystem. Engineers are among the first people involved in bringing clinical IoT services and devices to market. Their roles in development, as well as in product and systems' maintenance, make them key players in the clinical IoT ecosystem. Yet, most design of today's digital health solutions is driven by technical user-requirements and specific business objectives, without addressing the broader questions of trust and trustworthiness of the product. While engineers may meet specific functional requirements, they also bear interest, if not responsibility, for consequences downstream. In part, this is because stakes are much higher in medicine; a faulty insulin pump or pacemaker can have life or death consequences. Absent clear information to parse through and evaluate IoT applications, or standards to evaluate the quality of IoT technologies on behalf of consumers, engineers must take a more active leadership role in ensuring trust and the trustworthiness of their products.

In this chapter, we consider four key questions for engineers:

1. What is trust and why does it matter for engineers and developers of clinical IoT?
2. What are key ethical frameworks that engineers and developers of trustworthy clinical IoT can use to evaluate their own work and professional development?
3. How can high-profile cases from other areas of engineering, business, and healthcare inform efforts to build trustworthy IoT ecosystems?
4. How can engineers and developers become leaders who bring trustworthy products to market and promote the trustworthiness of clinical IoT ecosystems?

5.2   What Is Trust?

Trust has a variety of definitions depending on what field you are in, whether you are interested in trust between two people, trust in organizations, systems, or technologies. Social scientists have long regarded trust as a key, multidimensional component of interpersonal relationships, financial interactions, organizations, social networks, and in society more generally [8, 9]. In healthcare, seminal studies by David Mechanic [10, 11] and others have identified the importance of trust in the doctor–patient relationship, demonstrating that trust is critical for encouraging open and frank communication and promoting treatment compliance [12–14].

5.2.1   Dimensions and Definitions of Trust

Key terms that elucidate the dimensionality of trust include confidence, vulnerability, fidelity, integrity, dependability, and others (see Fig. 5.1). Trust can be defined as "the willingness of a person to be vulnerable to another for a given set of tasks" [15]. In this definition, trust is a form of implicit or explicit contract between two subjects. Expectations matter with respect to the perceived benefit of entering into the contract, as does the risk of loss. Trust may have a basis in prior experience, knowledge, or some other rationale, and is different from faith on the one hand and certainty on the other. Importantly, there is risk and uncertainty inherent in any trusting relationship, as connoted by the notion of vulnerability, but that risk is not a blind one as it can be when taking things "on faith." As an example, trust is often related to, if not equivalent to, privacy and security in technology circles. Privacy and security often mitigate concerns about risk and may create systems that are thus less reliant on trust. A system impervious to external threats or failure does not require vulnerability on the part of end-users. Unfortunately, such systems rarely (if ever) exist. Since the Office of the National Coordinator started monitoring large-scale health data breaches in 2009, the number of people with stolen health records has increased exponentially. Breaches of unsecured protected health information affected over 11,400,000 people in the U.S. in the year 2020 [16].

While addressing privacy and security is of critical importance in the engineering and development of clinical IoT, we argue that privacy and security are necessary

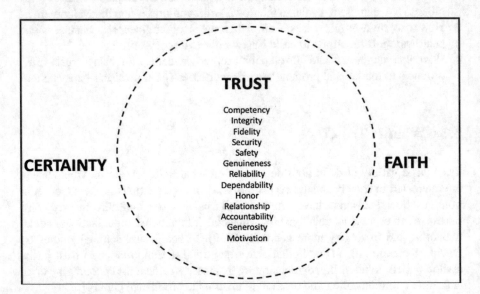

Fig. 5.1 Dimensions of Trust

but not sufficient conditions for trust in clinical IoT. Privacy and security are necessary because they are key components of the expectations with clinical IoT applications. Trust in clinical IoT, however, goes beyond privacy and security to include reliability, transparency, and utility [17]. By extension, engineering and development must go beyond privacy and security in order to build the bridge between trust, acceptance, broad adoption, and sustainable use.

5.2.2 Why Does Trust Matter to Engineers and Developers?

Trust is an important antecedent to accepting broad use of clinical IoT. While many engineers may be distant parties to the clinical encounter, the devices and software they develop can figure prominently in the health and well-being of patients and the people that care for them. This makes the engineer one of the first to engage in a set of actions that brings clinical IoT to patients, each of which relies on trusted relationships. The efficacy, reliability, and trustworthiness of clinical IoT products start with the engineer. Trust is a key factor not only in the market-based transactions that drive adoption of clinical IoT, but also in the ethics of care that define the clinical encounter. Failure in clinical IoT devices—some of which can cause real harm to patients—reflects on the personal integrity and professional ethics of the engineer and the other actors in the clinical IoT ecosystem.

There are a number of ways the engineer might think about their role in the ecosystem of trust. In the next two sections, we consider this role as a matter of professional ethics. We describe core ethical principles from business ethics, bioethics, research, public health, and data ethics as well as case studies from a variety of relevant settings that demonstrate the promise and peril of clinical IoT. These principles and cases can guide engineers as they define their role ensuring trust across the clinical IoT ecosystem. Then in the final section, we articulate a family of leadership roles that engineers can cultivate to promote trustworthy clinical IoT.

5.3 What Are Key Ethical Frameworks that Engineers and Developers of Trustworthy Clinical IoT Can Use to Evaluate Their Own Work and Professional Development?

A variety of ethical frameworks offer helpful guidance to engineers and managers developing trustworthy healthcare IoT and associated systems. In addition to codes of engineering ethics, these include general strategies for moral reasoning, as well as ethical frameworks from business ethics, bioethics, research, public health, and data ethics. At the same time, IoT challenges the adequacy of these frameworks. Developments in biotechnology and data analytics are pressing development of new, more systems-oriented ethical paradigms that encompass connections between the venues of clinical care, research, population health, and data management.

In this section, we present several of these ethical frameworks. We will draw upon conceptual lenses offered by these frameworks to explore cases and analogies to IoT in the subsequent section.

5.3.1   Engineering Codes of Ethics

Both the U.S. National Society of Professional Engineers (NSPE) and the international Institute of Electrical and Electronics Engineers (IEEE) have developed codes of ethics for their members (see Table 5.1). These codes emphasize the duty of engineers to safeguard the health and welfare of the public. They also stress the relationship between technical competence and ethical engineering, and engineering aims to be socially useful. The NSPE includes attention to engineers' obligation to their clients, whereas the IEEE managerial focus is on obligations among colleagues and teams.

Other professional societies also offer resources for engineering ethics. The U.S. National Academy of Engineering's Center for Engineering Ethics and Society (CEES) maintains a special focus on integrating ethics education in engineering training [20]. The Association for Practical and Professional Ethics (APPE) includes attention to engineering ethics cases and commentary in its endeavors and annual meeting [21].

What do engineering codes of ethics mean to developers of IoT? The NSPE and IEEE codes locate their endeavors within broader contexts of professional identity, and of the humanistic aims of engineering. Codes such as these become meaningful when they are incorporated into the development of:

- Key performance indicators
- Hiring, evaluation, and promotion procedures
- Board engagement
- Professional discourse on ethical challenges

Table 5.1 Codes of Ethics: National Society of Professional Engineers[a] and IEEE[b]

National Society of Professional Engineers	IEEE
Fundamental Canons Engineers, in the fulfillment of their professional duties, shall:	We do hereby commit ourselves to the highest ethical and professional conduct and agree:
1. Hold paramount the safety, health, and welfare of the public. 2. Perform services only in areas of their competence. 3. Issue public statements only in an objective and truthful manner. 4. Act for each employer or client as faithful agents or trustees. 5. Avoid deceptive acts. 6. Conduct themselves honorably, responsibly, ethically, and lawfully so as to enhance the honor, reputation, and usefulness of the profession.	I. To uphold the highest standards of integrity, responsible behavior, and ethical conduct in professional activities. 1. To hold paramount the safety, health, and welfare of the public, to strive to comply with ethical design and sustainable development practices, to protect the privacy of others, and to disclose promptly factors that might endanger the public or the environment. 2. To improve the understanding by individuals and society of the capabilities and societal implications of conventional and emerging technologies, including intelligent systems. 3. To avoid real or perceived conflicts of interest whenever possible and to disclose them to affected parties when they do exist. 4. To avoid unlawful conduct in professional activities and to reject bribery in all its forms.
1. Engineers shall be guided in all their relations by the highest standards of honesty and integrity. 2. Engineers shall at all times strive to serve the public interest. 3. Engineers shall avoid all conduct or practice that deceives the public. 4. Engineers shall not disclose, without consent, confidential information concerning the business affairs or technical processes of any present or former client or employer, or public body on which they serve. 5. Engineers shall not be influenced in their professional duties by conflicting interests.	5. To seek, accept, and offer honest criticism of technical work, to acknowledge and correct errors, to be honest and realistic in stating claims or estimates based on available data, and to credit properly the contributions of others. 6. To maintain and improve our technical competence and to undertake technological tasks for others only if qualified by training or experience, or after full disclosure of pertinent limitations. II. To treat all persons fairly and with respect, to not engage in harassment or discrimination, and to avoid injuring others. 7. To treat all persons fairly and with respect and to not engage in discrimination based on characteristics such as race, religion, gender, disability, age, national origin, sexual orientation, gender identity, or gender expression. 8. To not engage in harassment of any kind, including sexual harassment or bullying behavior. 9. To avoid injuring others, their property, reputation, or employment by false or malicious actions, rumors, or any other verbal or physical abuses.

(continued)

Table 5.1 (continued)

National Society of Professional Engineers	IEEE
6. Engineers shall not attempt to obtain employment or advancement or professional engagements by untruthfully criticizing other engineers, or by other improper or questionable methods.	III. To strive to ensure this code is upheld by colleagues and co-workers. 10. To support colleagues and co-workers in following this code of ethics, to strive to ensure the code is upheld, and to not retaliate against individuals reporting a violation [18].
7. Engineers shall not attempt to injure, maliciously or falsely, directly or indirectly, the professional reputation, prospects, practice, or employment of other engineers. Engineers who believe others are guilty of unethical or illegal practice shall present such information to the proper authority for action.	
8. Engineers shall accept personal responsibility for their professional activities, provided, however, that engineers may seek indemnification for services arising out of their practice for other than gross negligence, where the engineer's interests cannot otherwise be protected.	
9. Engineers shall give credit for engineering work to those to whom credit is due, and will recognize the proprietary interests of others [19].	

[a]Reprinted by Permission of the National Society of Professional Engineers (NSPE) www.nspe.org
[b] © 2021 IEEE. Reprinted with permission of the IEEE

5.3.2 Markkula Center for Applied Ethics Framework for Ethical Decision-Making

Professional codes of ethics are helpful statements of ideals and commitment. Between the lines, they presume ethical tensions and institutional power dynamics that may complicate or challenge ethical decision-making. One venue that encourages explicit attention to such endemic ethical tensions is Santa Clara University's Markkula Center for Applied Ethics (MCAE). The Center has devised accessible materials to guide both general ethical decision-making and ethical decision-making for engineers more specifically. MCAE has developed a general framework that encourages people to deliberate ethical challenges through pluralistic moral orientations, including consequentially focused, rights-focused, justice-focused, virtue-focused, and relationally focused paradigms [22].

The MCAE framework provides an architecture for articulating competing moral claims. It does not explicitly address mechanisms for negotiating tradeoffs among those claims. Some engineering ethicists have advocated using weighted decision matrices for such tradeoff negotiation [23]. In the contemporary healthcare environment, the overarching goal of achieving high *value* (significant impact at economical cost) warns against treating diverse ethical aims of the system as independent variables. A new movement to apply "lean design" to healthcare seeks to simplify health systems in order to identify and encourage value [24].

What does the MCAE framework mean for developers of IoT? It reminds them that many modes of ethical reasoning, aiming at different moral ends, are relevant to their work—and encourages them to think about their own role from the perspective of all those moral orientations.

5.3.3   Business Ethics: Duties to Stakeholders Amidst Pressure from Shareholders

Contemporary business ethics has moved well beyond economist Milton Friedman's famous 1970 exhortation that since "the business of business is business," the only social responsibility is the maximization of profit for shareholders [25]. Today, we recognize that business affects a much broader group of stakeholders than the shareholders who own stock [26]. Stakeholders include consumers, workers, creditors, communities, government, and the environment. In healthcare, patients, populations, and third-party payers are important stakeholders [27]. Figure 5.2 shows this relationship between shareholders and stakeholders, the former being a subset of the latter. Business ethics strategies aim to:

- Include stakeholder perspectives in business development
- Negotiate tensions between stakeholder and shareholder interest
- Align stakeholder and shareholder interest

All of these strategies foster individual and institutional habits of resistance to undue or distorted pressure from shareholders, while recognizing legitimate financial interests of shareholders. The literature encompassing these strategies is sometimes tagged "stakeholder theory."

What does stakeholder theory mean for developers of clinical IoT? Stakeholder theory pushes engineers and engineering managers to inculcate habits of mindfulness regarding broad stakeholder interest, and the ability to question business directives that may pose potential harm to stakeholders. Applying stakeholder theory to the business of clinical IoT leads one to ask questions about: What parties are impacted by your work? How do they stand to gain or lose?

Fig. 5.2 Shareholders are a
subset of stakeholders

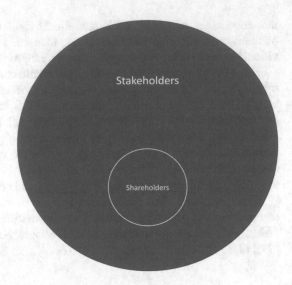

5.3.4 Bioethics: From Patient Rights to Bioethics Beyond Individualism

As clinical IoT enters the realm of the clinic, it will be judged by the principles and frameworks of bioethics. We dive more deeply into this area given our assumption that some engineers may not have deep knowledge of the ethical landscape of healthcare. We also posit that the opportunities and success of clinical IoT will rely on successful navigation of this landscape.

Each of the bioethical frameworks summarized in Table 5.2 offer analogically helpful guidance to engineers and engineering managers developing medical IoT.

5.3.4.1 Principles of Bioethics

In the USA, the development of bioethics historically was aligned with mid-twentieth century civil rights movements underscoring ethical respect for individuals regardless of gender or race. Civil rights movements in the political sphere fomented the rejection of undue paternalism in medicine, challenging previous ethical paradigms that could be summarized as "doctor knows best."

Following the work of seminal thinkers Tom Beauchamp and James Childress, clinical ethics is often summarized as comprised of four principles [28] as follows:

- Respect for patient autonomy
- Non-maleficence (do no harm)
- Beneficence (do good)
- Justice (treat similar cases similarly, ethically)

Table 5.2 Summary of bioethical frameworks

Framework	Question(s) it seeks to answer	Elements	One key source
Principles of Clinical Medical Ethics	How can medicine treat patients as moral agents? How can medicine explore the complexity of, balance among, and negotiate tradeoffs between important elements of ethical clinical care?	**Principles of:** Respect for Patient Autonomy (includes informed consent and respect for privacy) Non-maleficence (Do no harm) Beneficence (Do good) Justice (Treat like cases similarly)	Tom Beauchamp and James Childress, *Principles of Biomedical Ethics*
Research Ethics	How can human research participants be treated as ends in themselves, not only as means to the end of scientific knowledge-production?	**Ethical constraints on research:** Respect for human persons Protection of vulnerability (vs. "Guinea pigs") Informed consent for research, with understanding that intervention is experimental Oversight by Institutional Review Boards (IRBs)	*Belmont Report*
Public Health Ethics	How are bioethical challenges similar/different when the patient is a population? How can the promotion of population health negotiate among the best interests of individuals, subgroups of the community, and the population as a whole?	**Values to be Integrated:** Trust (professional transparency) Health and safety Health justice and equity Reciprocity and solidarity Human rights and civil liberties Inclusivity and engagement	American Public Health Association, *Public Health Code of Ethics*

Like the MCAE framework, the principles encourage thinking through an ethical challenge from the perspective of diverse ethical goals—while they explicitly highlight tensions among the goals.

The principles are most robustly understood as infrastructure to organize sophisticated ethical conversation around topical families of ethical challenges. Respect for patient autonomy requires upholding patient dignity in several ways: maintaining privacy and confidentiality; educating patients on treatment options; and honoring their informed choices regarding treatment or decline of treatment.

Attention to benefits and harms of potential interventions requires that risks as well as potential benefits, and the unintended as well as intended effects of treatment be considered. It also requires that potential benefits and harms to therapeutic relationships and healthcare institutions be evaluated. Justice requires that relevant ethical criteria governing medical decision-making be distinguished from pernicious biases or caprice, and applied consistently.

Beauchamp and Childress consider each of the principles as equally ethically binding. At the same time, they recognize that the values expressed in the principles can tragically conflict. To take a classic example, from a clinician's perspective a competent Jehovah's Witness' decline of a potentially life-saving blood transfusion poses a dilemma between the clinician's desires both to respect patient autonomy and to be medically beneficent. One intended use of the four-principle framework is to organize ethically nuanced negotiation of tradeoffs among the principles. At the extreme, this would include articulating a defense of prioritizing one principle over another in a truly dilemmatic case and minimizing infringement of the disfavored principle.

When well-used as a conceptual infrastructure, the principles beg questions about how to *avoid* ethical dilemmas. For example, many Jehovah's Witnesses now develop advance directives to clarify their general aversion to transfusion; whether they would want transfusion in a life-threatening situation; and whether in an emergency they would be open to treatment with derivative blood products (the acceptability of which is a matter of debate within the tradition). By articulating benefits and harms from patients' points of view, advance directives help healthcare physicians consider best alignments of autonomy and beneficence.

Increasingly clinical medicine is moving beyond the encouragement of advance directives to promote a more robust model of "shared decision-making" between medical professionals and patients. Shared decision-making is a dynamic process that incorporates patient value-solicitation into ongoing evaluation and treatment [29].

The principles of bioethics have been institutionalized through the development of hospital ethics committees, state medical society ethics committees, and ethical committees of medical professional organizations. Each of these forums may offer analogies to the development of ethical oversight of clinical IoT.

What do the principles mean for engineers of IoT? Bioethical principles remind developers of medical IoT to keep the vulnerability of end-users "front and center" though the developers may never meet those individuals. After all, the clinicians' "patients" are the engineers' "users." The principles challenge engineers to consider how users' values may be solicited and incorporated into design. They also press engineers to consider deliberately ethical tradeoffs that implicate design. For example, maximizing the ability of IoT users to adaptively use a technology may be in tension with legitimately "paternalistic" constraints on such use aimed at patient safety. A major disanalogy is that unlike clinicians, IoT developers rarely have ongoing personal relationships with patients using their products. The simultaneous distance and intimacy—their creations are embodied by patients—creates a relational paradox.

5.3.4.2 Research Ethics

In the USA, research ethics were born of scandal. In the historical wake of the Nuremberg trials of Nazi doctors who had experimented on Jews and others in concentration camps, Americans were horrified by revelations of gross exploitation of vulnerable people in American medical research such as the Tuskegee syphilis study and the Willowbrook hepatitis study. Conducted by the U.S. Public Health Service from 1932 to 1972, the Tuskegee study examined the life cycle of untreated syphilis in poor uneducated African-American men—who knew neither that they were being used as research subjects, nor that existent penicillin could cure their illness [30]. The Willowbrook hepatitis study, conducted in New York State throughout the 1950s, deliberately infected severely disabled institutionalized children with hepatitis A for experimental research [31].

In 1976, the National Commission for the Protection of Human Subjects of Biomedical and Behavioral Research published the Belmont Report delineating principles of ethical research [32]. The Belmont Report extends the notion of informed consent to research: researchers should ensure potential human research subjects understand the difference between treatment and research and knowingly choose to participate in research. The Belmont Report recognizes that some groups of people may be particularly vulnerable to exploitation and deserving of special protection, especially given the de facto power of medical institutions. The Belmont Report catalyzed the development of Institutional Review Boards, or IRBs. IRBs of research-sponsoring institutions such as hospitals, universities, and government agencies ethically review all research proposals involving experimentation on humans.

What does research ethics mean for engineers of IoT? Research ethics requires engineers to be mindful of the extent to which their products may be experimental, and the end-users de facto may be research subjects as well as patients seeking therapeutic treatment. Research ethics demands that IoT developers disconcertingly but proactively ask themselves: "What might a Tuskegee or Willowbrook of IoT look like, and how could it happen?" It asks engineers to consider how protection of experimental subjects might be worked into design, and what kinds of evidence should be collected and analyzed to validate or call into question the overall benefit of the product.

5.3.4.3 Public Health Ethics

Populations are also "patients." The goal of public health is to prevent illness and promote health in populations. Increasingly, ethical thinkers reflecting on public health recognize the limits of ethical frameworks based on individual rights to address population health. Public health ethics must negotiate tradeoffs when individual rights conflict with public health initiatives, or when the interests of different groups within a population are in tension. Recently, the American Public Health Association (APHA) published a code of public health ethics, highlighting core values and ethical frameworks to promote the common good while attending to individual and group interests [33].

Significantly, the APHA identifies the first core value to be engendering trust through transparent professionalism. Other values identified are: health and safety; health justice and equity; reciprocity and solidarity; human rights and civil liberties; inclusivity and engagement. The code directs reflective public health officials to analyze comparative effectiveness, consider proportionality, and discern responsible use of resources in meeting their public charge.

What does public health ethics mean for engineers of IoT? Public health ethics asks engineers to be mindful that ultimately end-users may include communities and populations, not just individual patients. It asks them to consider proactively the challenges of scaling, breadth of usability, and production economies that could promote or thwart health equity.

5.3.4.4 Data Ethics

The rise of healthcare data analytics offers the opportunity for research, clinical care, public health, and healthcare quality-improvement to inform each other continuously in "knowledge-loops." While the erasure of rigid boundaries between those nodes of healthcare offers great potential for innovation, it also poses ethical challenges. Each of those domains encompasses a different set of primary ethical commitments. Creating dynamic ethical systems as well as data systems—reflective infrastructures that adequately honor each domain-defining ethical commitment while allowing data to flow between the domains—is a new challenge. Large-scale biobanks, health informatics data repositories, and "learning health systems" are working to develop process-oriented ethical frameworks to govern dynamic inter-related systems. These ethical pioneers often focus on governance models, and the representational mechanisms for stakeholders embraced by those models, that enable ongoing negotiation of ethical tensions within and between linked systems.

Several frameworks have been developed to articulate elements of trust in complex data systems, including: the FAIR principles, the TRUST principles, and the CARE principles (see Table 5.3).

All three frameworks share an emphasis on the preciousness of data that comes from human bodies or human experience. Taken together, the combination of FAIR, TRUST, and CARE principles urge those working within data systems to consider simultaneously the ethical interests of data providers and data users, as well as the integrity and sustainability of the data itself.

What do data ethics mean to engineers of IoT? Data ethics remind engineers that they must retain bi-focal ethical lenses on data. One lens enables continuous attention to the integrity of the data as such. The other fosters continuous recognition that data comes from people and encodes identify-conferring aspects of themselves and their life experiences. Keeping both lenses de-fogged results in an ethically appropriate sense of the preciousness of data, which in turn promotes deliberate attention to its accurate and ethical collection, cleaning, and maintenance.

Table 5.3 Samples of frameworks for ensuring trust in complex data systems

Framework	Question it seeks to answer	Elements	Who articulated
FAIR	How can we make data reusable?	**Data** must be: **Findable Accessible Interoperable Reusable**	The FAIR International round-table of data-using stakeholders [34]
TRUST	How can we maintain trustworthy digital data repositories over time?	**Data repositories** must embrace: **Transparency Responsibility User Focus Sustainability Technology** (Infrastructure)	International round-table of data users [35]
CARE	How can communities maintain control of, and direct the use of, data from their members?	**Data managers** must seek: **Collective benefit** (to those who gave data) **Authority** (to community which gave) **Responsibility** (Response-ability) **Ethics** (Broadly understood)	Global Indigenous Data Alliance [36]

5.4   How Can High-Profile Cases from Other Areas of Engineering, Business, and Healthcare Inform Efforts to Build Trustworthy IoT Ecosystems?

This section pairs paradigmatic ethical case studies from other engineering, business, and healthcare settings with emerging challenges of developing trustworthy clinical IoT. The juxtaposition is intended both to invite application of the ethical frameworks, and to encourage analogical comparison. Analogical thinking encourages direct confrontation with risks posed by new technologies, as well as explicit recognition of ethical tradeoffs and their transparent negotiation.

5.4.1   The Boeing 737 Max Catastrophes

Consider an example of catastrophic capitulation to undue shareholder pressure from a non-medical venue. In October 2019 and March 2019, two disastrous commercial jet crashes in Indonesia and Ethiopia killed 346 people. Both airplanes were Boeing 737 Max jets. The 737 Max was Boeing's most recently inaugurated fleet (2017). Boeing's initial insistence that the first crash was a result of pilot error became untenable after the second. With the plane's software system implicated in the crashes, Boeing 737 Max jets were grounded worldwide and the company's CEO, Dennis Muilenburg, was fired.

An over-narrow focus on shareholder interest had subverted the fundamental safety mission of the enterprise, in the end proving disastrous to shareholders as well as to hapless air passengers. Responding to its competitor Airbus' development of a new plane, Boeing had designed and marketed the 737 Max in record time. To do so, it retrofitted many adjustments to its designs for planes smaller than the 737 Max. Both the retrofitting and the compartmentalization of responsibilities surrounding it contributed to disaster.

Investigations after the crashes criticized many factors: over-cozy relationships between Boeing and the US government's airline safety regulator, the Federal Aviation Administration (FAA); inadequate pilot instruction on the software system in the plane's pilot manual; the squelching of internal communications flagging a potential problem; and the ignoring of negative simulation results [37]. Of particular interest to engineers is a key design issue that was pilloried in retrospect after the crash: the use of software to try to compensate for a fundamental structural design flaw [38]. The aerodynamics of the plane caused periodic nose-up stalls; the problematic software system aimed to right those stalls by pushing the nose down when needed. The software system was developed as a work-around for a design problem that in fact was too dangerous to let stand in the first place. The Boeing case cautions engineers of IoT to consider:

- How the technical problem they are being asked to solve relates to other aspects of a project and overall mission
- How to solicit and attend mission-critical feedback
- Who is endangered by, and owed information about, problems

Echoes of the Boeing case are evident in lethal failures with two kinds of clinical IoT, insulin pumps and pacemakers, that have been the subject of regulatory action and/or industry recall. Defects need to be clearly differentiated from user error just like in all software.

Reconciling the design methodologies, skill sets, and build approaches of both hardware and software is a challenging endeavor. The ability to avoid harm in product development will depend on the commitment to drive understanding between different kinds of engineers working in tandem on product development and the development and maturation of a well understood, transparent, auditable testing methodology to validate the relationships between the different work streams.

The medical community complained that defects in one cardiac pacemaker were not only acknowledged belatedly. In addition, their implications for patients who already had the device implanted, and the physicians managing their care, went unattended by the manufacturer and the FDA [39]. After all, pacemakers are not like car seats—one cannot do a simple switch-out after a model is recalled. Clinicians are beginning to consider risk communication to patients who have implanted IoT devices with known flaws. For example, the University of Michigan Hospital and the Cleveland Clinic developed brochures for patients who learn that they have implanted cardiac devices that have been the subject of recall [40, 41].

5.4.2 Self-Driving Cars: A New Trolley Problem?

Innovations in self-driving cars created an ethical dilemma that many have compared to the classical philosophical hypothetical case called "the trolley problem." The trolley problem posits that a runaway trolley is barreling down the tracks toward five people left tied to the tracks [42]. The imagined moral reasoner is at a switching station that could divert the trolley to a sidetrack, saving the five. However, there is one person on the sidetrack likely to be killed by that switch. Should the moral agent divert the trolley, thus becoming the proximate cause of one person's death in the attempt to save a greater number?

Technologists highlight that development of self-driving cars requires programming answers to the trolley problem in accident-avoidance algorithms [43]. What should the car do in situations where some accident seems unavoidable? For example, should it prioritize protecting the driver who bought the car, or others? One major developer of self-driving cars faced criticism for insisting that in such situations, the driver must override and make the decision [44]. Critics argued that a major rationale for developing self-driving cars is to reduce accidents, the majority of which are caused by human error. To insist that humans take over the car in potentially lethal situations appears a liability-evasion that undermines the reason for developing self-driving cars in the first place.

In response to the trolley problem posed for self-driving cars, MIT developed an interactive website called "Moral Machine" that went viral [45]. The designers of the site presumed that ethical, not only technical, criteria inevitably must be worked into the algorithms governing self driving cars. They thought the most defensible ethical algorithms would be (a) publicly transparent and (b) representative of consensus ethical views. They invited the public to weigh in, registering what they would want a self-driving car to do in simulated situations where complete avoidance of death or injury was impossible. Seventy thousand people from 42 countries participated in the simulations. Strong majorities among the participants thought cars should favor the well-being of humans over animals, young over old, and greater numbers over lesser without privileging the driver [46]. At the same time, there were marked cultural differences in responses (e.g., participants from Eastern countries were more likely to favor old potential victims), and apparent class biases (many favored the well-dressed over the apparent homeless potential victim). Germany, the first country to develop rules for such algorithms, prohibits favoring any human demographic. The judge who played a key role developing the guidelines was unimpressed by the Moral Machine mass simulations, noting that Germany's past warns against assuming prevalent social biases are ethically defensible [47].

The "trolley problem" of self-driving cars underscores that ethical, not only biophysiological, algorithms may be required for the development of some forms of health IoT. The ethical presumptions embedded are likely to be more defensible the more transparent they are. Consider shutting off a pacemaker, for example. The ethical right of patients to turn off their pacemaker as burdens outweigh benefits is well established. When patients reach a point when they are in a dying process, the pacemaker's continued efforts to stimulate the heart can become a form of torture. What if a patient is no longer able to make or communicate a judgment? Currently, the decision to turn off or leave on the pacemaker would fall to the patient's legal surrogate decision-maker. But should a "self-driving" pacemaker ever be allowed to make the decision to shut off based on combined biophysiological data and embedded ethical algorithms reflecting wider social input? What if the self-driving decision and the surrogate decision conflict? Which would best represent or advocate for the patient? Indeed, assessing the degree to which algorithms versus surrogates should be used for decision-making on behalf of patients in medical *extremus* might become part of future advanced care planning and the formulation of advance directives. Conversely, a failure to acknowledge that any ethical presumptions are embedded in the complex data and feedback systems governing health IoT could inherently rob patients of autonomy, or could invidiously impose untested social values on patient pools.

5.4.3   The SUPPORT Study

A recent controversy in bioethics poses a particularly relevant analogy to ethical challenges of IoT because it involved a device connected to vulnerable patients' bodies, albeit not an IoT device: the SUPPORT study (Surfactant, Positive Pressure, and Oxygenation Randomized Trial). The SUPPORT clinical trial examined oxygenation levels for premature babies regulated by a continuous positive airway pressure (CPAP) machine used in conjunction with the drug surfactant. Due to inadequately developed lungs, premature babies often need pressurized oxygen supplementation to survive. However, over-oxygenation can adversely affect eye development in premature babies, causing blindness. Decisions about oxygenation level thus presented a high-stakes balancing act. The study sought to ascertain the best oxygenation level. Between 2005 and 2009 approximately 1300 babies at 22 major hospitals participated in the study, by consent of parents [48, 49]. The study randomly assigned premature infants to be treated at higher or lower levels of oxygen saturation. It found that babies oxygenated at the lower end of the scale were more likely to die, while those at the higher end were more likely to be blinded. The study generated intense ethical controversy. In 2013, the U.S. Department of Health and Human Resources Office of Human Research Protection found the study violated federal regulations for ethical research [50].

Defenders of the study argued that attacks on it undermined basic aims of comparative effectiveness research, which by definition seeks experimental means to determine which of several extant treatment strategies is superior [51]. They insist that the undue risks and associated incomplete informed consent alleged by critics could only become known through the research itself [52]. Opponents, however, criticized the informed consent process, the standard of care presumed, and the study design.

The most frequently voiced criticisms were of the informed consent process. Critics claimed that by focusing on the explored relationship between oxygen level and vision risk, the consent process obfuscated the basic tradeoff at stake between two different risks: risks of death due to pulmonary failure and risk to vision due to treatment—leaving parents unable to assess the true risk of participation in research. Other critics argued the problem was not only in the consent process, but in the actual research design and analysis. Study design treated the two possible negative outcomes, death or blindness, equally despite the vast qualitative difference between them [53]. The draconian tradeoff at stake also made assertions about standards of care fraught [54]. Disagreements about whether a standard of care had been settled before the study contributed to opposition by some physician groups within participating hospitals.

SUPPORT raises ethical questions that predictably may arise in the development of clinical IoT. How much should the machine–body interface be controlled by patients (or their advocates), physicians, institutions, or programmers? How much do each of those parties need to know to participate with both scientific and ethical integrity? How much, and what kinds, of evidence are needed to support or challenge standards of care in practice and how can that evidence be attained? Many kinds of treatments may cause intended good effects, unintended but predictable negative effects, or unintended and unpredicted negative effects. How should tradeoffs among those potential effects be negotiated, and by whom?

A contemporary development in clinical IoT that raises parallel challenges is the use of deep brain stimulation (DBS) in patients with Parkinson's, brain injuries, chronic pain, extreme depression, or obsessive-compulsive disorders. This experimental therapy requires the implanting of electrical nodes in the brain through surgery, and then the control of electrical currents applied through mechanisms outside the body. Many patients receiving DBS report significant symptom improvement. At the same time, there are serious risks, including inherent risks of surgery on the brain as well as risks of node displacement or lead leakage. Moreover, the long-term effects of DBS are unknown. The tradeoff between potentially large benefits and potentially large harms is particularly acute, challenging both research standards and informed consent processes for patients—who often are desperate when they consider the therapy [55]. Some applications of DBS can fundamentally change personality, a result that may be viewed positively, negatively, or both at once. Given the stakes, the question of who should control the electrical dosage bears on complex questions of autonomy, authority, and expertise. An engineer working on the development of DBS mechanisms should be ethically aware of how her design will or will not be integrated within current standards of care, informed consent processes, and research strategies.

5.4.4   The Havasupai Case: Genetic Alliance (GA) and Genetic Alliance Registry and Biobank (GARB)

In 2010, Arizona State University settled out of court a landmark case brought against it by the Havasupai tribe of Native Americans [56]. The Havasupai live in a remote region at the base of the Grand Canyon. During the 1990s, researchers at Arizona State collected blood from the Havasupai in order to study diabetes, which has a dramatically high prevalence among the Havasupai. In 2004, the Havasupai discovered residual blood samples had been used to study schizophrenia and tribal origin. The Havasupai protested that this research was unconsented. They claimed that in addition to the intrinsic violation of dignity in the lack of consent, the research tangibly harmed the tribe by associating them with the stigma of mental health disorders and by challenging the tribe's own origin myths. Arizona State University agreed to pay $700,000 in damages and to participate in the ritual return of the blood samples to the tribe.

In an age when systematized biorepositories enable continued use of many kinds of tissue samples, as well as the linking of biosamples to other health databases, the Havasupai case stands as a stark warning. It reminds scientists and researchers of the intimate connections between biological samples and human identity, and thus connections to issues of consent, control, and authority.

Fortunately, there are also positive examples of biobanks or learning health systems striving self-consciously to embody ideals of research ethics and data ethics. One organization that has worked self-consciously to embody many of the TRUST, FAIR, and CARE principles is the Genetic Alliance (GA). This non-profit organization supports research and clinical translation for rare genetic diseases. While it does not specifically work with the development of IoT, GA's mission shares some of the ethical challenges of medical IoT. Its creative responses to those challenges provide inspiring fodder to medical IoT designers.

Genetic Alliance is an umbrella organization whose membership is comprised of diverse disease-advocacy non-profit organizations sharing an interest in genetic research [57]. While the historical codification of ethical principles for data registries proceeded from TRUST to FAIR to CARE, the Alliance began from a commitment to redressing power imbalances that are the focus of CARE. GA sought to rectify what it considered non-patient-focused incentives, funding, and foci of scientific research on genetic diseases. From GA's point of view, priorities of the research "establishment" had become both scientifically and ethically distorted.

In contrast, GA sought to put those most impacted by genetic disease in the "driver's seat" of research and development [57]. The experience of patients and families afflicted by rare genetic diseases orients the member disease-specific organizations of the Alliance. The simultaneously charismatic and visionary long-time CEO of GA, Sharon Terry, is the mother of two sons with a rare genetic disease.

How to make data reusable (the FAIR challenge) in sustainable repositories (the TRUST challenge) is of critical import in research on rare genetic diseases. By definition, the patient pool is relatively small and diffuse, while being acutely affected. Commercial pharmaceutical companies may direct resources where there are more convenient research clusters or clearer expectations of financial returns. GA realized the scientific preciousness of biosamples and medical data collected from many of their clients for clinical care were not being tapped in more systematic research. In 2003, the Genetic Alliance founded its own Genetic Alliance Registry and Biobank (GARB) for biosamples and associated data.

GA's commitments link a governance structure focused on stakeholder engagement to a systematic strategy fostering data reusability and repository-maintenance. The Alliance seeks to make stakeholders, those affected by genetic disease, shareholders of the research enterprise in several ways [58]. Voluntary contributors of genetic samples and data to the biobank, both organizations and individuals, make up the advisory and governance boards of the biobank. Decisions about what research GA should fund, and about what outside-funded research can collaborate with GARB, are thus made by the impacted patients and families whose data enables that research. Moreover, participants who contribute samples and data to the biobank permanently own their own data. GA has developed sophisticated systems that create a continuous loop of participant affirmation of research values and consent to use their data, coupled with continuous opportunity to withdraw. It also has developed robust educational and training programs so that lay research participants can understand research enterprises, and so that lay participants who wish to become involved in governance roles can become effective stewards.

The warnings of the Havasupai case and the efforts of GA to embody TRUST, FAIR, and CARE rubrics have significant implications for the development of health IoT. Health IoT devices increasingly will collect research data from the patient— initially to inform clinical care of the patient. However, that data could also be used for many other purposes, including serving population health goals or commercial goals of the manufacturer. What informed consent means, then, for health IoT users may go beyond how data collected by the device will be used in their own care. The extent to which the device renders them a research subject, and how their intimate data will be submitted to or become fodder for artificial intelligence (AI) algorithms, may be legitimate ethical interests of patients. Since the increasing complexity of health data systems may preclude patients' complete control over their own intimate data, ethical models of governance for IoT health systems merits deliberate ethical creativity.

5.4.5 Algorithmic Bias Against African-Americans in US Healthcare

Transparent public critique of the data algorithms used to allocate healthcare resources is often limited by the proprietary nature of many of the algorithms. However, a landmark 2019 study published in *Science* dramatized how enormous the magnitude of data bias can be, and how dramatically that can exacerbate health disparities and impede health equity [59, 60]. The study was inspired by the puzzlement of the clinician-investigators who had noticed their black patients received systematically lower risk scores from their institution than white ones with similar medical profiles.

The study analyzed by patient-race the effects of a commercial algorithm used by health systems that provide services to 200 million people. It concluded that a wrongful choice of proxy-metric in the algorithm reduced the eligibility of African-American patients for intensive medical management by 50% compared to similarly medically situated white Americans. The algorithm sought to identify patients with complex medical needs who could benefit from "high risk care management" programs. These programs invest intensive proactive medical staff time and structured healthcare team-coordination for the benefit of such patients. The algorithm used healthcare costs per patient in the previous year as a proxy for medical vulnerability of the patient. However, in fact black patients on average had received less care than white counterparts in the past. So the proxy simply magnified pre-existing health inequities, eliminating black patients from appropriate care because they had previously received less care. The Obermeyer study galvanized public discussion not only because of the extremity of the bias it revealed in one algorithm, but because it highlighted the degree of bias that may be hidden through the untransparent use of algorithms lacking adequate critical review throughout the healthcare system.

The Obermeyer study cautions developers of health IoT because even the most elegantly honed integration of data algorithm with IoT design could result in harm if the data used to develop the algorithm was biased. For example, if a patient pool used to develop device-driving algorithms was skewed by unrecognized selection bias, use of the product on wider populations could have unintended negative consequences.

5.4.6   Health Hacking: Kidnapping Hospitals for Ransom

In both the United States and Germany, cyberattacks on hospital information systems were launched during the fall of 2020. These malware attacks cripple hospital information systems while ransom is demanded by cybercriminals. In September, German police launched a negligent homicide investigation following the death of a Cologne woman in critical care [61]. When a ransomware attack on her hospital forced an emergency transfer to a hospital 20 miles away, she did not survive the journey. In October 2020, American hospitals in Oregon, Vermont, and New York were simultaneously crippled, and some had to postpone surgeries and radiological cancer treatments [62]. The US Federal Bureau of Investigation issued a warning citing Russian cybercriminal rings, but specific actors were never verified or brought to justice.

Cybersecurity experts increasingly worry that health IoT could become a lethal new terrain for health-hackers [63]. In 2017, the FDA recalled 500,000 pacemakers due to hackability concerns. The agency oversaw the development of a security patch that could address the issue for the already-implanted devices [64]. In 2020, the FDA warned that a widely used telemetry station, a critical-care device communicating patients' vital signs to integrated systems, was vulnerable to attack [65].

Cases of health hacking for ransom warn developers of IoT to consider how bad actors could intersect with IoT systems, rendering them vulnerable to ideological terrorists or criminal opportunists. Designing against possibilities for human error by good-faith actors is necessary but not sufficient to overall protective design.

5.4.7 Confronting Risk: A Cross-Cutting Theme of Analogies

All of these analogies urge explicit attention to risk, not only desired benefit, of technologies under development. What are the arrays of risks associated with development and with use? Who will bear those risks? How are they distributed? Are the potential bearers of risk and benefit the same people, or different? How can risks be reduced? How can they be fairly allocated?

Addressing such thorny questions about risk explicitly and proactively is a fundamental challenge for ethical engineering management and business development of health IoT. Meeting that challenge will require not only frankness about endemic risks, but explicit deliberation of the negotiated tradeoffs that determine how much risk, of what types, will be borne by whom.

5.5 How Can Engineers and Developers Become Leaders Who Bring Trustworthy Products to Market and Promote Trustworthiness of Clinical IoT Ecosystems

As the previous cases demonstrate, trust is a key factor in the ethics of care within the clinical encounter. Trust is also, however, a key factor to consider in the market-based transactions that will drive the adoption of clinical IoT in practical terms. In this section, we consider what you as an engineer can do, what your company can do, and what the engineering community can do to ensure trust and trustworthiness of products and actions. Specifically, we focus on three key activities: (a) talking to people: engaging patients to improve awareness of product use and consumer need; (b) fostering trust within your organization as a business leader; and (c) engaging in policy and standards development.

5.5.1   Talking to People: Engaging Patients to Improve Awareness of Product Use and Consumer Need

Being trustworthy is not only "doing the right thing." It is also being reflective and knowledgeable about how your work impacts the world. Patient engagement has long been a tool for public health and healthcare practitioners as a way of doing just that: understanding stakeholder interests and building trust. There are several methodologies that people use to engage patients and other stakeholders, such as interviews, focus groups, and social media. The fundamental commonality across these methods is that they all involve engaging with people, asking questions, and using the responses to inform future work. In Fig. 5.3, we offer a set of sample questions you might use in engaging users of clinical IoT, and patients in particular. In adapting these questions to your own use, consider why you are asking the questions—is it to gather new information about something you don't already know? Are you asking for feedback on something in development? How will you use the answers to the questions you are asking? To maintain engagement over time, best practices in patient engagement suggest a single interview should be a part of a relationship that gets built over time. After an interview is conducted, summaries may be returned to the participant, as well as some communication about how the input you receive is ultimately applied to product development [66].

---

1) Tell us a little about your experience as a patient and the device you use. How did you come to this decision? (including: who was involved? (doctor, family, other?))

2) What were the deciding factors in deciding to use the device? What were the questions you had before making a decision?

3) How confident do you feel about making the decision to use the device? What makes you feel this way?

4) Do you think you were provided enough information about how your device would be maintained and/or serviced? Were there questions you had that didn't get answered? What went well?

5) What advice would you give other patients about using a device such as yours? Are there people who should NOT use a clinical IoT device such as yours?

6) What do you think engineers need to know about patients to develop trustworthy products? What do patients need to know about engineers / engineering of clinical IoT to trust products?

Fig. 5.3 Questions for engaging patients about their user experience

5.5.2   Fostering Trust Within Your Organization: Your Role as a Business Leader

Medicine has its own culture—its own norms, values, social structures, policies, and economy. Your role as an engineer—as a team member or business leader—will require ambassadorship. While technology designers, developers, and engineers need not obtain medical degrees, a solid comprehension of care processes and goals, care settings, and roles that contribute to the practice and administration of medicine would be desirable. This is in particular for those in a leadership position for the companies that are designing and building technologies intended to be deployed in medical workflows.

Current medical training often does not emphasize effective inter-professional teaching that transcends recent historic silos [67]. That makes it all the more important for leaders in healthcare technology to possess relevant skills. Design leaders must be able to develop and lead interdisciplinary teams that can synthesize technological innovation with medical science. Bridging communities of professional practitioners as well as scientific domains is essential to solve real health problems for patients, families, and communities. Ideally, leaders of teams and companies developing healthcare technology should have a deep understanding of the specific disease burden their product seeks to redress. Understanding the constellation of medical devices, data tools, and pharmaceutical products currently in use or in research for treatment of the target disease would also be desirable. So too would a broad view of how their technology in development fits within a broad context of prevention, diagnosis, treatment, symptom-reduction, and whole-patient care.

An understanding of healthcare organization and financing is also a desirable, if not requisite, asset. Ideal healthcare technology leaders are effectively interacting with policy-makers as technical resources and subject matter experts within the health system. They should understand the policy drivers that determine the provision of medical resources. They should also understand the ecosystem of academic medicine, industry, and policy-makers that determine the trajectory and future for the practice of medicine, as well as where their design solutions complement emerging practice. Healthcare technology leaders must hone a diverse set of skills and engage patients and healthcare professionals since both are equally important in the development and dissemination of clinical IoT.

Leadership is also about understanding and shaping the future. Today's most respected leaders in healthcare technology are actively engaged in the learning about ethics, and are working toward the implementation of ethics into practices, standards, and operations. This includes institutionally tying continuous ethical deliberation to board of directors-level governance within their organizations. The impetus is more than a moral imperative; it is also a practical eye for real risks and liabilities, and an understanding for where international policy priorities will settle.

Trustworthiness, then, is integral to corporate culture and needs to be cultivated. D.J. Patil, who served as President Barack Obama's chief data ethics officer, urges organizations to be able to answer the question, "How does this organization build trustworthiness?" Equally, he urges engineers to ask this question of potential employers, and, if they don't have any answer, choose not to work there.

5.5.3   Engaging in Policy and Standards Development

Regulations are one mechanism for protecting consumers and ensuring safety and trust in clinical applications. In the USA, the FDA as an agency was born from a chaotic marketplace where effective medications were sold while many peddled snake oil and labeled products as miracle cures. At best, snake oils and miracle cures did no harm, at worst, they caused disease or death. Similarly, some clinical IoT applications and devices can be highly effective at reducing medical errors and improving health outcomes, while others offer little marginal benefit or can be actively harmful to patients. Regulatory oversight for clinical IoT is uncertain. The role of the FDA, for example, is limited to diagnostic tools such as Software as a Medical Device (SaMD). Other federal agencies with potential jurisdiction over aspects of clinical IoT include the Federal Trade Commission, a consumer protection agency, that tracks and reports large-scale data breaches, and the Centers for Medicare and Medicaid Services (CMS) that decides whether clinical IoT devices are covered by insurance. The Office of the National Coordinator (ONC) for Health Information Technology, part of the Department of Health and Human Services, is a key agency incentivizing and setting a national health IT agenda, including issuing and enforcing rules for practices such as information blocking, as required by law. There can be a lack of clarity around who is responsible for regulating clinical IoT partly because of the complex nature of clinical IoT development and implementation, and also because the technology for clinical IoT and related technologies are far outpacing the capacity for regulatory regimes to regulate them.

Registries such as the Manufacturer and User Facility Device Experience (MAUDE) database and the National Evaluation System for Health Technology (NEST) program are part of the assessment of the FDA's post-market surveillance for the safety of medical devices. Such programs can be greatly enhanced when used in conjunction with corporate registries that monitor their own products, though this strategy also opens questions of conflicts of interest. Can corporations fully meet their responsibility to account for the harm of their products when their business incentive is to solely promote the benefits of their products? How should such partnerships be regulated?

Beyond regulation, another mechanism available to ensure trust in clinical IoT is standards. Standards are key infrastructure that can be used to "hardwire" trust into clinical IoT. They are not necessarily legislated or part of formal governmental rule-making, but are rather part of professional norms, and are negotiated among stakeholders in the clinical IoT infrastructure uniting multiple "communities of practice" that are part of the IoT ecosystem. As a process of norming, standards create path dependence as organizations and individuals come to rely on an infrastructure instantiated by standards and adapt [68]. Efforts such as the IEEE/UL P2933 Standard for Clinical Internet of Things (IoT) Data and Device Interoperability with TIPPSS (Trust, Identity, Privacy, Protection, Safety, and Security) working group, and others, will generate a set of recommendations for the clinical IoT field that would ensure trust is an integral part of technical and process standards for clinical IoT development and use.

Policy-making is a public process. For engineers and developers, being engaged in policy-making, or at least being aware of rules and regulations, will help you communicate with and ask questions of legal teams. Engagement with policy also has real and impactful meaning on the parameters for the development of high-quality and trustworthy clinical IoT. We propose here two ways for you to be involved in policy that impacts your work, regardless of where you are in your career and your leadership role within your organization. First, become involved in professional organizations that engage in the policy process. Organizations such as IEEE engage the engineering and policy communities directly. Professional organizations outside of the typical purview of engineers that address issues in healthcare ethics such as the American Public Health Association (APHA) and the American Society of Bioethics and Humanities (ASBH) are increasingly engaged in assessing the policy and ethics of technologies such as clinical IoT. These organizations often help provide the expertise that informs policy-making nationally and internationally.

Second, know your federal agencies: The Food and Drug Administration (FDA), Federal Trade Commission (FTC), Office of the National Coordinator for Health IT (ONC), Centers for Medicare and Medicaid Services (CMS), and others are all likely to have an impact on the marketplace for clinical IoT. When making new policies, these agencies will often issue calls for public input. The Twenty-First Century Cures Act, for example, went through a public comment period that generated nearly 500 responses when considering policy for information blocking and data sharing that generated considerable dialog in the media and in professional communities. This input was critical in shaping the final rule.

Policy can be the formal outcome of a regulatory process, part of professional consensus making, or the operating procedures of your organization. Each of these is an implicit reflection of the values of the people involved in decision-making, be they a specific community, public, or elite [69]. Whether that action is to do nothing, with consumers at the whim of caveat emptor, or to create legal accountability for safety and efficacy, speaks volumes about how you value public good and social responsibility. Knowing your own personal values will help you shape opinions and articulate your participation in the policy-making process that impacts your work.

5.6   Conclusion

Currently, mistrust is high and growing—fast-paced health IT has made great advances, but has also contributed to physician burnout and is running against a current in which trust in medicine is declining [70, 71, 72]. Furthermore, the non-health interests of the technology sector often lie in direct conflict with the needs of patients. The unintended consequences of mistakes in engineering and development can have spillover effects on trust throughout the ecosystem. Engineers like you can work to redress and build trustworthiness. Doing so can build confidence in your profession and its partnership with healthcare. Ensuring trustworthiness can also reduce the need for complex regulation and lead to greater professional autonomy. In this chapter, we outlined several frameworks for you to think about what trust means, how it applies to your work, how ethics plays a role in the scope and impact of your work, and a few ways to engage the wider ecosystem within which engineers operate to bring clinical IoT to market. Ultimately, we encourage you in this chapter to ask yourself as an engineer two self-reflective questions: How do I affect the world? How does the world affect me?

References

1. Fernández-Caramés TM, Froiz-Míguez I, Blanco-Novoa O, Fraga-Lamas P. Enabling the internet of mobile crowdsourcing health things: A mobile fog computing, blockchain and IoT based continuous glucose monitoring system for diabetes mellitus research and care. *Sensors.* 2019;*19*(15):3319. doi: https://doi.org/10.3390/s19153319
2. Gowrishankar S, Prachita M, Prakash A. IoT based heart attack detection, heart rate and temperature monitor. Int. J. Comput. Appl. 2017;*170*(5): 26–30.
3. Serdaroglu K, Uslu G, Baydere S. Medication intake adherence with real time activity recognition on IoT. In: 2015 IEEE 11th International Conference on Wireless and Mobile Computing, Networking and Communications (WiMob), Abu Dhabi. 2015; 230-237. doi: https://doi.org/10.1109/WiMOB.2015.7347966.
4. Bates DW, Landman A, Levine DM. Health apps and health policy: what is needed? *JAMA.* 2018; 320:1975–1976
5. Lagan S, Sandler L, Torous J. Evaluating evaluation frameworks: a scoping review of frameworks for assessing health apps. BMJ open. 2021 Mar 1;11(3):e047001.
6. Medtronic recalls MiniMed insulin pumps for incorrect insulin dosing [Internet]. U.S. Food and Drug Administration. 2020 Feb 12 [cited 2021 July 20]. Available from https://www.fda.gov/medical-devices/medical-device-recalls/medtronic-recalls-minimed-insulin-pumps-incorrect-insulin-dosing
7. Burke LE, Ma J, Azar KM, Bennett GG, Peterson ED, Zheng Y et al. Current science on consumer use of mobile health for cardiovascular disease prevention: a scientific statement from the American Heart Association. Circulation. 2015 Sep 22;132(12):1157-213. https://doi.org/10.1161/CIR.0000000000000232
8. Giddens A. The Consequences of Modernity. 1st ed. John Wiley & Sons; 2013
9. Luhmann N. Familiarity, confidence, trust: problems and alternatives. In: D. Gambetto (Ed.) [Internet]. Trust: Making and Breaking Cooperative Relations (Electronic edition), University of Oxford. 2000; 94-107. Available from http://citeseerx.ist.psu.edu/viewdoc/download?doi=10.1.1.23.8075&rep=rep1&type=pdf

10. Mechanic D. The functions and limitations of trust in the provision of medical care. J. Health Polit. Policy Law. 1998; 23 (4): 661e686. https://doi.org/10.1215/03616878-23-4-661.

11. Mechanic D, Meyer S. Concepts of trust among patients with serious illness. Soc. Sci. Med. 2000; 51 (5):657e668. https://doi.org/10.1016/S0277-9536(00)00014-9

12. Maxwell K, Streetly A, Bevan D. Experiences of hospital care and treatment seeking for pain from sickle cell disease: qualitative study. Br. Med. J. 1999;318(7198):1585e1590. https://doi.org/10.1136/bmj.318.7198.1585.

13. Rogers WA. Is there a moral duty for doctors to trust patients? J. Med. Ethics. 2002;28 (2):77e80. https://doi.org/10.1136/jme.28.2.77.

14. Thom DH, Wong ST, Guzman D, Wu A, Penko J, Miaskowski C, et al. Physician trust in the patient: development and validation of a new measure. Ann. Fam. Med. 2011 Mar; 9 (2): 148–154. doi: https://doi.org/10.1370/afm.1224

15. Hall MA, Camacho F, Dugan E, Balkrishnan R. Trust in the medical profession: conceptual and measurement issues. Health Serv Res. 2002 Oct;37(5):1419-39.

16. U.S. Department of Health & Human Services - Office for Civil Rights. Accessed April 6, 2022. https://ocrportal.hhs.gov/ocr/breach/breach_report.jsf

17. Richardson JE, Middleton B, Platt JE, Blumenfeld BH. Building and maintaining trust in clinical decision support: Recommendations from the patient centered CDC learning network. 2020 Apr; 4(2):e10208. https://doi.org/10.1002/lrh2.10208

18. IEEE advancing technology for humanity, code of ethics [Internet]. IEEE. 2020 [cited 2021 August 16]. Available from https://www.ieee.org/about/corporate/governance/p7-8.html.

19. NSPE Codes of practice for engineers [Internet]. National Society of Professional Engineers. 2019 [cited 2021, July 15]. Available from https://www.nspe.org/resources/ethics/code-ethics.

20. National Academy of Engineering Center for Engineering Ethics and Society (CEES) [Internet]. 2020 [cited 2021 January 5]. Available from https://www.nae.edu/26187/CEES.

21. Association of Practical and Professional Ethics (APPE) [Internet]. [Cited 2021, January 5]. Available from https://www.appe-ethics.org

22. A Framework for ethical decision-making [Internet]. Santa Clara University Markulla Center for Applied Ethics. 2015 [updated 2020, cited 2021, January 10]. Available from https://www.scu.edu/ethics/ethics-resources/ethical-decision-making/a-framework for-ethical-decision-making/.

23. Wise G, Keat W, Balmer R, Kosky P. Systematic approach to ethical decision making using matrices. In: 2008 38th Annual Frontiers in Education Conference [Internet]. IEEE. 2008 November [cited 2021 January 10]. Available from https://doi.org/10.1109/FIE.2008.4720292.

24. Ward A. Lean design in healthcare: a journey to improve quality and process of care. New York: Routledge Taylor and Francis Group; 2019.

25. Friedman M. The business of business is to increase profits. New York Times. 1970 Sept 13:SM7.

26. Laplume AO, Sonpar K, List RA. Stakeholder theory: reviewing a theory that moves us. J Manage. 2008; 34(6):1152-1189. https://doi.org/10.1177/0149206308324322

27. Werhane PH. Business ethics, stakeholder theory, and the ethics of healthcare organizations. Camb Q Healthc Ethics; 2000 Spring; 9 (2):169-181. doi: https://doi.org/10.1017/s0963180100902044

28. Beauchamp T, Childress JF. Principles of biomedical ethics. 8th ed. Oxford University Press; 2019.

29. Elwyn G, Frosch D, Thomson R et al. Shared decision making: a model for clinical practice. J Gen Intern Med. 2012; 27(10):1361-7. https://doi.org/10.1007/s11606-012-2077-6

30. The U.S. public health service syphilis study at Tuskegee [Internet]. U.S. Center for Disease Control. 2021 April 22 [cited 2021 July 20]. Available from https://www.cdc.gov/tuskegee/timeline.htm

31. Krugman S. The Willowbrook hepatitis studies revisited: ethical aspects. Rev Infect Dis. 1986; 8(1):157-62. https://doi.org/10.1093/clinids/8.1.157.

32. The Belmont report: Ethical principles and guidelines for the protection of human subjects of research [Internet]. Bethesda, Md. National Commission for the Protection of Human Subjects

of Biomedical and Behavioral Research. Department of Health, Education and Welfare. 1979, April [cited 2021 July 15]. Available from https://www.hhs.gov/ohrp/regulations-and-policy/belmont-report/read-the-belmont-report/index.html

33. Public health code of ethics [Internet]. American Public Health Association. 2019[cited 2021 Jan]. Available from https://www.apha.org/-/media/files/pdf/membergroups/ethics/code_of_ethics

34. Wilkinson M, Dumontier M, Aalbersberg I, et al. The FAIR guiding principles for scientific data management and stewardship. Sci Data. 2016; 3:160018. https://doi.org/10.1038/sdata.2016.18

35. Lin D, Crabtree J, Dillo I, et al. The TRUST principles for digital repositories. Sci Data. 2020; 7:144. https://doi.org/10.1038/s41597-020-0486-7

36. Care principles for indigenous data governance [Internet]. Global Indigenous Data Alliance, 2019 [cited 2021 Jan]. Available from https://www.gida-global.org/care

37. U.S. Congress House Committee on Transportation and Infrastructure, Final committee report: The design, development, and certification of the Boeing 737 Max [Internet]; 2020 Sept. Available from https://transportation.house.gov/imo/media/doc/2020.09.15%20FINAL%20737%20MAX%20Report%20for%20Public%20Release.pdf

38. Herkert J, Borenstein J, Miller K. The Boeing 737 MAX: Lessons for engineering ethics. Sci Eng Ethics. 2020; 26(6):2957-2974. https://doi.org/10.1007/s11948-020-00252-y

39. Sengupta J, Storey K, Casey S, et al. Outcomes before and after the recall of a heart failure pacemaker. JAMA Intern Med. *2020;180(2):198–205*. https://doi.org/10.1001/jamainternmed.2019.5171

40. What to do if your cardiac device is recalled [Internet]. University of Michigan Health System. 2020 [cited 2021 Jan 18]. Available from https://www.uofmhealth.org/health-library/abk4204.

41. Heart device and pacemaker recalls: what you need to know [Internet]. Cleveland Clinic. 2018 [cited 2021, June 10]. Available from https://health.clevelandclinic.org/heart-device-and-pacemaker-recalls-what-you-need-to-know/

42. Thomson JJ. Killing, letting die, and the trolley problem. The Monist. 1976; 59(2):204-217.

43. Bonnefon JF, Shariff A, Rahwan I. The social dilemma of autonomous vehicles. Science. 2016;352(6293):1573-6. https://doi.org/10.1126/science.aaf2654.

44. Lin P. Robot cars and fake ethical dilemmas. Forbes [Internet]. 2017 April 3 [cited 2021 July 18]. Available from https://www.forbes.com/sites/patricklin/2017/04/03/robot-cars-and-fake-ethical-dilemmas/?sh=2e51d99213a2

45. The moral machine [Internet]. Massachusetts Institute of Technology (MIT). 2016 [cited 2021 June 10]. Available from https://www.moralmachine.net/

46. Maxmen A. Self-driving car dilemmas reveal that moral choices are not universal. Nature. 2018 Oct 24.469-470. https://doi.org/10.1038/d41586-018-07135-0

47. Lester C. A study on driverless car ethics offers a troubling look into our values. New Yorker. 2019 Jan 24[cited 2021 Jan 24]. Available from https://www.newyorker.com/science/elements/a-study-on-driverless-car-ethics-offers-a-troubling-look-into-our-values

48. SUPPORT Study Group of the Eunice Kennedy Shriver NICHD Neonatal Research Network. Target ranges of oxygenation saturation in extremely pre-term infants. N Engl J Med 2010; 362:1959-1969. https://doi.org/10.1056/NEJMoa0911781.

49. U.S. National Library of Medicine. Surfactant positive airway pressure and pulse Oximetry trial (SUPPORT) [Internet]. 2020 [cited 2021 Aug 10]. Available from https://clinicaltrials.gov/ct2/show/NCT00233324

50. The Office for Human Research Protections' evaluation of the Surfactant, Positive Pressure, and Oxygenation Randomized Trial [Internet]. U.S. Department of Health and Human Services, Office of Inspector General. 2014 Report (OEI-01-14-00560). 2014 Sep 15 [cited 2021 Jun 15]. Available from https://oig.hhs.gov/oei/reports/oei-01-14-00560.asp

51. Hudson KL, Guttmacher AE, Collins FS. In support of SUPPORT: The View from the NIH. N Engl J Med. 2013; 368:2349-2351. https://doi.org/10.1056/NEJMp1306986.

52. Magnus D, Caplan AL. Risk, consent, and support. N Engl J Med. 2013; 368:1864-1865. https://doi.org/10.1056/NEJMp1305086.

53. Merz JF, King N. Rapid response to U.S. Study criticized for experimentation on premature infants. BMJ. 2013; 347:f4198. https://doi.org/10.1136/bmj.f4198
54. Shepherd L. The SUPPORT study and the standard of care [Internet]. Hastings Center Bioethics Forum. 2013; May 17 [cited 2021 August 14]. Available from http://www.thehastingscenter.org/Bioethicsforum/Post.aspx?id=6358&blogid=140.
55. Shermer M. Ethical issues in deep brain simulation. Front. Integr. Neurosci. 2011 May 9; 5:17. https://doi.org/10.3389/fnint.2011.00017
56. Harmon A. Indian tribe wins right to limit research on its DNA [Internet]. New York Times. 2010 Apr 21 [cited 2021 June 5]. Available from https://www.nytimes.com/2010/04/22/us/22dna.html
57. Advocacy-led research [Internet]. Genetic Alliance. [cited 2020 Dec 10]. Available from http://www.geneticalliance.org/programs/advocacy-led-research.
58. Terry S, Horn E, Scott J. Genetic Alliance Registry and Biobank: a novel disease-advocacy driven research solution. Per Med. 2011; 8(2). https://doi.org/10.2217/pme.11.1.
59. Obermeyer Z, Powers B, Vogeli C, Mullainathan S. Dissecting racial bias in an algorithm used to manage the health of populations. Science. 2019; 366(6464):447-453. https://doi.org/10.1126/science.aax2342.
60. Ledford H. Millions of black people affected by racial bias in health-care algorithms. Nature 2017 Oct; 574: 608-609.
61. Ralston W. The untold story of a cyberattack, a hospital, and a dying woman [Internet]. Wired. 2020 Nov 11[cited 2021 Dec 10]. Available from https://www.wired.co.uk/article/ransomware-hospital-death-germany.
62. Volz D, McMillan R. Hackers hit hospitals in disruptive ransomware attack [Internet]. Wall Street Journal. 2020 Nov 11 [cited 2021 Jul 13]. Available from https://www.wsj.com/articles/hackers-hit-hospitals-in-disruptive-ransomware-attack-11603992735.
63. Boudko S, Abie H. Adaptive cybersecurity framework for healthcare internet of things. In: *2009 13th International Symposium on Medical Information and Communication Technology (ISMICT) [Internet]* 2019 [cited 2021 June 10]. pp. 1-6. https://doi.org/10.1109/ISMICT.2019.8743905.
64. Hern A. Hacking risk leads to recall of 500,000 pacemakers due to patient death fears [Internet]. The Guardian. 2017 Aug 31 [cited 2021 Jul 18]. Available from https://www.theguardian.com/technology/2017/aug/31/hacking-risk-recall-pacemakers-patient-death-fears-fda-firmware-update.
65. Stephenson J. FDA warns that some GE healthcare telemetry servers, health information stations are vulnerable to cyberattack. JAMA Health Forum. 2020;1(2): e200161. https://doi.org/10.1001/jamahealthforum.2020.0161.
66. Bombard Y, Baker GR, Orlando E, Fancott C, Bhatia P, Casalino S, et al. Engaging patients to improve quality of care: a systematic review. Implement Sci. 2018 Jul 26;13(1):98. doi: https://doi.org/10.1186/s13012-018-0784-z.
67. Salari S, Klapman S, Fry B, Hamel S. Interprofessional education: in silo, ineffective. Med. Sci. Educ. 2017 Dec;27(4):831-3.
68. Edwards PN, Jackson SJ, Bowker GC, Knobel CP. Understanding infrastructure: Dynamics, tensions, and design. Report of a workshop on "History & Theory of Infrastructure: Lessons for New Scientific Cyberinfrastructures" [internet]. 2007 Jan. [cited 2021, July 18]. Available from. https://deepblue.lib.umich.edu/bitstream/handle/2027.42/49353/UnderstandingInfrastr?sequence=3
69. Buse K, Mays N, Walt G. Making health policy. McGraw-hill education (UK); 2012 May 1
70. Patel RS, Bachu R, Adikey A, Malik M, Shah M. Factors related to physician burnout and its consequences: a review. Behavioral sciences. 2018 Nov;8(11).98.
71. Baker DW. Trust in Health Care in the Time of COVID-19. JAMA. 2020 Dec 15;324(23):2373-5.
72. Meyer SB, Ward PR. Differentiating between trust and dependence of patients with coronary heart disease: furthering the sociology of trust. Health Risk Soc. 2013;15 (3):279e293. https://doi.org/10.1080/13698575.2013.776017

Chapter 6
The Hospital of the Future and Security: An Arranged Marriage

Alexis Diamond and Joanna Lyn Grama

Contents

Throughout history, many societies have practiced arranged marriages, and many still do today. Literature notes that arranged marriages are not forced, where the bride and groom have no say in the choice of the marital partner. Rather, arranged marriages are careful and conscientious negotiations between families to form alliances for mutual benefit. (Rubrio, Gabriella. "How Love Conquered Marriage: Theory and Evidence on the Disappearance of Arranged Marriages." University of California, Merced. 2014.) This chapter uses the notion of careful and conscientious negotiations and mutually beneficial alliances as a metaphor for the relationship that must be developed between the Hospital of the Future and the practice of information security.

A. Diamond · J. L. Grama (✉)
Vantage Technology Consulting Group, El Segundo, CA, USA
e-mail: Alexis.Diamond@VantageTCG.com; Joanna.Grama@VantageTCG.com

© Springer Nature Switzerland AG 2022
F. D. Hudson (eds.), *Women Securing the Future with TIPPSS for Connected Healthcare*, Women in Engineering and Science,
https://doi.org/10.1007/978-3-030-93592-4_6

6.1 Introduction

The future often spawns ideas of far off times, when boundaries and truths have evolved beyond today's comprehension. Every industry hopes to embrace the future as new concepts, products, and general thinking emerge in the world's ever-changing environment. The healthcare industry faces arguably the most obstruction in adapting to new ideas due to governmental regulations, patient risks, high construction costs, low margins, etc. To reduce the risk of being outdated, healthcare facilities concentrate on building the *Hospital of the Future* (HotF) with every capital and construction project. However, the HotF is not a programmable concept or an end-state; it is a notion of functionality. The program of the HotF transforms depending on historical time and environment because the HotF comes from a desire to provide the highest quality of care.

Yet, an inherent conflict exists when thinking about the promise of the HotF and how to protect the vast amounts of patient data that will be created, used, transmitted, and stored in technologies designed to optimize processes, workflow, and information. Internet of Things (IoT) devices figure prominently into discussions about the HotF. The myriad of connected things (sensors, tags, monitors, cameras, devices, etc.), where each device may contain multiple connected elements that talk to other devices in the HotF ecosystem, presents a tremendous opportunity to improve the quality of care. Consider, for example:

- A comprehensive Electronic Health Record (EHR) that moves beyond the point-in-time digital charting represented by an Electronic Medical Record (EMR).[1]
- Observation/non-contact sensors in each patient room can monitor the patient's temperature, breathing rate, and other vital signs, reducing physical connections (e.g., wires and other such invasive monitors) to the patient. For example, these types of sensors could detect a patient is sleeping and alert clinical or cleaning staff not to enter the patient room.[2]
- Incorporating video analysis, algorithms can monitor a patient's facial cues and movements to analyze pain levels.
- Infrared image depth sensors can be used as a bed-monitoring system that detects a patient exiting a bed or falling.
- Tracking systems can be used to monitor the real-time location of patients, clinical staff, visitors, medications, specimens, and supplies across the hospital campus.[3]

---

[1] An EMR is best understood as the digital version of a patient's chart when they are receiving care from a single healthcare provider. An EHR is a patient's records from multiple encounters and potentially multiple care providers. An EHR is understood to provide a holistic view of a patient's comprehensive health.

[2] Sleep is an important part of the healing process.

[3] These real-time location systems (RTLS) can be either passive or active systems that use Wi-Fi, Bluetooth, RFID, Ultrasound, Infrared, and/or GPS technologies to track and monitor things. Passive systems include non-powered tags that need to be scanned for information, while active

- In-room one-way camera systems[4] can be used to monitor psychiatric patients, critical care patients, patients prone to seizures or receiving treatment for seizures, or other patients whose condition and treatment require constant monitoring.
- In-room video conferencing systems can be used to enhance patient/provider, patient/family, and care team communications, conversations, and interactions. The use of cameras and video conferencing within healthcare facilities has expanded universally, and its use during the 2020 coronavirus global pandemic is well documented.

And, of course, the HotF makes quick use of the data generated from all of these devices—analyzing it and transmitting it to an operational command center and the patient's EHR in real-time or near real-time for use by the patient care team. The influx of data and connected devices presents the information security technologist with the thorniest of issues—how to protect some of the most sensitive personal information there is while not hindering or obstructing patient care or healthcare processes and workflow. Information security concepts, that is, protecting the confidentiality, availability, and integrity of information used with the HotF, cannot be considered an add-on. Instead, they must be considered upfront in the design of the HotF, with the care and review of a deliberately arranged marriage.

This chapter introduces IoT use cases for the HotF, outlines some of the information security and privacy concerns that technologists have about IoT use in the HotF, introduces the information security and privacy lexicon that most healthcare providers and healthcare IoT visionaries should be familiar with, and defines a path forward to ensure a successful long-term relationship between healthcare IoT and information security and privacy in the HotF.

6.2   The HotF: Designed to Improve Quality of Care

A hospital's quality of care is founded on the empowerment and safety of patients and staff. Patients' empowerment derives from their ability to understand and participate in their care. Meanwhile, healthcare staff's empowerment expands from their ability to deliver patient care effectively. However, the ability to deliver and understand a patient's care relies significantly on an optimal and transparent flow of information. Since the EHR began to standardize nearly two decades ago,

---

systems include powered tags that actively report locations to the system. Tracking tags for active systems are expensive and used to track patients, staff, and live critical equipment, while tracking tags for passive systems are comparatively inexpensive and can be used on supplies, medications, specimens, and materials.

[4] Some of these camera systems might be configured in a "video sitter" manner. Video sitter refers to a non-recording patient facing-camera streaming to a display monitored by a nurse that only watches approximately 16 beds in 2-hour shifts.

technology has been the cornerstone of this information flow. The transparency of this flow and analysis of the information has empowered patients and staff's safety and satisfaction while allowing for optimization and efficiency.

As technology continuously advances, so too the HotF concept evolves. While previously information security has been an afterthought to technology selection, the information generated, used, stored, and transferred has become too monumental and too critical to a facility's success to be an afterthought. Fundamentally, the HotF comes to fruition and matures through a constant drive towards providing the highest quality care. To do this, the HotF needs to prioritize unprecedented transparency (access to information and efficiency of information security), participation from patients and staff (in both patient care and information security), and the safety of patients and staff (physically and virtually).

As we think about the HotF and how to use IoT technologies within it, focusing on the quality of care forces the questions to change from *what is the technology?* to *what does an optimized process or flow look like, and how does technology enable this functionality?*

Connected Healthcare Devices

The use of IoT devices in healthcare is not new, but its use is growing [1]. Once the stuff of science fiction, today's healthcare IoT devices include:

- Blood glucose monitors that can measure and wirelessly transmit the patient's glucose levels to the healthcare provider's smart device allowing the provider to make changes to the patient's treatment plan.
- Cardiac pacemakers that monitor a patient's vital signs and can adjust the device settings, either automatically or with provider intervention, according to the patient's activity level.
- Smart orthopedic braces that can sense and measure the progress that a patient is making after joint replacement surgeries and allow a physical therapist to modify rehabilitation exercises to improve mobility.
- Ingestible medical devices (aka the electronic pill) that are swallowed by the patient and contain wireless imaging sensors that can take pictures of the patient's gastrointestinal (GI) tract for diagnostic purposes.
- Bionic implants and prosthetic limbs that can be monitored and adjusted to restore and improve functionality and ability [2].

Perhaps more than any other industry, the healthcare industry leans on the usefulness of storytelling, through use cases, to discuss scenarios and define priorities with patients and staff. The next sections set out use cases for the HotF and IoT technologies.

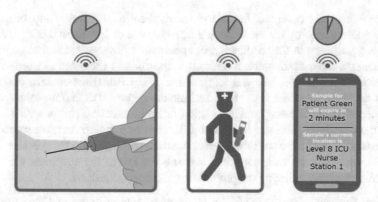

Fig. 6.1 Chain of Custody Graphic. (Courtesy of Vantage Technology Consulting Group)

6.2.1   Automation to Improve Chain of Custody

A common theme of HotF use cases is targeting the reduction or elimination of staff members' low-value tasks. These tasks require lengthy, typically repetitive, and possibly tedious manual input or effort to accomplish. If a workflow or process holds repetitive low-value tasks, a solution may be in a use case for automation. In addition to eliminating time spent on low-value tasks, automation creates additional benefits in coupling time-monitored tasks with technology's ability to log activity.

Critical to the automation use case is the notion of Chain of Custody, as depicted in Fig. 6.1. In the healthcare context, the chain of custody refers to the continuous log of staff members that have handled a medical item such as medication, a specimen, or a particular supply. It holds an enormous weight in any facility due to the laws and guidelines outlining time, personnel, and procedural requirements related to providing patient care. Any possible violation of these requirements can be grounds for litigation. Automation use cases involving medications and specimens, or supplies, hold particular significance for improving the chain of custody.

Specimen and Medications HotF lab and pharmacy departments are particularly ripe environments for time-monitored automation. Laboratory and pharmaceutical workflows embody the movement of small items through transportation and authentication processes. In this use case, the medication or specimen would be passively tracked throughout its journey through a passive Real Time Location System (RTLS). As the appropriate department handles the medication or specimen, the building's systems[5] passively track the item's location, staff member interaction, and any other pertinent information (such as room temperature) without any manual input.

---

[5] This type of tracking could also happen between buildings or clinical locations.

The system also compares the flow of the medication or specimen to the expected flow, as determined by the medication's intended use or specimen's intended test. If there is a variation in the medication or specimen's flow, outside of an appropriate contingency, the system alerts a relevant authority and escalates as needed. Some specimens, for example, have a strict time-sensitivity from time of extraction to time of testing. If the specimen is not tested within the approved time frame, the specimen must be redrawn, reducing patient satisfaction and increasing staff workload. In this case, the tracking of the specimen and affiliation of the staff member would allow the system to inform the staff member of the time remaining on the specimen's time frame throughout the transportation, alerting the lab of the specimen's estimated time of arrival and reducing the probability of a needed redraw.

Medical Supplies This same RTLS technology, which tracks and logs the movement of specimens and medication, can help manage supplies and materials. Typically supplies are tracked manually, which relies on memory and regular scheduling to maintain Periodic Automatic Replenishment (PAR) levels for the room or unit. With a passive RTLS, the technology can manage par levels for each storage location, including the central storage, allowing the technology to create purchase orders as supplies are needed automatically. The 2020 global coronavirus pandemic has highlighted a need to more closely monitor the levels of general supplies such as gloves and masks due to the unusual increase in demand and increase of theft of these supplies [3].

6.2.2 Visualization to Alleviate Information Overload

Information overload and alarm fatigue is a massive failure of technology in hospitals today. Clinical staff members are bombarded with notifications of changes in each of their patient's states throughout their shift. Staff can miss important pieces of information that get drowned out in the noise of simple updates. All of the information is important, so the use cases for the HotF utilize multiple ways of conveying information to staff to optimize information flow and reduce alarm fatigue. Through visually implied triage and streamlined dashboards, clinical staff can more easily understand the urgent or necessary information at the right time instead of trying to know all of the information all of the time.

Door Overlays This use case is founded in the current use of nurse call dome lights above patient rooms/beds. The lights typically show a combination of one to four solid or blinking colors to indicate codes, doctor-in-room, and other basic room status notifications. In this case, a department head wanted to "look down a hallway and see what room I need to be in" or to see the status of the department.

This use case explores the integration of an additional simple color scheme through visual door frame overlays to indicate each room's patient care status. For example, the patient rooms with patients meant to be discharged that day may have a green overlay, while patients that have just received test results have an orange

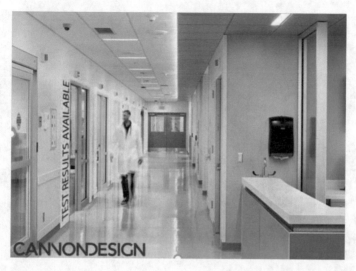

Fig. 6.2   Door Overlay Graphic. (Courtesy of Vantage Technology Consulting Group and Cannon Design)

overlay (Fig. 6.2). These overlays would simplify the clinical staffs' workflow and reduce the number of notifications sent to their mobile devices.

Patient Room Interfaces   Within a patient room today, several clinical screens and interfaces show the clinical staff the patient's medical status, acquired from all the sensors built into the patient room. Before or upon entering a patient room, care team staff typically need to hunt for pertinent information through a charting computer and surrounding clinical monitors before being able to fully examine the patient.

A use case for the HotF integrates all of the needed information into one interface near the patient's head, allowing staff to look at or near the patient as much as possible while still visualizing all necessary information to facilitate care (Fig. 6.3).

The amount of information on each patient stretches from vital monitoring and physiological patterns, through medications and pain levels, to a previous night's sleep assessment. Several sensors capture this information and can transmit it to the patient room interface. As technology understands clinical staff preferences and a patient's care plan, the information presented on the patient interface can be streamlined to allow clinical staff to immediately know the patient's vital signs and any other information particular to that patient. This quick view reduces clinical staff frustration in hunting for the most pertinent information across multiple sources and enhances staff focus.

The visibility of patient vital information is equally helpful outside of the room. Some facilities are moving towards interactive real-time signage outside of the patient's room. Critical information such as fall-risk notifications, allergy warnings, and isolation restrictions are displayed prominently and clearly outside of the room to inform clinical staff of essential care instructions.

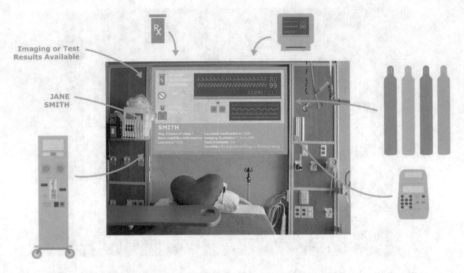

Fig. 6.3 Patient Interface Graphic. (Courtesy of Vantage Technology Consulting Group)

Today, this type of information is manually placed on a patient's room signage either as an integrated physical sliding mechanism or through velcro and tape. The manual placement does not guarantee the information is correct or updated promptly for an individual patient. Automated digital signage relieves nurses of the low-value manual task of changing and updating signs. In the HotF, nurses and physicians alike will use these interfaces to request basic room services, share information, and review important patient care information.

6.2.3 Care Team Interface to Reduce Provider Burnout

The healthcare huddle is a common sight at hospitals. They are daily meetings between care teams to discuss patients and their care plan and review insights gleaned since the last huddle. These huddles can happen at the start of a shift or before a care team goes into a patient's room. Depending on the number of rooms being evaluated, huddles grow very large, especially in teaching hospitals. The huddle can clog a hospital hallway with a collection of workstations on wheels and staff looking for flat surfaces to take notes on paper or their individual electronic devices.

The HotF supports mobile collaboration through a use case involving clinical mobility and effortless charting, embracing the mobility of the care team and the need for interdisciplinary huddles. A mobile device is assigned to each care team member. This device allows the care team member to document or evaluate any necessary action or assessment for each patient through a Care Team interface for care team members' visibility and collaboration. The device simplifies the note-taking, medication delivery, assessments, or specimen retrieval actions into passive actions for the staff member. Instead of sitting at a charting computer, hours after-the-fact, to recount events, the device and building take an educated guess, with minimal manual input through voice transactions, simple location-based logic, or proximity, at what likely happened with each patient encounter, then requests confirmation from the clinical staff at a comfortable and appropriate time for the staff member. This "One-Click" charting model allows the staff member to focus on patient care instead of documentation or charting, empowering the clinical staff and reducing burnout.

Since the outbreak of the coronavirus, the mobile empowerment of clinical staff has become even more vital to increase collaboration, reduce travel across hospital campuses and buildings, and decrease hallway congestion. Offices have moved from feet to miles from the patient, forcing care team members to communicate virtually. As interdisciplinary processes have brought new insights and perspectives care teams have begun to rely on, the pandemic has accelerated the need for a next-generation Care Team interface to increase collaboration. In the HotF, interdisciplinary care teams interact with the Care Team interface as they would with their care team collaborators. They can inquire and report nuanced information from the Hospital's interface effortlessly, enabling swift progression in planning and developing patient care plans.

As the virtual move to collaboration empowers the clinical staff collaboration, a side effect becomes patient empowerment. The regular update and interaction with the virtual care plan allow the ability to share real-time considerations with the patient. As a patient's care plan changes with each step of a patient's treatment, a patient's care plan is regularly changing. Traditionally, this places a significant burden on the care team to keep the patient and patient's family up to date with each change. By moving the patient's care plan from discussions in a hallway to documented private and privileged discussions within the care team's interface, the system can keep both the provider and patient up to date with any perceived changes.

For example, one of the most common questions the physicians regularly answer regards the estimated discharge time frame. The transparency of this time frame has an enormous impact on patient satisfaction, especially if there are contingencies. Informing the patient of a prerequisite checklist or outstanding tasks for discharge via a Patient Interface, through data entered by a provider in the Care Team Interface, allows the patient to understand the terms of discharge and gives them goals and targets in their treatment.

6.2.4   Patient Interface to Promote Transparency and Control

In the HotF, this information comes to the patient through the Patient Portal or Patient Interface. The interface formalizes the checklists, care plan, treatments, imaging and testing appointments, and estimated physician and clinical appointments into a Patient Care Schedule. The schedule is full of expectations and assumptions updated in real time because the interface must inform the patient, not only of prerequisites for discharge[6] but all insights and aspects of their care. The patient would be aware of when to expect their physician or specialist to visit through the assumptions the technology infers from the physician or specialist's typical patterns. Transparent views of time frames for the patient's care empower the patient and approved family members to make informed decisions on visits and conversations.

The Hospital of the Future may alleviate some of the anxiety and uncertainty patients typically experience in their vulnerable state in a hospital. The HotF Patient Interface will allow for improved patient control of the patient's environment. Any person, especially staff, entering a patient's room is introduced to the patient through the interface. As staff enter, the interface relays the staff's reason for visit and role in the patient's care. When discussing the patient's care, a physician or nurse may push content to the Patient Interface for further explanation or understanding of the patient's condition or treatment recommendation. The Patient Interface allows the patient to explore and experience their environment and care in their native language and should provide translation services as needed. The Patient Interface would ideally connect with a Voice Assistance[7] system to answer medical questions about the patient's condition and care. While also functioning in the patient's native language, the Voice Assistance system would allow the patient to explore their care and control their environment through questions and commands as easily as fingers and pillow speakers. The Patient Interface empowers the patient to engage with their care, environment, and entertainment, such as Patient TV, video streaming services, etc.

With the empowerment of the Patient Interface, patients can proactively integrate themselves into their comprehensive care. The interface would allow the patient to: personalize their information and how they view it and interact with it, integrate social media updates and notifications, and import pictures of loved ones or favorite places as background or looped slideshows. The Patient Interface should be a "one-stop-shop" for patient education, entertainment, and engagement.

6.2.5   Hospital at Home

The HotF reaches further than the confines of the hospital walls. The HotF's digital presence, such as the Patient Interface, allows the facility to expand the reaches of care outside of the physical inpatient building, reducing the facility's spacial

---

[6] To be discharged, patients typically must hit certain milestones or goals, such as bending their elbow at 90° or reaching a specific blood pressure.

[7] Ideally, the Voice Assistance system would be able to answer medical questions about a patient's condition and care.

needs outside of the physical inpatient building. As wearables and IoT sensors become cost-effective and more accurate, healthcare facilities are empowered to treat patients within their own homes, where they may recover faster and safer than within the healthcare facility. As everyday wearable technology gains medical accuracy and becomes more of an integral part of the clinical information flow, predictive analytics can apply an overlay to day-to-day living, giving physicians insights into possible future problems and even preempting emergency situations. These wearable technologies allow patients to interact with their health through applications on their smartphones and smart devices.

As the digital presence of the HotF, the HotF's application (App) would allow for the connection of the patient's wearable technology as well as engagement with the patient's past, present, and future care. The App would enable a patient to video conference a registered nurse or physician to help triage before the patient visits the facility. The App could redirect them to urgent care or the emergency room if necessary.

Video Triage and telemedicine have become a staple of many healthcare facilities in 2020, accelerating their deployment since the outbreak of the coronavirus pandemic. After triaging the patient, a nurse or physician may be able to check the patient into the department or facility and alert the department or facility of the patient's estimated arrival time. The App, through the Patient Interface, can then give driving directions to the patient to a reserved parking spot near the patient's destination. As the patient exits the car, the App changes to walking directions to the patient's assigned exam room or patient room, without the need for a waiting room or registration desk. The rest of the experience is within the room itself.

6.3   The HotF: Promise or Peril?

The use of IoT devices in the HotF use cases to improve patient quality of care shows tremendous potential benefit for patients and healthcare providers. Yet, for the technologist focused on information security and privacy protections, the dangers also seem tremendous—and those questions come into play only after interoperability issues have been addressed[8] and the various regulatory processes have deemed a device and software safe for medical use.[9] Questions a technologist might ask about the information security and privacy status of IoT innovations noted

---

[8] Issues of interoperability are not trivial. In 2019, the IEEE established a standards committee and working group to develop a standard for Clinical Internet of Things (IoT) Data and Device Interoperability with TIPPSS—Trust, Identity, Privacy, Protection, Safety, Security (P2933). The project is intended to improve healthcare outcomes and protect patient privacy and security by enabling secure data sharing in connected healthcare. The work of the project is expected to be completed in 2023. To learn more, visit: https://standards.ieee.org/project/2933.html#Working

[9] In the United States, the Food and Drug Administration regulates the sale and safety of medical devices. Medical device classifications, regulations, and authorities vary by country.

in HotF use cases focus both on the security of the IoT devices and sensors, as well
as the data that those devices create.

6.3.1 Information Security and Privacy Questions on HotF Use Cases

While the healthcare industry leans on use cases to discuss scenarios and define
future possibilities for quality patient healthcare, most information security and
privacy professionals, particularly those in the healthcare industry, live in FUD
(fear, uncertainty, and doubt) influenced reality where the stakes are high for a
misstep concerning information security or privacy controls.[10] Thus, technologists
have many questions about the use of healthcare IoT devices and the data that they
generate.

Chain of Custody
- What are the digital chain of custody controls that must be put in place to make
  sure that the locations of people, specimens, and medications are not tampered
  with?[11]
- How can the system be manipulated by someone intent on wrongdoing to harm
  a patient or hospital staff member? Or, to steal supplies or medication from the
  hospital?
- What alerting mechanisms must be put into place to address situations where a
  person, specimen, medication, or supplies are leaving permitted HotF campus
  areas? What response activities need to be put in place and how do those change
  based on the type of item being tracked?
- What is the backup system that must be put in place to track people, specimens,
  and medications if the primary digital chain of custody system is offline?
- What type of administrative controls must be put in place to limit data analysis[12]
  and protect the privacy of patients and hospital staff that are tracked?

Digital Doorway, Integrated Patient Displays
- How do door and room sensors authenticate a patient or provider and limit access
  to unauthorized people?
- How can the system be manipulated to harm a patient?

---

[10] The stakes are also high for healthcare—literally life and death. Failing to implement information security and privacy controls that are end user friendly will cause healthcare professionals to
engage in practices that bypass those controls.

[11] Distributed ledger technologies, like those represented by blockchain, may be of particular
usefulness in addressing this question.

[12] The HotF may wish to limit data analysis because the cost of data storage and analytics tools
can be prohibitive as data sets get very large, and collecting and storing more data than one needs
is generally thought of as a poor privacy practice.

- How are all the IoT devices and sensors physically secured so that they cannot be tampered with? What alarms exist to alert medical staff to devices and sensors that have been tampered with?
- What happens when these systems are not available and how does that impact healthcare delivery?
- How does the HotF comply with state and federal laws related to the security and privacy of patient data, e.g., HIPAA in the United States?
- How does the system differentiate between a typical, responsive patient and one who shouldn't see certain data types because of fragile health? How should this be implemented?
- How does the system know when patients and healthcare providers are in the room as opposed to visitors who should not see patient data?
- How much control does the patient have over the data that is shown in the room?
- Similar to conventional door icons and patient door signs/indicators, how much data is potentially exposed to a visitor who knows the meaning behind the color codes and icons?

Mobility (Includes Clinical Mobility, Patient Interfaces, Hospital at Home)
- What are the digital chain of custody controls that must be put in place to make sure that devices used for mobile charting are not lost, stolen, or tampered with? How is the integrity of the data transmitted via those devices ensured?
- Are the video conferencing tools used in the HotF environment secure and safe from digital eavesdropping? How do hospital staff and patients authenticate identity prior to the use of video conferencing?
- How are the end-point devices that the patient uses to access their data secured?
- How much control does the patient have over which clinical data to share in the hospital at home environment?
- What happens when these systems are not available and how does that impact healthcare delivery?

6.3.2 Securing Healthcare Big Data

The currency of the HotF is data. IoT devices used for healthcare purposes will generate, transmit, analyze, and store large amounts of data that are specifically designed to provide useful and reliable information about a patient's medical state and healthcare outcomes. These data can also be combined for research purposes that review hospital operations and treatment outcomes, and design for future medical therapies that benefit humankind.

"Big data" is a term used to define large, complex electronic data sets, usually gathered from multiple sources, as well as the transactional data and metadata related to these data sets, which in turn must be analyzed together. The big data produced by the HotF can help provide:

- Performance Monitoring, Trending, and Reporting: Allowing reporting and analysis of the facility's historical status and current performance in areas such as sustainability and patient throughput.
- Real-time Response and Actions: Allowing automation to take over low-value cause-effect tasks such as automated reordering of supplies or automated maintenance requests.
- Predictive Analytics, Modeling, and Simulation: Allowing the facility to simulate changes to processes, workflows, and services such as simulating the addition of more examination rooms or changing the timing of the nurses' shifts, and predicting the potential impact of the changes.

While the potential seen in such large data stores is great, its use is not without risk. Due to their size and complexity, these HotF data sets require a concerted inquiry into how information security and privacy will be maintained across and within them. Heightened security and privacy concerns about HotF big data include questions of volume and sensitivity. This includes both the amount of data that is collected, which calls into question issues of identification of patients and healthcare providers, even when data are de-identified or anonymized, as well as the sensitivity of the data elements collected and potential sensitivity variations between different systems collecting data. This concern is especially acute for systems and devices collecting healthcare data. Access issues also come into play, as robust identification, authentication, and authorization mechanisms need to exist to permit persons or entities with permitted access to query the larger data collections.

Volume The volume of personal data being collected, stored, and used by multiple parties is a common concern with big data. There are two issues at play when we discuss volume. The first is the number of records included in a big data collection. The question asked in this context is "How much information do you have?" The second aspect is the number of data elements collected per individual, potentially translating into "How much do you know about me?". In the HotF scenario, the answer to both questions might be "A lot."

Even when used for a purpose that has a direct patient benefit, like the provision of healthcare, such large collections of data, and the insights that they can reveal, are often viewed with suspicion, particularly if personally identifiable information (PII) is included among the collected data. The very act of matching data from different sources may also lead to the creation of a new data set that contains sufficient data elements to identify underlying individuals; in such instances, additional privacy protections are required to protect individuals.

Sensitivity The sensitivity of data in big data collections is also a concern. There are two related sensitivity issues. The first is acknowledging that big data sets may include different categories of data in any number of combinations. This is complicated in the healthcare environment where some types of patient data may be protected by state and federal laws. The second issue is understanding that different categories of data may need markedly different security and privacy protections because of the sensitivity of that data or the ability of that data element to identify an individual in multiple different data collections. In the United States, the government-issued Social Security number is a data element used to access multiple public and private data collections. As a data element, it is quite sensitive and must be protected accordingly.

Access Finally, the widespread availability of personal data being collected and stored within the HotF, and the near-global availability of data through the Internet and via personal mobile devices, poses unique access concerns for healthcare data collections. These collections are almost always designed to be accessed by multiple entities, from various locations, and for different purposes. Many of those different access options were described in the use cases presented previously. Yet, ubiquitous access raises pervasive concerns about how to control that access.

Access concerns fall into two broad categories: (1) external threats—protecting data from external actors without legitimate access to the data; and (2) internal threats—protecting data from internal actors such as individuals with legitimate access to systems who intentionally exceed the scope of their pre-approved authority, who access data from unapproved devices, or who make mistakes and accidentally disclose data. In the HotF vision, multiple IoT devices and Information Technology (IT) systems and their data are linked and communicating simultaneously. This means that data sets from multiple owners are combined into shared systems. As a result, information security controls are necessary to not only secure the data from external interference but also to implement access control policies for legitimate medical staff members, patients, and their families.

6.4 Understanding Information Security and Privacy Concepts in the HotF

Overcoming the IoT device and data security and privacy questions posed by the HotF use cases requires not only technologists to understand the healthcare use cases, but also requires healthcare design professionals to understand basic information security and privacy concepts. Only when technologists and healthcare design professionals come together with a common lexicon about use cases and information security and privacy, the vision of the HotF can be realized.

6.4.1 Information Security

Information security refers to the mechanisms that protect information technology (IT) devices, including IoT devices, and the data contained on those devices. Information security is not only the technical controls implemented into IT systems. It includes the study and practice of protecting data in all its forms, whether stored in an IT system, on a personal device, in an EMR/EHR, on paper, or another physical medium. Information security includes protecting technologies and data from all types of threats, whether those threats are perpetrated by outsiders planning malicious activity, or by individuals with legitimate access to IT systems and data. The practice of information security includes three distinct concepts: confidentiality, integrity, and availability.

Confidentiality means protecting data, in any form, from unauthorized access throughout its entire lifecycle, from data creation to storage to data destruction. Unauthorized access includes access by individuals not affiliated with the underlying healthcare entity storing the data, for example, criminals and hackers. It also includes access by individuals within an organization who purposefully exceed their scope of authority in accessing information. This could be, for example, individuals looking up the records of celebrities or other targeted individuals when they have no professionally legitimate reason to do so [4]. For many of the HotF use cases, confidentiality also encompasses questions of maintaining the confidentiality of care team members, as well as the patient and their family members. The information security concept of confidentiality is most often implicated when an organization experiences a data breach.

Integrity means ensuring that data used, stored, and processed within IT systems are accurate. It means that the systems themselves have internal controls to make sure that users enter and process data correctly and that conflicting data elements are identified and resolved. Integrity also requires that only authorized users can change, move, or delete certain types of data files. When data have integrity, they are considered accurate and can be relied upon for decision-making. This is a critical concern when providing patient care.

Availability means ensuring that data are available when needed and that IT systems are operating reliably. Stakeholders can ensure data availability in several ways, such as designing IT systems that are "redundant," meaning that they are designed and installed in such a way that a failure of one component will not cause an entire system to fail. The systems and data contained therein must also be resistant to attacks and must be backed up regularly. When ransomware attacks occur in the healthcare industry, whether to steal data, change data, or reduce data and system access, they are thwarting the information security concept of availability [5]. For the HotF, business continuity and disaster recovery safeguards that ensure availability are life and death considerations.

To reduce IoT HotF risks to the confidentiality, integrity, and availability of IT systems and data, controls from the following general information security areas must be considered:

- Asset management, which focuses on how IoT devices and sensors, the IT systems that they connect to, and the data that they create, analyze, and store, are managed throughout their lifecycle from creation or acquisition to destruction.
- Identification, authentication, and access control, which relate to how authorized users, including patients and hospital staff, are identified, authenticated (prove their identity), and given access to IoT systems and/or data within those systems.

- Operational security, which pertains to how IoT devices and sensors, the IT systems that they connect to, and the data contained within them are operated, protected from threats, and tested for vulnerabilities. Ransomware and malware protection, system logging and monitoring, data backups, and vulnerability management are all included in this general category.
- Communications security, which pertains to how IoT devices and sensors, the IT systems that they connect to, and the data within those systems are protected when data move between networks or across IT systems, both within a single organization or among multiple organizations. This may be an interesting area to explore further as patients move across different healthcare and insurance organizations for care.
- Physical and environmental security, which relate to how IoT devices and sensors, the IT systems that they connect to, and the data contained within them are protected from physical loss, mechanical failure, and environmental damage. This includes protecting IT systems from the risk of theft or loss; natural disasters such as fires, floods, and tornados; intentional vandalism; and power loss, or other mechanical failures.
- Incident response, which pertains to how organizations identify, respond to and recover from information security incidents involving IoT devices and sensors, the IT systems that they connect to, and the data within those systems.
- Business continuity and disaster recovery, which pertain to the response and recovery controls that an organization must implement for different types of events like a global pandemic, a ransomware attack, a physical loss of system access such as from a natural disaster or terrorist attack, or loss of network connectivity. Depending on their severity, ongoing information security incidents can push organizations into a business continuity response activity.
- Training and awareness, which relate to how organizations train their employees and other IT users and spread awareness about how the organization promotes good information security practices. Training and awareness are important because employees and other trusted individuals, even with the best of intentions, can unknowingly compromise the security of IT systems and the data contained within those systems.

The Health Data Regulatory Landscape

This chapter very deliberately does not focus on the regulatory requirements that will affect the Hospital of the Future (HotF). Laws such as the U.S. Health Insurance Portability and Accountability Act (HIPAA) [6], the 1976 Medical Device Amendments to Federal Food, Drug, and Cosmetic Act, and state laws relating to consumer privacy and data breaches, could occupy a chapter of their own, and many of the chapters in this book touch on the complicated nature of the regulatory landscape.

Nonetheless, the role of HIPAA does bear mention when talking about the security and privacy of health information. This law is best known for its rules that protect the privacy and security of personally identifiable health information. HIPAA dictates how covered entities, like the HotF, may use protected health information (PHI). PHI is any individually identifiable information about the health of a person. It includes past, present, or future information regarding patient health, including mental and physical health data. The Privacy Rule dictates how covered entities must protect the privacy of PHI. The HIPAA Security Rule states the administrative, physical, and technical rules for how covered entities must protect the confidentiality, integrity, and availability of electronic PHI. Most of the general information security controls discussed in this section are also addressed by the HIPAA privacy and security rules.

The U.S. Department of Health and Human Services, via its Office for Civil Rights, oversees compliance with the HIPAA Privacy and Security Rules. A HIPAA Security or Privacy Rule violation can result in a maximum fine of USD$1.5 million per year. Minimum fines range from $100 to $50,000 per violation. HIPAA criminal sanctions are possible if a person criminally obtains or discloses PHI in violation of HIPAA. Criminal violations of HIPAA are pursued by the U.S. Department of Justice.

6.4.2 Privacy

The rise in the use of IoT devices and sensors and the ease of creating, collecting, and storing IoT generated data leads to increased concern about the privacy of that data. Privacy is a simple term used to explain concepts that apply both to individuals and society at large. For individuals, privacy means the right of a person to control their data and to control or direct how those data are collected, used, and shared.

The notion of patient control is foundational to the discussion of the HotF use cases. For instance, data from HotF IoT devices and sensors should be collected lawfully and in ways that seek to affirm a patient's or a healthcare provider's[13] individual privacy rights. This means that collecting entities, whether the HotF or device manufacturer, should seek permission whenever possible before collecting individually identifiable data and should only collect the minimum amount of data necessary to achieve specific healthcare goals. Establishing a set of privacy principles will be instrumental in helping protect patient and healthcare provider privacy. Adherence to these principles will promote transparency, accountability, and trust within the HotF ecosystem.

One privacy framework to consider might be the Fair Information Practice Principles (FIPPs). The FIPPs are part of the U.S. federal Privacy Act of 1974 [7] and have been influential in shaping U.S. privacy law. They were designed to address privacy concerns arising from larger digital collections of personal data,

---

[13] As healthcare providers could also easily be inadvertently tracked in the HotF through their access and interaction with patient IoT systems, or deliberately tracked from RTLS embedded in a hospital identification badge, ensuring provider privacy is also a consideration in the HotF.

and thus provide a good model for considering IoT-related privacy issues within the HotF. The FIPPs consist of eight privacy principles:

1. Purpose Specification: Organizations should tell individuals why data are being collected, and for which uses, before the data are collected.
2. Collection Limitation: Organizations should collect only the data that they need and must obtain those data by lawful means or with notice and consent from the individual.
3. Data Quality: Organizations should only collect accurate data and should have a process that an individual can follow to correct inaccurate data.
4. Use Limitation: Organizations should only use data for the purposes specified when the data are originally collected or otherwise permitted by law.
5. Security Safeguards: Organizations should protect collected data from unauthorized access (e.g., confidentiality), destruction (e.g., availability), and modification (e.g., integrity).
6. Openness: Organizations should be transparent and provide individuals with information about their data collection activities.
7. Individual Participation: Individuals should be able to find out if data about them have been collected by an organization, and they should have access to any such data.
8. Accountability: Organizations that collect data must be held accountable for adhering to these privacy principles.

6.5   Conscientious Negotiations: Marrying Healthcare IoT in the HotF with Information Security and Privacy

Marrying IoT in the HotF with information security and privacy is not an insurmountable task. It means understanding that the HotF isn't really about the technology at all. Instead, it's about raising the quality of patient care, improving the delivery of healthcare services through the optimization of workflows and processes, and enhancing healthcare staff satisfaction.

To successfully arrange a marriage between the HotF and information security and privacy, several guiding principles must be agreed to and embraced:

- The perspective of the individual, whether patient or healthcare provider, must be absolute when thinking about the healthcare IoT. From the patient perspective, we must understand how the individual wants to receive healthcare and the level of control that the individual wants with respect to their healthcare data. For healthcare providers, we must understand how they wish to interact with their patients and how they wish to participate in HotF workflows and processes.

- Healthcare IoT device vendors and healthcare design visionaries must consider an information security and privacy "by design"[14] approach, as these concepts do not bolt-on well after a technology is already in place.
- Information security and privacy technologists cannot stop the forward march of the healthcare IoT, and our approach to securing the healthcare IoT and data within the IoT must move beyond the visible horizon of compliance requirements.

Safety, patient and staff participation, and unprecedented transparency, access and efficiency are hallmarks of the HotF that can only be achieved by incorporating information security and privacy controls into the design of the IoT technologies used in the HotF.

References

1. IEEE, Internet of Things: Today and Tomorrow (May 2018), https://ieeexplore.ieee.org/document/8400064
2. Opening Eyes to a Frontier in Vision Restoration, Monash University, Melbourne, Australia, September 14, 2020. Available from https://www.monash.edu/news/articles/opening-eyes-to-a-frontier-in-vision-restoration
3. Frustrated Nurse Urges To Stop Stealing Supplies from Hospital, CNN, David Williams, March, 27 2020. Available from https://www.cnn.com/world/live-news/coronavirus-outbreak-03-27-20-intl-hnk/h_1b7d0da61e02d8ba6c8159761b87b25b
4. Six people fired from Cedars-Sinai over patient privacy breaches. Los Angeles Times, July 12, 2013. Available from http://articles.latimes.com/2013/jul/12/local/la-me-hospital-security-breach-20130713
5. Woman Dies During a Ransomware Attack on a German hospital, The Verge, September 17, 2020. Available from, https://www.theverge.com/2020/9/17/21443851/death-ransomware-attack-hospital-germany-cybersecurity
6. Health Insurance Portability and Accountability Act of 1996 (HIPAA), U.S. Code, vol. 42, sec. 1320d.
7. Privacy Act of 1974, Pub. L. No. 93-579, 88 Stat. 1896, codified at U.S. Code Vol. 5, sec. 552a.

---

[14] "By design" systems engineering approaches to information security and privacy advocate that these concepts be included and considered in early stages of the technology/engineering design lifecycle.

Chapter 7
The Right Not to Share: Weighing Personal Privacy Threat vs. Promises of Connected Health Devices

Jenny Colgate and Jennifer Maisel

Contents

7.1 Introduction

Connected health devices and applications (hereinafter "connected health devices") offer tremendous promises in healthcare management and delivery by shifting medical care outside of the doctor's office or hospital setting directly into the hands, homes, and everyday lives of patients. As we currently find ourselves dealing with the Coronavirus pandemic, doctors and patients alike have been forced to become rapid adopters of connected health devices. There is no question that the changes that are happening today are going to significantly impact the future of healthcare and increase the use of remote healthcare. Changes that have happened because of COVID have likely propelled us years, if not decades, into the future.

While the future (and present) promises a lot of things to a lot of people, there are tradeoffs. In the case of connected health devices, the tradeoffs concern information privacy and data protection. The more you get—the more convenient and personal

J. Colgate · J. Maisel (✉)
Rothwell, Figg, Ernst & Manbeck PC, Washington, DC, USA
e-mail: jcolgate@rothwellfigg.com; jmaisel@rothwellfigg.com

© Springer Nature Switzerland AG 2022
F. D. Hudson (eds.), *Women Securing the Future with TIPPSS for Connected Healthcare*, Women in Engineering and Science,
https://doi.org/10.1007/978-3-030-93592-4_7

the healthcare—the more you give up about yourself. To your doctors. To medical device companies. To drug companies. To the world, including those that wish to exploit your information.

The problem is that there is no comprehensive law regulating the collection and use of personal information in the United States. Nor is there a single law regulating "health-related data" in the United States. Instead, there is a patchwork system of *hundreds* of federal and state laws and regulations. Thus, some consumers may simply decide not to share his or her health-related data or use connected health devices without clear guidance as to what, exactly, he or she is giving up. Of course, some customers may also not be aware of the privacy and safety issues and just blindly agree to use connected health devices, and share their data, without understanding the risks.

In this chapter, we will discuss the future (and now) of connected health devices, the promises and personal privacy threats associated with connected health devices, the state of the law as it relates to these devices, and best practices for "bridging the gap" between the personal privacy threats that exist under the current legal regime and promises of connected health devices.

7.2 The Future of Connected Health Devices

The market for connected health devices was approximately $14.9 billion USD in 2017 and is expected to grow to $52.2 billion USD by 2022 [1]. Meanwhile, the global IoT market size was about $170.6 billion USD in 2017 and is expected to reach $561.0 billion USD by 2022 [2]. This means that connected health devices are currently accounting for about 10% of the IoT market.

One key to the projected explosive growth of the IoT and connected health devices is the large-scale adoption of 5G (the fifth generation of wireless communication technologies supporting cellular data networks). 5G is important to the growth of IoT and connected health devices because it expands the frequencies on which digital cellular technologies transfer data, which allows for the connection of more devices within the same geographic area [3]. More specifically, 4G can support about 4000 devices per square kilometer, whereas 5G can support around one million [4].

With the large-scale adoption of 5G will come not only an explosive growth of IoT and connected health devices, but also an explosive growth in the data being generated by those devices and subsequently analyzed by companies that get their hands on it (referred to as "big data"). Market intelligence and advisory firm International Data Corporation (IDC) has forecasted that connected IoT devices will generate 73 zettabytes (ZB) of data in 2025 or, put differently, 73 trillion gigabytes (GB) [5]. To put this in context, in 2010, the total amount of data on earth exceeded 1 ZB; by the end of 2011, the number grew to 1.8 ZB; and in 2020 the number was expected to reach 35 ZB [6]. If the 10% market calculation referenced above carries over into data generation, that would mean that by 2025 connected health devices alone would generate almost 8 ZB (or 8 trillion GB) of data.

So, who cares? What good is the data, and why should you care about data generation, who has access to it, and what they are doing with it? We will cover that in the sections that follow—Sects. 7.3 and 7.4. Table 7.1 has examples of connected health devices, some of which are referenced throughout this chapter.

7.3   Promises of Connected Health Devices

Connected health devices offer a lot of promise to individuals and their loved ones, healthcare professionals, medical device companies, and pharmaceutical companies. Indeed, the name of the game in connected health devices appears to be aimed at providing *better healthcare*: earlier detection, monitoring of loved ones, data-driven results, better adherence to treatment, increased convenience, more comfort, and healthier lifestyle. We discuss some of these benefits below.

Earlier detection and prevention. One of the most prevailing promises offered by connected health devices is early detection, and possibly prevention, of adverse health issues. For example, ordinary smartwatches that monitor blood pressure have saved people's lives from heart attacks. One of these people is 28-year-old New York-based podcast producer James T Green, whose Apple watch told him his heart rate was higher than normal, leading him to seek medical advice and get a CT scan, which revealed a pulmonary embolism [7]. Numerous other connected health devices have similar prevention goals. Connected glucose monitoring and connected contact lenses (which monitor glucose through tears) can be used to more regularly test glucose levels of diabetics, which can be life-saving. More constant monitoring, particularly during different "events" in one's day or life (meals and snacks, exercise, sleeping, nighttime, sickness, routine changes, new medications) [8], can prevent complications and adverse health conditions that are caused by glucose levels getting too high or too low, such as diabetic ketoacidosis (DKA), hyperosmolar hyperglycemic nonketotic syndrome (HHNS), heart disease or heart attack, stroke, kidney damage, nerve damage, eye damage, or skin problems [9]. Connected ear inserts are aimed at early detection of issues affecting the heart, brain, or lungs [10]. The ITBra is aimed at early detection of breast cancer [11]. Connected tampons are aimed at early detection of endometriosis, sexually transmitted infections, and cancer (uterine, cervical, and ovarian) [12]. And facial scan technologies and voice analyses are currently being studied as ways for early detection of Parkinson's disease [13] and Alzheimer's disease [14].

Monitoring of loved ones. Another promise of connected health devices is aimed at providing greater independence to a patient in exchange for allowing others to remotely monitor his or her well-being. For example, the Apple Watch's fall detection technology contacted a man's emergency contacts, as well as emergency services, when he fell off his bicycle and was rendered unconscious [15]. A teenager from Georgia created a mental health application, called NotOK, that operates like a digital panic button and alerts family and friends to your exact location via text message [16]. The Embrace smartwatch is expected to be a game changer for families with children suffering from epilepsy. Not knowing when a seizure will happen is a huge reason why children with epilepsy are oftentimes forced to lead modified lifestyles—not swimming in deep water; not taking baths unattended; teens not driving; parents sleeping on the floor in their children's bedrooms. The Embrace smartwatch could change some of these practices, as it will send an alert to caregivers, along with GPS data on where the wearer can be found, when it suspects a seizure. Because it also tracks data on subjects, such as sleep and activity patterns, it could also help health professionals and caregivers understand the triggers of a particular individual's seizures [17].

Data-driven results. Connected healthcare applications promise improved health outcomes by collecting data that provides a more accurate or complete picture of a person's health or lifestyle. For example, Parkinson's patient monitoring, using a watch-like device, is expected to lead to better treatment because data can be recorded real-time, instead of relying on patients to remember and answer questions correctly when they are at doctor appointments. A study performed by Cedars-Sinai Medical Center in Los Angeles comparing the patient monitoring device with patient self-reports found that patients were not very good at determining what constituted abnormal movements and often forgot or skipped making note of them, whereas they wore the watch consistently. One of the doctors in the study, Dr. Tagliati, reported, "People tend to tell the doctor that they are well even when they are not. And when they are not doing well, due to the day-to-day variability of their fluctuations, it is difficult to finely adjust their medications. The Parkinson's KinetiGraph (PKG) device gives us information we just didn't have before" [18]. There are also a number of medical devices that are intended to provide better, more personalized information to users within the privacy of their own homes. For example, while the data obtained from connected period trackers and breast pumps could certainly be shared with medical professionals in some instances, these devices—much like a lot of the data obtained from Fitbits and smartwatches—are intended for personal information, use, and betterment. For example, just as a smartwatch may help someone stay on an exercise schedule, a connected period or fertility tracker could help couples conceive, and a connected breast pump could help mothers stay on a breast pumping schedule [19].

Better adherence to treatment. Yet another common goal of connected health devices is to help afflicted individuals better understand and adhere to treatment plans. One example concerns connected inhalers. Research suggests that inhalers are commonly misused; however, it is unclear which inhalers have the highest misuse rates and what steps are causing the most difficulty for patients [20]. Teva's connected inhaler is expected to solve some of these issues [21]. Similarly, ingestible sensors are expected to improve issues with patients forgetting to take medication, forgetting to fill a prescription, and actively discontinuing or modifying a regimen. For example, in November 2017, the FDA announced its approval for the first time of an existing drug (aripiprazole tablets, which are used to treat schizophrenia) that utilizes a digital ingestion tracking system (Abilify MyCite system). The system works by containing an ingestible event marker (IEM) sensor embedded in each tablet, and a wearable sensor patch that detects the signal from the IEM tablet sensor after ingestion and transmits data to a smartphone application and web-based portal. The system, and corresponding data, allows healthcare professionals and caregivers to track drug ingestion and adherence [22].

Increased convenience. Another promise of connected health devices is convenience, which oftentimes is centered around the concept of being able to do at home or from anywhere things that previously required a trip to a doctor's office or a lab, or other times is centered around the concept of having technology do for you automatically what previously required manual effort. Roche's CoaguCheck Vantus is one of many examples of connected medical devices alleviating the need for multiple lab visits, as it allows one to test blood coagulation from home and the results are transmitted wirelessly to a healthcare provider [23]. Connected contact lenses—to automatically measure glucose levels, thereby alleviating the need for diabetics to prick and test their fingers multiple times daily—are another example of connected healthcare providing increased convenience, and making automatic efforts that used to require manual effort [24].

More comfort. Yet another promise of connected health devices is comfort—both comfort in performing required medical procedures, as well as improving one's health/comfort. For example, the aforementioned connected contact lenses may alleviate the need for diabetics to prick their fingers [24]; connected breast pumps may alleviate the need for bulky external breast pumps [19]; and connected temperature monitors/adjusters designed to warm and cool your body may alleviate you from getting too hot or too cold [19].

Healthier or happier lifestyle. Finally, while a lot of devices in the connected health space are focused on treatment and early detection, there are several focused on maintaining a healthier and/or happier lifestyle. Indeed, this is largely the focus of general smartwatches and Fitbits. It is also the focus of a number of condition-specific smartwatches and apps, such as Embrace smartwatches, which allow epileptics to live more normal, comfortable lifestyles including swimming, driving, and sleeping alone [25]; smartwatches, like the Apple Watch 5, with fall detection, which allow some elderly people to live alone, and some athletes to train alone [26]; and wearable mental health devices and applications, which allow individuals suffering from depression, bipolar disorder, and other mental illnesses to have comfort in knowing that loved ones are able to monitor them, but without having to sacrifice independence [27].

7.4   Personal Privacy Threats

Of course, as with most things in life, where there are promises there are also pitfalls. When it comes to connected health devices, a lot of the pitfalls concern threats to personal privacy. We have summarized just some of these threats below, and then in the section that follows we explain the laws that are currently in place and how they operate (and in some cases fail to operate) to keep these privacy threats in check.

Hacking. A large number of connected health devices, including smartwatches and Fitbits, work by communicating data over a network to other devices, such as smart phones, doctors' offices, application servers, and other devices in the network. The problem with these network connections is that they make the medical device susceptible to hacking. For example, a hack could take the form of installing a virus on your smartwatch and having your smartwatch pass that virus to your phone. A ransomware attack could take control of your router and spread malicious code to every device connected to your Wi-Fi—including your Wi-Fi-enabled medical devices. A hacker could know when you are out on a run, based on data from your smartwatch, and choose that time to rob your home. A hacker could identify your emergency medical contacts based on data in your fall detection or mental health applications and send false emergency alerts to your medical contacts. Perhaps a hacker could send false medical reports to your doctor. Maybe a hacker could alter data in your account, leading to a misdiagnosis or a change in treatment protocol down the road.

Studies show that patients are aware of these security risks that accompany the promises of connected health devices. For example, according to research conducted by Bespak, a global market leader in the design, development, and manufacturer of drug delivery devices, 63% of surveyed COPD (chronic obstructive pulmonary disease) patients believed that a connected inhaler would help in preventing the worsening of their respiratory condition, but 59% voiced that they did not want a connected device, with the majority identifying security/fear of data hacking as the primary reason [28].

Sharing of sensitive information. Let's face it, there are some things people just do not want to share with anyone, even their healthcare providers, and even close family members. Even if sharing the information can help them. For some people, certain information is just *too* private. Shouldn't individuals have a say in where to draw this line?

Data Ownership and Unauthorized Access Issues. Another personal privacy pitfall associated with connected health devices is data ownership. That is, who should own data that a connected inhaler, connected contact lens, connected hearing aid, connected breast pump, or connected tampon records about you? [28]. Moreover, how does one prevent the stealing of data and use of stolen data? For example, even if a contract provides that the patient owns the data associated with a connected hearing aid, how can that patient ever know if someone else— like the device manufacturer or his healthcare provider, or some rogue employee at either—has the data and is using it in unauthorized ways?

Unauthorized Data Sharing. Data sharing is another privacy threat. While from a privacy perspective individuals may be unwilling to share data obtained from monitoring every crook and crevice of their body, the upside with data sharing is the more you share, the more you get. Sharing data with your loved ones may allow them to monitor you and your condition. Sharing data with health providers may allow them to better diagnose, treat, and prevent illnesses. Sharing data with medical device companies may allow them to improve designs and offer better functionality. Sharing data with insurance companies could help lower premiums. But with all this sharing comes the risk that someone uses a person's data in an unauthorized manner. Moreover, the more entities with whom a person shares data, the harder it is to prove—in the event of misuse—who is responsible. For example, what if suddenly advertisers appear to know about your medical condition, even though you never authorized anyone to share your personal information with advertisers? Or what if an insurance company denies you coverage, or charges you higher premiums, based on personal information they have amassed about you?

Lost Devices. Another threat comes from the ability to lose devices. With so many devices connected, there is a concern that if any device in the network—be it your wearable tracking device, your smartphone, your loved one's smartphone to whom alerts are sent—is inadvertently left in a doctor's office, coffee shop, or airport, then your data and the entire network could be at risk.

Processing Without Consent. In many instances, the law does not require an end-user to affirmatively consent to a company's use and processing of their data from a connected health device. If the device is used personally by someone, unconnected to the healthcare system, and does not concern children under 13 years of age, then US law may not require notice and consent. This scares a lot of people—just the idea that entities out there have their very personal information, and they have no idea who has it and how they are using it.

Access and Deletion Issues. Related to the concern of processing without consent is the concern that individuals cannot even find out what data entities are processing information about them. It is a black box that is out of their control. And, one step further, in many cases individuals have no right to tell entities to delete their personal health information in the United States.

Changed Dynamics in the Healthcare Space. Yet another threat related to personal privacy is the threat that healthcare dynamics will change if personal health information is shared. For example, patients may have different expectations of clinicians if they believe the clinicians are monitoring their data on a regular basis. Changes in patient expectations may cause patients to skip or deprioritize routine appointments in the belief that the doctor will reach out to them if there is an issue. Insurance companies may also expect greater performance from clinicians, based on the data to which they have access. Data could also lead to additional evaluation/performance measures, resulting from all of the data (i.e., data on conditions, outcomes, treatments) [22].

7.5   Information Privacy and Data Security Protections of IoT Health Data

The US Supreme Court Justice Louis Brandeis famously referred to the right to privacy as the "right to be let alone" [29]. Notwithstanding Justice Brandeis's early recognition of the importance of the right to privacy, the United States does not have a comprehensive privacy law. Nor does the United States have a comprehensive privacy law that applies to the data we are talking about here—health-related data. Rather, there are numerous privacy and security-related laws that could apply to health-related data in the United States depending on a variety of factors such as: the individual from whom the data is being collected, the categories of data being collected, the type of entity collecting and processing the data, and the type of device collecting the data.

In the sections that follow, we first provide a quick primer on the concepts of "information privacy" and "data protection," and then we explain some of the laws concerning connected health data, giving you a sense of just how complicated the legal landscape is.

7.5.1 Background on Privacy and Data Protection

In the United States, individual privacy is protected by the constitution, common law, and most commonly, by statutes. In the context of IoT data and the connected health devices discussed above, our primary focus will be on the legal concepts of "information privacy" and "data protection" as governed by statutes. Information privacy concerns the rules regarding the collection, use, disclosure, retention, and disposal of personally identifiable information, as well as any rights an individual has to determine how his or her personally identifiable information is collected, used, disclosed, retained, and destroyed. Data protection concerns the rules regarding the handling, storing, and management of personal information.

While there are numerous statutory definitions of personal information (PI) or personally identifiable information (PII), such definitions generally encompass information that can be used to distinguish or trace an individual's identity. Personal information may include information such as a name, social security number, biometric records, and the like, alone or when combined with other personal or identifying information which is linked or linkable to a specific individual, such as a date and place of birth, and the like. Heightened privacy and security limitations may be afforded to certain categories of sensitive personal information, such as passport numbers, license numbers, social security numbers, tax identifiers, financial information, medical records, racial or ethnic origin, political opinions, religious or philosophical beliefs, genetic data, and biometric data, to name a few. Nonpersonal data may include anonymized or aggregated data where the data elements that identify an individual have been removed. Pseudonymized data may include data that detaches the aspects of the information attributed to the specific individual, such as replacing the name of an individual with an artificial identifier or token.

In the United States, there is a patchwork system of federal and state laws and regulations governing information privacy and data protection, and there is currently no comprehensive federal law regulating the collection and use of personal information. Historically, many information privacy and data protection laws were drafted to cover fairly specific industries and types of data, and most of these laws were aimed at (1) providing transparency regarding what data was collected and/or (2) providing or restricting access to the information collected. Most were not aimed at restricting the collection or processing of information.

7.5.2 Relevant Statutes Concerning IoT Health Data

The natural place to start when discussing health data is the "Health Information Portability and Accountability Act" (HIPAA). But as we explain below, HIPAA only applies to *some* connected health data, notably health*care* data (i.e., data collected and processed by the healthcare system) and does not apply to other health data, such as information that you track on your own. Other industry-specific statutes, such as biometric and genetic information privacy laws, IoT security laws, and children's privacy laws close some but not all of the gaps left open by HIPAA.

HIPAA (Healthcare Data) The Health Insurance Portability and Accountability Act (HIPAA), 29 U.S.C. § 1181 *et seq.* establishes national standards for the administration and protection of individuals' health information, including blocking medical providers from giving third parties "protected health information." HIPAA applies to organizations referred to as "covered entities," which include healthcare providers, health plans, and healthcare clearinghouses that conduct healthcare transactions electronically, as well as "business associates" that conduct healthcare transactions on behalf of such covered entities. The HIPAA Privacy Rule specifies safeguards to protect patient-identifying health information and sets limits on the uses and disclosures of such information without consent from a patient. The Privacy Rule also gives patients certain rights, such as the right to access and correct their health information. The HIPAA Security Rule specifies appropriate administrative, physical, and technical safeguards to protect the confidentiality, integrity, and availability of electronic health information. HIPAA violations can be quite expensive and can range from $100 to $50,000 USD per violation (e.g., per record) with a maximum penalty of $1.5 million USD per year.

In sum, HIPAA provides comprehensive protection for healthcare data. While it does not limit *what data* can be collected, it provides nearly everything else— limitations on sharing, transparency and access to recorded data, security measures to protect processed data, and hefty fines for violations. The problem is that it does not apply to all of your health data. Take, for example, your smartwatch. If your doctor gives you a smartwatch to monitor your blood pressure and you share that data with your doctor so your doctor can directly monitor your blood pressure, the data is likely covered by HIPAA. But if you buy the same smartwatch on your own and use it to monitor your blood pressure, that data (i.e., the same data, but not shared with a healthcare provider) is not covered by HIPAA. This distinction likely does not make sense in our current world of off-the-shelf connected health devices.[1]

A few other industry-specific laws close some of the gaps left open by HIPAA when it comes to health data, including those pertaining to biometric data, discrimination based on health data, IoT devices, and children.

BIPA (Biometric Data) The Illinois Biometric Information Privacy Act (BIPA) was enacted in 2008 and is the first and oldest regulation over biometric data in the United States. BIPA regulates the use of "biometric information" based on certain enumerated "biometric identifiers," such as a retina or iris scan, fingerprint, voiceprint, or scan of hand or face geometry. Five additional states, including Texas, Washington, California, New York, and Arkansas have passed their own biometric statutes or expanded existing laws to include biometric identifiers. BIPA is notable because it remains the only legislation to-date that provides an individual with a private right of action for violations of the statute. Additionally, Courts have more recently held that BIPA does not require individuals to show they actually suffered harm beyond a violation of their legal rights under the statute in order to bring suit [30]. As a result, there have been a flood of class action lawsuits filed under BIPA, several with massive settlement amounts, see, e.g., [31].

BIPA's definition of "biometric identifier" contains a healthcare setting exclusion so as to not conflict with HIPAA:

> Biometric identifiers do not include information captured from a patient in a healthcare treatment, payment, or operations under the federal Health Insurance Portability and Accountability Act of 1996. Biometric identifiers do not include an X-ray, roentgen process, computed tomography, MRI, PET scan, mammography, or other image or film of the human anatomy used to diagnose, prognose, or treat an illness or other medical condition or to further validate scientific testing or screening.

But think about a person using a facial scanning technology to explore plastic surgery ideas or a voice scan to detect Alzheimer's disease. If the person uses these scanning technologies on his or her own, the facial and voice data is likely not covered by HIPAA but may be protected under BIPA. But as soon as this data is shared with his or her doctor, then the very same scans are covered by HIPAA—and thus, are excluded from BIPA.

Discrimination Based on Health Information Laws including the Genetic Information Nondiscrimination Act (GINA), the Americans with Disabilities Act (ADA), and the Patient Protection and Affordable Care Act (PPACA) prevent various forms of discrimination based on medical information. GINA protects individuals from discrimination based on their genetic information in both health insurance and employment [32]. GINA sets a floor of minimum protection against genetic discrimination and does not preempt state laws with stricter protections. The ADA

---

[1] As a result, some legislatures have proposed laws, such as the federal Smartwatch Data Act, that instead aim to protect all health data generated by healthcare devices as protected health information, regardless of whether that data is shared with your healthcare provider.

prohibits discrimination based on disability, including both physical and mental conditions. Section 1557 of the PPACA prohibits discrimination on the basis of, inter alia, disability in certain health programs or activities. While these laws are well-intentioned, again, they are not comprehensive and do not generally cover all forms of discrimination based on health data.

IoT Security Regulations Another law that could potentially regulate devices in the IoT healthcare space is the California IoT law, Senate Bill 327, "Security of Connected Devices," signed into law on September 28, 2018, which specifies the security obligations of "manufacturers" of "connected devices." California's IoT law defines connected devices as "any device, or other physical object that is capable of connecting to the internet, directly or indirectly, and that is assigned an Internet Protocol address or Bluetooth address." Covered manufacturers must equip connected devices with a reasonable security feature or features. (Note: The California IoT law also has a HIPAA carve-out, but it is unclear whether it would even apply to most connected medical devices, as it would seemingly require a HIPAA covered entity or business associate to manufacture the medical device(s) at issue.)

Oregon has enacted similar legislation, OR House Bill 2395, "Relating to security measures required for devices that connect to the internet," and has a narrower definition of "connected device" as a device or physical object that connects to the internet and is used primarily for personal, family, or household purposes. Additional IoT law bills have been introduced, and we can expect to see increasing regulation in this area. These laws will likely provide a sense of security to connected health device users, at least with respect to security-related concerns.

Internet Service Provider Regulations Laws directed at internet service providers (ISPs) are also relevant to the connected healthcare space, as ISPs have access to the wealth of personal information concerning their customers that is transmitted over the Internet. A number of states, such as Maine, Nevada, and Minnesota [33], have privacy laws directed at ISPs, which prohibit providers from disclosing users' personal information unless the customer expressly consents to it. Other states, like California, similarly regulate ISPs, but a customer has to expressly request that the ISP protect the customer's information (it is not the default). There is a lot of pending legislation related to ISP privacy, and it is expected that many states will be adopting laws in this area soon.[2]

Information About Children Healthcare devices that are used by children or collect data about children will be subject to the Children's Online Privacy Protection Act (COPPA). COPPA puts parents in control of the online collection

---

[2] States began introducing ISP privacy regulations in 2017 in response to the repeal of the Federal Communication Commission's broadband privacy rules that required internet providers to obtain consent before using geolocation, financial, health, children's and web browsing history information for advertising and marketing purposes.

of personal information from children under age 13 and includes: (1) a disclosure requirement that companies have a privacy policy that clearly and completely discloses to parents what information is collected, how the collected information will be used, and what the parent's rights are with respect to modifying or deleting the information; (2) a requirement that companies obtain verifiable consent from the parent to the collected and intended use of the data; and (3) a requirement that companies take reasonable measures to protect the security and confidentiality of the obtained information.

One of the difficulties with COPPA is there is no "one size fits all" answer about what makes a site or product directed to children. The Federal Trade Commission (FTC) has identified the following factors to help determine whether COPPA applies: the subject matter, visual content, the use of animal characters or child-oriented activities and incentives, the age of models, the presence of child celebrities or celebrities who appeal to children, language and other characteristics of the site, whether advertising, promoting or appearing on the site, is directed to children, and competent and reliable empirical evidence about the age of the audience [34].

In summary, there are numerous industry-specific privacy laws in the United States that may apply to connected health devices and connected health device data. Consequently, determining which apply and when can get very complicated.

7.6   General Information Privacy and Data Protection Regulations

In addition to the aforementioned industry-specific laws, there are also a number of broader data privacy and protection statutes and regulations, which may be generally relevant to connected health devices—not necessarily because they are required in every context, but mostly because they are far-reaching enough and strict enough that they have become "de facto" standards. Below is a brief summary of some of the more relevant ones.

Europe's General Data Protection Regulation The European Union General Data Protection Regulation (GDPR) took effect on May 25, 2018 and protects the processing of personal data, free movement of personal data, and fundamental rights and freedoms of persons. The GDPR applies to controllers and processors established in the European Union, regardless of where the processing takes place, as well as controllers and processors outside of the European Union whose activities include offering goods or services in the European Union or monitoring behavior of data subjects within the European Union. Organizations must, among other requirements, implement privacy by design and privacy by default practices, maintain appropriate data security, conduct data protection impact assessments on new processing activities, report data breaches to regulators and data subjects, and get appropriate consent for most personal data collection and provide notification of personal data processing activities. The GDPR also provides consumers, or data subjects, with certain rights, such as the right to request that personal data be erased and no longer processed, the right to request a copy of all personal data and purpose of processing, the right to request a transfer of all their data, the right to object to certain automated decision-making processing, and the right to request correction of personal data. The GDPR is significant for its potential extraterritorial reach to entities outside of the European Union and for its penalties of up to 20 million Euros or 4% of annual revenues.

Because medical devices are often sold internationally, and companies often times do not want to make different devices for different parts of the world, or have different data practices for different parts of the world, GDPR sometimes ends up being a "de facto" worldwide privacy law, as it is generally thought to be the strictest privacy law. This is a benefit for US customers because, for example, such companies would seek consent before collecting personal data and would provide notification of personal data processing activities because this is the GDPR standard.

California Consumer Privacy Act   The California Consumer Privacy Act (CCPA) took effect in January 2020 and is a landmark privacy bill that has been compared to the GDPR due to its overarching approach and strong privacy protections. The CCPA applies to "covered businesses," including any for-profit entity that does business in California, collects personal information of California residents, determines the purpose and means of processing that personal information, and meets one or more of the following criteria: generates $25 million USD in annual revenue; holds the personal data of 50,000 people, households, or devices; or makes at least half of its revenue from the sale of personal information. Covered businesses must provide certain disclosures to consumers, including categories of personal information collected, description of consumers' rights and online privacy policy. Covered businesses that sell personal information must also include a special "Do Not Sell My Personal Information" (PI) button on their websites to make it easy for consumers to object to the sale of their PI. Consumers are also granted certain rights, including the right to request records of the personal information collected, the right to erasure and deletion of the personal information, and the right to opt-out of having personal data sold to third parties. The California Attorney General may issue a $7500 fine per violation, and the CCPA provides a private right of action for unauthorized access to a consumer's "nonencrypted or nonredacted personal information" at $100–$750 per violation.

Similar to GDPR being a "de facto" standard, CCPA also ends up being a "de facto" US standard because most companies do not want to have separate policies for California than for the rest of the country. This is a benefit to US customers because, for example, such companies allow customers to restrict the sale of their information to third parties, and to access and request deletion of their personal information.

But here again, just as with several of the industry-specific laws, there is a HIPAA carve-out. Section 1798.145(c)(1)(A) provides that CCPA does not apply to protected health information that is collected by a covered entity or business associate governed by HIPAA. While, again, this seems relatively straightforward, it can get complicated. For example, going back to the smartwatch with the blood pressure monitor, when the watch is purchased by a California resident and no data is shared with the doctor, the data may be protected just under CCPA. But if the California resident then shares some of the data with his or her doctor, and the doctor records the data in the patient's medical records, that data has now become PHI collected by a covered entity under HIPAA. But does that mean that only that one piece of shared data is governed by HIPAA and not CCPA, but the same exact data that is still on the smartwatch is governed by CCPA? Issues like this have yet to be resolved, and these issues matter because a user's rights are different, and the protection afforded to the data is different, depending on what laws apply.

Federal Trade Commission Act The Federal Trade Commission Act (15 U.S.C. § 41 *et seq.*) empowers the Federal Trade Commission (FTC) to bring enforcement actions to broadly protect consumers against unfair or deceptive practices and to enforce federal privacy and data protection regulations.[3] The enforcement actions— and resulting fines—have grown in recent years, and the FTC and the Department of Justice imposed a record-breaking $5 billion dollar fine against an entity for violating consumer's privacy [35]. "The FTC has been keeping a close watch on the Internet of Things since the Internet of Things became a thing to watch," and has taken law enforcement actions against entities alleged to have sold vulnerable connected devices that put consumers' sensitive information at risk [36]. One trend in the FTC enforcement actions against IoT manufacturers is that the manufacturers were alleged to have misrepresented to customers that they took reasonable steps to secure the data they collected from users [37, 38].[4] Other FTC enforcement actions focus on misrepresentations by companies regarding their privacy policies, for example, sharing information with third parties notwithstanding a privacy policy that indicates otherwise.

In addition to its authority to investigate law violations, the FTC also has federal rule-making authority to issue industry-wide regulations [39]. For example, one FTC regulation that is applicable to connected medical devices is the "Health Breach Notification Rule." Under this rule, companies that have had a security breach

---

[3] Section 5(a) of the Federal Trade Commission Act, 15 U.S.C. § 45 prohibits "unfair or deceptive acts or practices in or affecting commerce."

[4] For example, in 2019, a smart home products manufacturer agreed to make security enhancements in order to settle FTC allegations that the manufacturer misrepresented to consumers that it took reasonable steps to secure its wireless routers and Internet-connected cameras. https://www.ftc.gov/news-events/press-releases/2019/07/d-link-agrees-make-security-enhancements-settle-ftc-litigation. In 2020, another entity settled allegations that it deceived customers by falsely claiming that its Internet-connected smart locks were designed to be "unbreakable" and that it took reasonable steps to secure the data it collected from users. https://www.ftc.gov/news-events/press-releases/2020/05/ftc-gives-final-approval-settlement-smart-lock-maker

must: (1) notify everyone whose information was breached; (2) in many cases, notify the media; and (3) notify the FTC. The Health Breach Notification Rule does not apply to businesses and organizations covered by HIPAA, as HIPAA's breach notification rule applies instead, but it is otherwise widely applicable to businesses in the connected medical device space [40].

Every state in the United States also has an unfair and deceptive acts and practices ("UDAP") law that is generally mirrored off of Section 5 of the FTC Act. Under these statutes, state attorneys general often bring actions similar to those brought by the FTC, for example, misrepresentations to consumers regarding reasonable security measures, and misrepresentations to consumers regarding data privacy practices.

Just as GDPR and CCPA create "de facto" standards, FTC Section 5 and state UDAP laws create "de facto" standards also—requiring companies to be truthful in their representations to consumers regarding security and privacy practices.

7.7 Best Practices

While connected health devices offer tremendous promises in healthcare management and delivery, some consumers may choose not to use connected health devices because of the privacy and security risks. An *uncomplicated* legal system that offers consumers basic protections with respect to all health-related information—regardless of whose hands it is in, where the involved persons and entities are located, and what type of data it is—would likely go a long way in building consumers' trust to use these attractive technologies. But as explained above, we aren't quite there yet.

Because we are not there yet, medical device companies should do their best to bridge the gap between the security, protection, and control that consumers want, and what the laws require. Creating a culture of transparency is key. Transparency builds trust, and without trust, people will not be comfortable sharing their most personal information, such as their DNA, facial scans, voiceprints, and women's information about their menstrual cycles, milk production, and breast tissue temperature. Let's face it, some people may never be comfortable recording this information. But for others, it's about trusting the system to realize the benefits that the technology has to offer.

We set forth below some practical guidance.

Reasonable Practices "Reasonable" information privacy and data protection measures will ultimately be decided in the eyes of the beholder. At minimum, and as reflected in a study conducted by the United Nations Conference on Trade and

Development (UNCTAD) [41], entities should consider core information and data privacy principles, including:

1. Openness and Transparency. Entities must be open about their personal data practices.
2. Limitations on Collection. Collection of personal data must be limited, lawful, and fair, usually with knowledge and/or consent.
3. Purpose specification. Specify the purpose of collection and disclosure at the time of collection.
4. Use limitation. Use or disclosure must be limited to specific purposes or closely related purposes.
5. Security. Personal data must be subject to appropriate security safeguards.
6. Data quality. Personal data must be relevant, accurate, and up to date.
7. Access and correction. Data subjects must have appropriate rights to access and correct their personal data.
8. Accountability. Data controllers must take responsibility for ensuring compliance with the data protection principles.

Privacy and Security Program After you identify the necessary steps to comply with applicable regulations, there still remains the question of what more do you want to offer. We suggest walking through the steps identified below and focusing not just on compliance, but also on trust-building and risk-management.

1. Inventory personal data. Create "data maps" for understanding how and what personal information is being collected and tracking its flow, i.e., collection, use, processing, storage, sale, and/or deletion.
2. Establish corporate rules. Determine the rules for the data being collected based on laws, regulations, contracts, and best practices.
3. Assign responsibility. Establish governance structure and assign responsibility within the organization to ensure policies and practices are compliant with corporate rules.
4. Data privacy policies and notices. Develop privacy policies that accurately communicate your privacy and security practices to your customers.
5. Individual rights management. Be prepared to manage requests from individuals pertaining to information privacy rights, such as providing information on the type of personal information collected or sold, providing a copy of the personal information collected, and maintaining and honoring consent preferences.
6. Vendor/Third Party Management. If personal data is being shared with vendors, service providers, and other third parties, entities must establish oversight to ensure that those third parties are complying with legal and regulatory requirements.
7. Training and Awareness. Everyone who manages personal information, including decision-makers, should receive training in the organization's privacy programs and policies.

8. Data privacy breach management program. An entity should define an organized approach to managing the occurrence and aftermath of a data privacy incident, security breach, or cyberattack.
9. Continuous compliance monitoring. Entities should define a compliance monitoring framework to support current and new operational practices, address future laws, and demonstrate ongoing compliance.

Data Rights Is there an intellectual property interest in the data? For example, perhaps a competitor will be able to reverse engineer an algorithm used in a novel sensing device by analyzing the sensor's measurements and data taken over time. Perhaps the data is creatively enhanced or arranged in a manner that may be afforded copyright protection. Who owns the data being collected? Does your contract provide that you own the data, but at the same time you provide individuals with the right to delete the data and object to your sharing the data with third parties? Are you legally permitted to analyze the data you collect for purposes of your own discoveries? It is critical to establish how to navigate different interests in the data collected by connected health devices, especially when those interests intersect or conflict.

Decision-Making Based on Data What decisions, if any, are being made about the data, and by whom? Perhaps the data will be sent directly to a physician for prescribing treatment, or to a machine learning application that automatically and dynamically determines an appropriate dosage to administer from an insulin pump. In the case of automated decision-making in healthcare, there are a number of safety and security considerations at stake. For example, how is harm and liability defined (e.g., if a patient manipulates data), what is the standard of care for an automated system, who or what is responsible when an accident occurs, and what are the ethical, legal, and social implications?

7.8 Conclusion

While the field of connected health devices may have leaped years, if not decades, into the future in view of the current Coronavirus pandemic, the law in the United States has remained largely as it was—a confusing patchwork of state and federal regulations. It is up to companies to develop information privacy and data security programs that focus on concepts like trust, transparency, and reasonable practices in order to ensure that connected health devices have a beneficial place in the future of society.

Table 7.1 Examples of connected health devices

Device	How it works
Smartwatches	
Fitbits and smartwatches	Fitbits and smartwatches are worn on user's skin to monitor health and exercise data, such as heart rate, calories burned, steps walked, blood pressure, sleep monitoring, and time spent exercising.
Medical alert smartwatches (e.g., Embrace smartwatch)	The Embrace smartwatch tracks generalized tonic-clonic seizures and aids in epilepsy management by, inter alia, alarming family members and caretakers that a tonic-clonic seizure is occurring [42].
Apple Watch 5	The Apple Watch 5 is able to detect falls. Once the watch detects what it considers to be a fall, it asks if you fell, dropped the Watch, or need emergency assistance. If it can detect movement, it will wait for input; however, if it does not detect movement, it will automatically call 911 to get you assistance [43].
OMRON HeartGuide	The OMRON HeartGuide was the first blood pressure monitoring clinically approved (i.e., highly accurate readings), which captures blood pressure data and relays it to an associated app, which can be used to share the information with a medical professional [43].
Mental Health Apps	
Cognition Kit	Cognition Kit is a collection of cognitive tests that can be licensed to pharmaceutical companies to collect real-world data on study participants via smartphones and smartwatches. Indicators such as how much time you are staying at home, what you are eating, how much exercise you are getting, your blood pressure, and your social media use can all be indicators of your current mental health.
Mind.me	Mind.me works passively in the background on one's smartphone, collecting data online and offline, and works to prevent a depressive episode by, inter alia, alerting a user's trusted circle of loves ones if it thinks something is amiss [27].
Connected Glucose Monitoring	
Guardian™ Connect Continuous Glucose Monitoring System	The Guardian™ Connect Continuous Glucose Monitoring System consists of a glucose sensor, which measures users' interstitial glucose levels every 5 min, and a transmitter, which sends those readings to users' mobile devices running the associated application. This results in users receiving 288 readings every day, as compared to 6–10 readings a day using the traditional finger-prick, blood glucose monitor. Additionally, the application provides the data that is collected in easy-to-read reports [44].

(continued)

Table 7.1 (continued)

Connected Inhaler	
Teva's connected inhaler	Teva's connected inhaler will track how often patients use their inhaler for "maintenance therapy" (e.g., is the inhaler being used the prescribed number of times per day), as well as if the inhaler is being used properly (e.g., proper technique). Both of these metrics can be shared with a healthcare professional, thereby providing information that was never previously available, which could be useful for healthcare management [45].
Connected Contact Lenses	
Glucose Monitoring Lenses	A team at Purdue University, as well as teams at Microsoft and Google, have been researching how to combine contact lenses with glucose monitors to assist diabetics, the idea being that tears—instead of pricking one's finger for a drop of blood—can be used to analyze glucose [24].
Pressure-Sensing Lenses	A team at Columbia University Medical Center has been developing smart contact lenses that monitor eye pressure with the hope of being able to more accurately gauge the speed at which one's glaucoma (the leading cause of blindness in the United States) develops. The pressure-sensing contact lenses could provide much more data, as they would allow for constant monitoring, including while one sleeps, whereas currently eye pressure is only monitored during regular ophthalmologist visits [46].
Connected Ear Sensors	
Ear-worn sensors to monitor heart, brain, and lung function	A research team at the Imperial College of London is researching the use of ear-worn sensors to monitor heart, brain, and lung function. Among the uses is the ability to identify and manage heart conditions by using an electro-mechanical sensor to detect dilation and constriction of blood vessels in the ear canal, thereby acting as a convenient, longer term, accessible "mini-electrocardiogram" (ECG) [10].
Connected Blood Coagulation Testing	
CoaguChek Vantus	A couple of years ago, Roche Diagnostics, Inc. launched the CoaguChek Vantus, a Bluetooth-connected device for testing blood coagulation. The system allows patients undergoing Vitamin K antagonist therapy to self-monitor their blood coagulation with a finger-prick, and then send those results wirelessly to their care provider, thereby saving patients days of waiting and repeated lab appointments [47].

(continued)

Table 7.1 (continued)

Parkinson's Patient Monitoring	
Wearable sensors on Wrist and Chest	Currently, most healthcare providers monitor Parkinson's symptoms by asking questions of patients during hospital visits and rating patients, based on their answers, on something called the Movement Disorder Society (MDS) Unified Parkinson's Disease Rating Scale. For example, questions ask about cognition, hallucinations and psychosis, mood (depression), anxiety, apathy, and features of dopamine dysregulation syndrome (i.e., unusually strong urges that are hard to control) [48]. Research is being done in the area of wearable sensors (worn on the wrist and chest) that pair with smartphone applications, which measure things like physical movements and tremors, paired with questionnaires that are completed throughout the day [49].
Digital facial scans	Studies have been done to validate the reliability of a tool that objectively captures and identifies the masked face and other early-stage facial express impairments and micromovements associated with Parkinson's disease [13].
Alzheimer's Detection	
Voice scans and handwriting analyses	Rhoda Au, the director of neuropsychology at Framingham Heart Study (FHS), has been looking at how researchers can improve diagnostic tests used to predict who will develop Alzheimer's, including the use of digital voice recordings and digital pen writings to aid in detection [14].
Ingestible Sensors	
Schizophrenia	Ingestible sensors are used with schizophrenia patients, to ensure they take their antipsychotics [50].
Cancer	Ingestible sensors are being used with cancer patients, to monitor when and how much medication is being taken [51].
HIV prevention	Ingestible sensors have been used in drug studies, such as a 2019 study regarding the HIV prevention drug Truvada for pre-exposure prophylaxis (PrEP). PrEP is a preventative drug designed to be taken by people who do not have HIV but are at risk for the condition, and it must be taken every day, according to the Centers for Disease Control and Prevention [52].
Cancer Detection	
Breast Cancer—ITBra	A research team, comprised of Cisco and Circadia Health, is developing a bra that could help detect early signs of breast cancer. Known as the ITBra, it would track changes in the temperature of the breast tissue over time to identify atypical patterns, which could signal increased risk [53].
Connected Fertility Trackers	
Ava Bracelet	The Ava bracelet is referred to as "the Fitbit for fertility," and it tracks five different physiological markers in order to accurately pinpoint when a woman is most likely to be fertile, including temperature, resting heart rate, heart rate variability, respiratory rate, and perfusion. According to a May 2019 study carried out by the University Hospital of Zurich, Ava can detect 5.3 fertile days in a woman's menstrual cycle with 89% accuracy [19].

(continued)

Table 7.1 (continued)

Connected Breast Pumps	
The Willow Pump	Willow's hands free, connected breast pumps debuted in 2017 and consist of two pumps that fit underneath a regular bra. The product connects to an app and can be used to track milk volume, pumping time, and past pumping sessions [19].
Connected Temperature Monitors/Adjusters	
Embr Wave	Embr Wave is a heating and cooling bracelet designed by a Massachusetts Institute of Technology (MIT) spin-off startup that warms and cools your body via your wrist [19].
Grace	Grace focuses just on cooling—but its claim to fame is that it does not simply track and adjust body temperature; it can actually preempt menopausal hot flashes [19].
Connected Tampons	
NextGen Jane	A company called NextGen Jane is researching the use of smart tampons that can analyze for genomic signals and cells in order to diagnose endometriosis and other conditions in the future [19].
COVID Detection	
COVID-detecting facemask	Scientists at Harvard and MIT created a sensor that emits a fluorescent light when activated by the Coronavirus, which can be embedded in a facemask or other materials to aid in COVID-19 detection [54]. We imagine it would only be a matter of time before the same mask would also be able to transmit messages to an application, which could alert your recent contacts and doctor's office.

References

1. https://www2.deloitte.com/content/dam/Deloitte/global/Documents/Life-Sciences-Health-Care/gx-lshc-medtech-iomt-brochure.pdf at 12 (citing MarketsandMarkets).
2. https://www.marketsandmarkets.com/Market-Reports/internet-of-things-market-573.html.
3. https://www.verizon.com/about/our-company/5g/iot-future-5g-communications.
4. https://www.raconteur.net/technology/4g-vs-5g-mobile-technology.
5. https://www.idc.com/getdoc.jsp?containerId=prAP46737220#:~:text=IDC%20predicts%20that%20by%202025,from%2018.3%20ZB%20in%202019.
6. https://www.researchgate.net/figure/Data-generated-from-the-Internet-of-Things-will-grow-exponentially-as-the-number-of_fig2_234017925.
7. https://www.weforum.org/agenda/2017/10/smartwatch-saved-man-from-heart-attack/.
8. https://www.mayoclinic.org/diseases-conditions/diabetes/in-depth/blood-sugar/art-20046628.
9. http://www.webmed.com/diabetes/uncontrolled-blood-sugar-risks.
10. https://www.hearingassociatesofnova.com/2018/01/29/future-tech-hearing-aids-that-can-monitor-vital-signs/.
11. https://www.scmp.com/lifestyle/health-wellness/article/2180728/hi-tech-itbra-breakthrough-asian-women-high-risk-breast.
12. https://www.verywellhealth.com/smart-tampons-4099042.
13. https://www.michaeljfox.org/grant/tool-identify-parkinsons-disease-using-digital-facial-expression-biomarkers.
14. https://www.beingpatient.com/voice-recognition-writing-alzheimers-test/.
15. https://www.medicalalertadvice.com/articles/apple-watch-fall-detection/.

16. https://www.marketwatch.com/story/this-teens-new-app-is-a-digital-panic-button-for-people-with-mental-illness-2018-04-05.
17. https://www.smithsonianmag.com/innovation/smartwatch-can-help-detect-seizures-kids-180971352/.
18. https://journals.lww.com/neurotodayonline/Fulltext/2019/08220/How_a_Watch_Like_Device_Is_Monitoring_Parkinson_s.8.aspx.
19. https://www.wareable.com/health-and-wellbeing/wearable-tech-for-womens-health.
20. https://www.ncbi.nlm.nih.gov/pubmed/28732842.
21. https://www.mobihealthnews.com/content/tevas-digital-inhaler-cleared-fda
22. https://www.uspharmacist.com/article/the-promise-and-pitfalls-of-digital-medication.
23. https://www.mobihealthnews.com/content/roche-launches-coaguchek-vantus-monitor-coagulation-levels-wirelessly/.
24. https://www.zdnet.com/article/how-smart-contact-lenses-will-help-keep-an-eye-on-your-health/.
25. https://www.neurologylive.com/view/embrace-smartwatch-gets-fda-goahead-for-seizure-monitoring.
26. https://www.techradar.com/best/best-medical-alert-smartwatches.
27. https://www.besthealthmag.ca/article/how-your-smartwatch-can-improve-your-mental-heath/
28. https://www.medicalplasticsnews.com/news/medical-devices/doubts-over-data-security-denting-smart-inhaler-potential.
29. https://www.brandeis.edu/now/2013/july/privacy.html.
30. Rosenbach v. Six Flags Entertainment Corp., 2019 IL 123186; Bryant v. Compass Group USA, Inc. (7th Cir.).
31. Facebook agrees to $550M BIPA settlement, https://www.chicagolawbulletin.com/facebook-agrees-to-550m-bipa-settlement-20200210.
32. Pub. L. No. 110–233, 122 Stat. 881 (2008) (codified in scattered sections of 26, 29, and 42 U.S.C.).
33. Maine – 35-A MRSA § 9301; Minnesota – Minn. Stat. §§ 325M.01 to .09; Nevada – NRS § 205.498.
34. https://www.ftc.gov/news-events/blogs/business-blog/2019/11/youtube-channel-owners-your-content-directed-children.
35. "FTC Imposes $5 Billion Penalty and Sweeping New Privacy Restrictions on Facebook," July 24, 2019, available at https://www.ftc.gov/news-events/press-releases/2019/07/ftc-imposes-5-billion-penalty-sweeping-new-privacy-restrictions.
36. https://www.ftc.gov/news-events/blogs/business-blog/2019/07/d-link-settlement-internet-things-depends-secure-software.
37. https://www.ftc.gov/news-events/press-releases/2019/07/d-link-agrees-make-security-enhancements-settle-ftc-litigation.
38. https://www.ftc.gov/news-events/press-releases/2020/05/ftc-gives-final-approval-settlement-smart-lock-maker.
39. https://www.ftc.gov/enforcement/rules.
40. https://www.ftc.gov/tips-advice/business-center/guidance/health-breach-notification-rule.
41. Data Protection Regulations and International data Flows: Implications for trade and development, available at https://unctad.org/en/PublicationsLibrary/dtlstict2016d1_en.pdf.
42. https://www.hcplive.com/view/fda-approves-embrace-smartwatch-for-seizure-monitoring.
43. https://www.techradar.com/best/best-medical-alert-smartwatches-2020.
44. https://www.medtronicdiabetes.com/products/guardian-connect-continuous-glucose-monitoring-system.
45. https://www.clinicalleader.com/doc/teva-develops-first-fda-approved-digitally-integrated-inhaler-0001;https://www.mobihealthnews.com/content/tevas-digital-inhaler-cleared-fda.
46. https://www.aao.org/eye-health/news/smart-contact-lens-glaucoma-patients.

47. https://www.mobihealthnews.com/tag/coaguchek-vantus;https://www.mobihealthnews.com/content/roche-diagnostics-launches-bluetooth-connected-self-testing-device-blood-coagulation.
48. https://www.movementdisorders.org/MDS/MDS-Rating-Scales/MDS-Unified-Parkinsons-Disease-Rating-Scale-MDS-UPDRS.htm.
49. https://parkinsonsnewstoday.com/2019/10/04/wearable-sensors-offer-way-of-ably-monitoring-day-to-day-movement-in-parkinsons-patients-study-says/.
50. https://www.wired.com/story/this-digital-pill-prototype-uses-bacteria-to-sense-stomach-bleeding/.
51. https://www.mobihealthnews.com/content/proteus-digital-pill-now-delivering-chemotherapy
52. https://mobihealthnews.com/content/etectrxs-ingestion-sensors-be-used-hiv-drug-study-brigham-and-womens-hospital.
53. https://www.iotforall.com/ai-and-iot-can-improve-cancer-treatment/.
54. https://www.theiotintegrator.com/health/sensors-that-detect-covid-19-could-be-in-your-next-face-mask.

Chapter 8
Ransomware: To Pay, or Not to Pay—That Is (One) Question

Melissa Markey

Contents

8.1   Introduction: Ransomware in Action

The day began much as any other. The morning shift arrived and began preparing for patients, checking schedules, preparing rooms, and planning procedures. Then, late in the morning of May 12, 2017, hospitals in the United Kingdom started reporting to the National Cyber Response Center that their information technology systems were inaccessible, locked by ransomware. The infections spread rapidly across the United Kingdom. By 4 p.m., the UK's National Health Service (NHS) declared a major incident and implemented its emergency management plan, shifting to

M. Markey (✉)
Hall, Render, Killian, Heath & Lyman, Heber City, UT, USA
e-mail: mmarkey@hallrender.com

© Springer Nature Switzerland AG 2022
F. D. Hudson (eds.), *Women Securing the Future with TIPPSS for Connected Healthcare*, Women in Engineering and Science,
https://doi.org/10.1007/978-3-030-93592-4_8

emergency operations to manage the operational changes required due to the massive ransomware infection. Over the course of approximately 8 h, the NHS had suffered an attack on their technology services that severely and adversely impacted operations for 1 week and had lasting repercussions for months. Even though cybersecurity researchers Marcus Hutchins and Jamie Hankins found a way to defang the ransomware within hours by sending it to a URL that was hard-coded in the exploit, which acted as a kill-switch and created a sinkhole, in the course of a single day over 200,000 computers worldwide had become infected. At least 80 of the 236 hospital trusts in the United Kingdom were impacted, either because they were infected, or because they had powered down technology to avoid infection [1]. In addition, 603 other NHS organizations were impacted, including 595 general practice physician offices [1].

The NHS had been hit by the WannaCry ransomware, which subsequent research indicated had significant commonalities in the techniques, tools, and infrastructure associated with Lazarus Group, a threat actor connected with North Korea [2]. While initially effective, the sinkhole didn't protect against the WannaCry attack for long. New variants were developed that didn't include the kill-switch. Since 2017, many new types of ransomware have been created; even today, ransomware remains a favored weapon of cybercriminals, and in 2021, ransomware gained front-page status as ransomware attacks took a major fuel pipeline offline, causing concerns about gasoline shortages, and hobbled operations at a major meat-processing company.

8.2   Ransomware in Healthcare

Even before these headline-grabbing attacks occurred, ransomware had been identified as a cyber threat of significant concern. While exact statistics vary, one security researcher noted an estimated sevenfold increase from 2019 to 2020 [3], while another reported a 50% increase in daily attacks in the third quarter of 2020 compared to the first half of 2020 [4]. The U.S. Department of Justice noted that ransomware attacks had increased from 1000 per day in 2015 to 4000 per day in 2016 [5]. In some sectors, ransomware is a predominant attack vector; Verizon reported in their 2020 Data Breach Investigation Report (DBIR) that approximately 80% of the reported cyberattacks in the education sector were attributable to ransomware [6]. Healthcare and government verticals are also often deliberate targets of ransomware threat actors.

In fact, ransomware as an attack vector had been posing an increasing threat to healthcare over the 3 years preceding the WannaCry attack [7]. Ransomware is commonly defined as malicious software that infects a computer or computer network and places that network, or the data stored on the network, under the control of a threat actor, either by locking the screen or by encrypting the data [8]. While some have characterized ransomware as not involving theft or sale of data [8], ransomware is becoming increasingly associated with exfiltration of data as a means of ensuring payment. Often referred to as "double-extortion," ransomware has become extortion enabled by cyber, as increasing numbers of threat actors are using data exfiltration and exposure to force payment of ever-higher ransom demands.

Healthcare is uniquely at risk of ransomware, for several reasons.

First, healthcare has highly valuable data, including a broad range of personal and corporate information. Basic patient demographic data is valuable on the dark web for purposes of identity theft; the addition of health insurance information increases the value, as medical identity theft is an even more profitable line of business. Healthcare data remains popular with cybercriminals due to the variety of data that is commonly included in the records, including data such as demographics, social security and national identity numbers, date of birth, and bank, credit card, health account, and other information. This data can be used for a variety of purposes, ranging from theft from the individual that is the subject of the record through access to accounts identified in the record, to opening lines of credit and bank accounts, tax fraud, and synthetic identity theft [9]. Because healthcare data can be exploited for a broad range of monetizable functions, the value of healthcare data is higher than the value of other stolen data [10]. Non-patient healthcare information is also valuable, for example, data related to physician licensure and billing information can be used for billing fraud.

Healthcare entities, particularly those that conduct clinical research, also frequently hold large amounts of intellectual property. As clinical research has expanded beyond academic medical centers to community health facilities and outpatient facilities, smaller hospitals and outpatient care locations with more limited budgets and resources for cybersecurity hold research data for innovations that hold great promise. Nation-states that are engaged in economic espionage may seek to access information about medical device and pharmaceutical innovations from the medical centers conducting the research, rather than the sponsoring company, on the theory that the healthcare provider will have less sophisticated defenses. Certain types of health information may also hold value for traditional espionage purposes, as bias persists regarding certain types of health conditions, and those in positions of confidence or trust may fear the disclosure of diagnoses.

Second, healthcare has a very low tolerance for loss of availability or integrity of data. Often when discussing cybersecurity in healthcare, the focus is on privacy and confidentiality of data. While confidentiality is undoubtedly important, integrity and availability of data are critical. Data privacy is necessary to ensure that patients confide freely to their healthcare providers regarding their health conditions and their habits. However, confidentiality, while often the focus of regulatory attention, is less likely to result in physical harm to a patient than in loss of integrity or availability. In recognition of the threats to integrity posed by ransomware, the National Cybersecurity Center of Excellence (NCCoE) at the U.S. National Institute of Standards and Technology (NIST) issued NIST Special Publication 1800-26, Data Integrity: Detecting and Responding to Ransomware and Other Destructive Events [11]. In this Special Publication, NIST noted that the NIST Cybersecurity Framework's functions of Identify, Protect, Detect, Respond, and Recover, can be used to quickly detect and respond to integrity attacks such as ransomware through the use of capabilities that focus on event detection, integrity monitoring, logging, reporting, mitigation, and forensics/analytics. A number of NIST standards and guidance were leveraged to develop a practice guide intended to support the development of plans to detect, respond to, and recover from data integrity events. The risk of incapacitation of operations and unauthorized changes to the data or assets of the entity merit implementation of technology, policies, and practices that focus on integrity.

Healthcare is also increasingly reliant on technology. As advances in technology unlock improved diagnostic and therapeutic capabilities, they simultaneously increase the risks associated with cybersecurity vulnerabilities. As a result, healthcare entities are often faced with a dilemma—to pay large amounts demanded as ransom, in hopes of receiving decryption keys that will unlock critically needed data, or to refuse to pay the ransom, revert to manual processes for recording data, and rebuild the entire system. Cyberattackers are attempting to remove any option by incorporating into the attack the exfiltration of sensitive data. One of the first cybercrime groups identified as using these tactics, techniques, and procedures (TTP) was Twisted Spider [12], the group primarily responsible for deployment of Maze ransomware [13]. Other cyber threat actors were not far behind. Not only does this provide additional sources of monetization to the attacker, it places pressure on the victim, by removing the possibility of simply restoring the system. Even if the victim has maintained pristine backups and is able to restore or rebuild a locked system without paying the ransom, the threat to publish data may well lead to a payment. The payment of the ransom, however, does not ensure that the exfiltrated data will not be exploited. There is no way to prove that the attacker has not created multiple copies, or already sold the data to one or more third parties who will further exploit the data. In some cases, entities that have paid the ransom in an attempt to buy silence find themselves extorted again; in some cases, where the victim failed to properly mitigate and remediate, the same threat actor has again exploited the vulnerability [14]. Alternatively, they may be notified by law enforcement at some future date that their data has been found on the dark web, offered for sale. As further evidence of the future monetization possibilities of the stolen data, new illicit marketplaces specializing in the sale of this data have been created, such as Marketo and File Leaks.

Maintaining the operational capabilities of healthcare is integral to orderly functioning of communities, and acts that bring into question the ability of healthcare to provide necessary services present a substantial threat not only to public health and safety, but to national security. Healthcare has been identified as critical infrastructure in the United States [15] and in the current Proposal for a Directive of the European Parliament and of the Council on the reliance of critical entities [16]; in the European Union, the European Union Agency for Cybersecurity (ENISA) also acknowledges healthcare as critical information infrastructure [17]. To ensure public health and safety, the public must have faith that the data held by healthcare entities—hospitals, clinics, physician offices, health insurers, pharmaceutical companies, and others—is safe, reliable, and protected from unauthorized access. Further, there must be confidence that healthcare services will be available when needed.

8.3 Technology and Policy Evolution

Ransomware, and approaches to prevent, defend against, and respond to ransomware, pose a complex technical and policy challenge. Cyber threat actors that engage in ransomware range from sophisticated nation-states to threat actors with limited skill and experience who have purchased ransomware and leverage the "ransomware-as-a-service" business model. The motivations of threat actors vary, from simply monetary, to economic espionage, to hacktivism. There is broad recognition that ransomware is a problem that must be solved; the economic and societal impact has reached global proportions. There is no simple solution. A comprehensive, policy-based approach is needed, which prioritizes the identification and prosecution of ransomware threat actors, imposes substantial penalties on threat actors and those that provide support to the threat actors, and provides support to ransomware victims. A fundamental requirement is the recognition that ransomware is not simply cybercrime committed for economic purposes. Ransomware has elements of state support, without which it would not be as successful, and which requires a broader public policy response than has been provided in the past.

Ransomware encompasses a broad range of variants, each of which has its own particular characteristics. The first known ransomware was created by an evolutionary biologist, Dr. Joseph Popp, who handed out software that purported to be a questionnaire regarding risk of infection with AIDS (Acquired Immunodeficiency Syndrome) at a World Health Organization (WHO) conference in 1989. When uploaded, the program hid files and changed names of files to strings of random characters, then demanded payment by mail. While the program was poorly written, it successfully disrupted the computers of AIDS researchers worldwide. However, ransomware didn't become big business for a number of years.

8.3.1 Technology Evolution

While there was some exploration of the concept of ransomware between 1995 and the early twenty-first century, it wasn't truly revived as an effective means of attack until about 2010. One of the challenges with early ransomware was creating an effective means of receiving the extorted money while providing pseudonymity and limiting traceability. The development of a viable cryptocurrency solution through the publication of *Bitcoin: A Peer-to-Peer Electronic Cash System* in 2008 [18] provided a relatively anonymous, transparent, internationally accessible method of payment that could be confirmed to permit immediate release of the decryption key. Suddenly, ransomware became scalable and easily monetized. Despite the development of other cryptocurrencies, bitcoin remains a favored form of payment for ransomware; however, it has become more difficult to completely obfuscate transactions and is increasingly subject to regulation. Know-your-customer, anti-money laundering, and other regulations may apply to transfers of cryptocurrencies [19], and cryptocurrency transaction analysis, such as provided by Chainalysis [20], permit visibility into currency transfers that help identify threat actors.

Further developments in technology, such as improvements in encryption and the development of ransomware-as-a-service [20], have further facilitated the growth of ransomware. There are estimates that a ransomware attack will occur every 11 s in 2021, with a cost of approximately $20 billion [20, 21]. Ransomware can infect almost every known type of computing device, including personal computers, laptops, mobile devices, and internet of things (IoT)/industrial control systems (ICS) [22, 23] including supervisory control and data acquisition networks (SCADA) that use programmable logic controllers (PLCs), and which are considered operational technology, rather than information technology [24].

8.3.2 Tactics, Techniques, and Procedures

Ransomware's evolution has affected its targets, its vectors of attack, and other tactics, techniques and procedures (TTPs). A common approach to evaluate the stages of a cyberattack is the cyber kill chain, which was developed by Lockheed Martin based on a military model. The idea of the cyber kill chain is that the attacker must complete all the steps in the chain to complete the attack; disrupting any of the steps stops the attack and prevents the accomplishment of the nefarious objective [25].

Different types of attacks have different cyber kill chains. Various analysts have described the ransomware cyber kill chain with varying stages and indeed, the kill chain may vary somewhat depending on whether the attack is targeted or general distribution, and whether exfiltration of data is involved. In general, however, the ransomware cyber kill chain will include common kill chain phases, such as:

- Reconnaissance (identification of targets)
- Weaponization (development of the ransomware, whether as a new variant or purchasing ransomware-as-a-service)
- Delivery (through phishing, waterhole, remote desktop protocol (RDP) attack, or other approaches)
- Exploitation (e.g., if a user-initiated action is required to trigger the attack)
- Installation (delivery of the infection to the target, which may include further spread through the network or to other, connected networks)
- Command and control (remote control of the infection)
- Delivery of the objective (delivery of the ransom note and/or exfiltration of data)

Not every ransomware variant implicates every phase of the cyber kill chain. For example, some ransomware requires a user-initiated action, such as a click on a malicious link or a visit to an infected website; others self-propagate like worms. Some, after they infiltrate the network, "phone home" to a command and control server for the encryption keys; others simply infect and encrypt. In those cases, the command and control phase may not be present. The importance of the cyber kill chain has traditionally been that each of the phases provides defenders an opportunity to intervene and disrupt the cyber threat actor. However, as valuable as the cyber kill chain concept is, it perpetuates the idea that this is solely a technical issue—that by implementing the proper safeguards or detection technology, the threatened entity can avoid becoming a victim. It disregards the impact of larger societal policies, such as tolerance of nation-state support of ransomware threat actors and lack of regulatory oversight of cryptocurrencies, in permitting threat actors to operate unencumbered.

Another useful analytical model is the MITRE ATT&CK model, which is a "...globally-accessible knowledge base of adversary tactics and techniques..." [26]. MITRE started the ATT&CK model to document adversary behaviors that were observed in the cyber investigations they conducted in the Windows operating environment. From there, it expanded to include techniques observed in attacks against macOS and Linux operating systems, and MITRE made the tool broadly available to the cybersecurity research community. This tool can be used to identify and classify techniques and tools used by threat actors, both to identify an attack, and to gain understanding of events and artifacts that may be identified in the environment [27]. ATT&CK also includes information about certain threat actors, which provides insight into preferred targets and motivations, and can be used in planning cyber defenses.

The U.S. Food and Drug Administration (FDA) worked with MITRE to leverage the ATT&CK tool to develop a standardized approach to using the Common Vulnerability Scoring System (CVSS) to conduct risk assessments for medical devices. The rubric for applying CVSS to medical devices [28] (the "CVSS Rubric") has been qualified by FDA as a medical device development tool (MDDT) [29], which indicates that the FDA has assessed the tool and, based on available evidence, has determined the tool works as intended and provides "...scientifically plausible measurements..." within the intended context of use [30]. The CVSS Rubric walks cybersecurity practitioners through a series of questions regarding the attack vector, attack complexity, privileges required, exploitability, impact (which includes considerations of confidentiality, integrity, and availability) as well as other considerations. The use of the CVSS Rubric provides a structured, standardized approach to the analysis of risks impacting medical devices. Through the use of the CVSS Rubric, a common language is provided that permits clear communication across the industry. This clarity, commonality, and standardization is valuable in information sharing and reporting; however, it may not be appropriate in all cases, and there is a learning and adoption curve.

In traditional analysis, ransomware is often viewed as simply a technical cybersecurity issue. The entity is responsible for implementing technology and administrative safeguards to protect against cyber threat actors. NIST has developed many resources that can be used to develop a program that assists with the cyber cycle established by the NIST Cybersecurity Framework of identify, protect, detect, respond, and recover [31]. To provide further direction, the Cybersecurity and Infrastructure Security Agency (CISA) created a "Bad Practices" website [32] intended to call out "exceptionally dangerous" practices, particularly for entities that are critical infrastructure or national critical functions. Originally focusing only on the use of unsupported or end-of-life software and use of known/default passwords, the "Bad Practices" is intended to focus on decisions that create "untenable risks" [33]. When a ransomware attack is identified, the focus is on the technical response—identification, containment, eradication, and recovery. The victim is blamed for not having implemented one or more security safeguards— or for inadequate training, or an employee's susceptibility to a phishing attack, or failing to withstand a brute force attack on remote desktop protocol. There is a belief that somehow, the victim of the cyberattack should have been able to prevent the attack—and that therefore, there should be a penalty imposed against the victim. As a result, there are regulatory requirements related to disclosure of the security breach, and at times, penalties are imposed.

8.3.3   Regulatory and Policy Evolution

Indeed, regulatory efforts to limit the impact of ransomware and other cyberattacks have traditionally focused solely on the entity that holds the data and manages the information security assets. As ransomware has increased in frequency and cost, law enforcement and health regulatory agencies in the United States, the United Kingdom, the European Union (EU), and globally, have increased regulatory requirements related to implementation of safeguards intended to protect data from the forced encryption and extortion that is the hallmark of ransomware. While there is no single privacy or cybersecurity law in the United States, most healthcare providers, health plans, and healthcare clearinghouses, the entities that contract with them to provide certain types of services, and certain other entities that are defined as "business associates" and handle health information, are required to implement technical, administrative, and physical safeguards to protect individually identifiable information under the Health Insurance Portability and Accountability Act of 1996 [34], as amended by the Health Information Technology for Economic and Clinical Health (HITECH) Act [35] and the implementing regulations [36] (collectively, HIPAA). These entities are also required to report most breaches of unsecured identifiable health information to the Office of Civil Rights. Other sources of cybersecurity and/or privacy requirements include the Gramm-Leach-Bliley Act [37], the Federal Trade Commission Act [38]; and the Fair Credit Reporting Act, as amended by the Fair and Accurate Transactions Act [39]. Finally, all 50 states have enacted breach notification laws, which have varying requirements regarding timing and whether there is a risk of harm. The General Data Protection Regulation (GDPR) [40] in the European Union also imposes breach notification requirements, as does the UK equivalent [41]. Most other countries have similar laws [1]. The

Regulation (EU) 2019/881 of the European Parliament and the EU Council of 17 April 2019 (the Cybersecurity Act) and the EU Network and Information Security (NIS) Directive impose further requirements for each Member State to develop cybersecurity for critical sectors, including health.

Despite the increasing regulatory requirements, and the fact that cybersecurity professionals have identified the risks to healthcare data from ransomware, including the loss or compromise of confidential patient information, loss of access to information critical to the care of patients and potential adverse impact on data integrity, entities in the healthcare sector continue to be victimized by ransomware. In the past 5 years, millions of health-related records have been encrypted by ransomware; hundreds of healthcare providers have been impacted and millions of dollars have been spent in mitigation and remediation efforts.

In one of the most detailed reviews of the impact of ransomware on healthcare, the Comptroller and Auditor General of the National Audit Office of the Department of Health in the United Kingdom issued the results of a thorough inquiry into the response of the NHS to the WannaCry cyberattack. During the week of May 12–May 18, 2017, the NHS confirmed that at least 6912 healthcare appointments were cancelled and estimated that more than 19,000 appointments were likely affected, based on the number of follow-up appointments that would likely have resulted from the original cancelled appointments. In five geographic areas, patients were unable to attend local emergency departments and had to travel further for emergency care. However, NHS did not collect data regarding the number of ambulances that were diverted, or the possible impact on patients of the diversion. An additional 92 NHS facilities were found to be infected, but not locked out of operation, by the ransomware; it was not clear whether these facilities remained operational due to the activation of the kill-switch that created a sinkhole. A total of 1220 diagnostic devices were identified as having been infected; and patient care was further disrupted as a result of isolating uninfected devices from the internet to avoid infection [1].

8.4   Data Integrity and Patient Safety

An underestimated threat from ransomware is the impact on data integrity and patient safety. While the focus of reporting related to ransomware often relates to the recovery of data, it is important to remember that ransomware also infects the functional technology that is critical to the provision of care. For example, ransomware can lock infusion pumps [42], and imaging machines such as magnetic resonance imaging (MRI) and computerized tomography (CT) machines. Further it can affect operational technology, such as heating, ventilation, and air conditioning (HVAC) machines, elevators, and lighting, further hindering basic, core functions necessary to daily operations. The inability to move patients between floors, to maintain tolerable ambient temperatures, and to provide necessary lighting for surgical suites can quickly bring a hospital to its knees; loss of freezers can ruin research and therapeutic products held by manufacturers and research universities. While most entities have generators to provide alternate sources of power, the control systems will be locked and unresponsive, and often disaster plans and incident response playbooks do not address this situation.

As automated processes in healthcare increase, the threats to data integrity and functionality also increase. Consider the potential patient safety impact if ransomware infected a surgical robot while the robot was in use, locking the robot until a ransom was paid or worse, threatening to disrupt the integrity of the operational data of the robot. In 2019, security researchers published a proof-of-concept (POC) ransomware attack, named Akerbeltz, against an industrial robot manufactured by Universal Robots, which had been demonstrated through penetration testing to have hundreds of vulnerabilities [43]. The POC attack could be accomplished through either physical access, via a Universal Serial Bus (USB) port, or via an adjacent network through exploitation of a buffer overflow vulnerability. The researchers were able to encrypt, disable the safety configuration, and block the mechanisms that had been created to permit re-establishment of normal operation, thereby locking the robot and triggering the display of a ransom demand. The security researchers indicated that further action to disable or damage the robot would be trivial [43].

While the Akerbeltz POC ransomware attack targeted an industrial robotic system, another team of researchers have already demonstrated that surgical robots are vulnerable to cybersecurity threats although this research did not focus on ransomware. In 2015, cybersecurity researchers at the University of Washington demonstrated the ability to hack a Raven II® [44] teleoperated research-capable surgical robot, which was designed to be operated remotely in austere environments [45]. Because this system is designed for austere environments, it can be operated using last-link wireless communication systems, which potentially increases attack vectors. Three types of possible attacks were identified: intention modification, where the attacker directly impacts the surgeon's intended actions by modifying packets in-flight; intention manipulation, where the attacker modifies the message transmitted from the robot to the surgeon, thus modifying the surgeon's response; and hijacking, in which the robot ignores the intended acts of the surgeon [45]. The success of these research-based attacks supports the possibility that ransomware could be transmitted to a surgical robot, overcoming the intended actions of the surgeon and potentially locking the robot, even in the midst of a surgical procedure [46].

These proof-of-concept robot attacks demonstrate vividly one of the potential risks of loss of availability when ransomware is leveraged against patient care technology. Similar losses of availability have been demonstrated in other known ransomware attacks that affected healthcare, including the WannaCry attack that impacted the UK's NHS, the Scripps ransomware attack of May 2021, which resulted in diversion of patients to other nearby healthcare facilities, and an attack in Germany which caused diversion of patients that initial reports indicated potentially contributed to a patient's death [47]. The threat to patient safety is relatively clear when one considers that technology relied on for safe treatment of patients that is vulnerable to ransomware ranges from surgical robots to ventilators, from intravenous infusion pumps to laboratory analytical instruments, and from imaging machines to life safety technology. Today's hospital is highly connected and technology-dependent, and the loss of availability of those resources can have an immediate and significant impact on the type and amount of care that can be safely provided.

When hospitals are faced with limitations in the care they are able to provide, they go on *diversion*—they notify Emergency Medical Services (EMS) agencies that they are unable to accept emergency patients and patient transfers, and divert those patients to other healthcare providers. In cases of ransomware, often the impact hospital will also have to cancel surgical cases and other appointments, and depending on the extent of the ransomware infection, in some cases patients that are currently being treated in the impacted hospital must be transferred to other facilities. These decisions are not made lightly. To divert an emergency patient that is facing a critical illness can potentially impact that patient's recovery and in some cases, the patient may not be able to tolerate the additional transport time. Cancellation of surgery and other appointments defers necessary medical treatment and increases the psychosocial burden on patients and caregivers. Transferring patients currently undergoing treatment at one facility to another facility is disruptive and can be psychologically and physiologically stressful. There are downstream impacts on the transporting agency and the receiving facilities as well. While the best option is to never suffer a ransomware attack, the next best option is to return to a stable operational status as quickly as possible.

The impact of data breach on patient safety was identified in a 2017 study conducted at Vanderbilt University's Owen Graduate School of Management. When outcome measures for acute myocardial infarction (AMI), as reflected in Medicare quality data, were compared for hospitals that had reported a data breach versus those that had not, hospitals that had suffered a data breach demonstrated an increase in 30-day AMI mortality rate, while non-breached hospitals showed a trend of decreased 30-day AMI mortality due to improvements in care [48]. Interestingly, the increase in the 30-day AMI mortality rate persisted for 2 years after the date the breach was reported [48]. Given that this study reflected data breaches that predated the increased occurrence of ransomware, the potential significance of ransomware on safety comes into sharper focus. The Healthcare and Public Health Sector Coordinating Councils of the U.S. Department of Health and Human Services (HHS), published *Health Industry Cybersecurity Practices: Managing Threats and Protecting Patients* [49] as the work product of the 405(d) Task Group established by the Cybersecurity Act of 2015. The Cybersecurity Practices document is intended to represent [50] voluntary principles, based on the consensus of the members of the Task Group, that are helpful to mitigate the five most significant cybersecurity threats facing healthcare, including ransomware. The Task Group specifically identified patient safety as a concern, including risks related to connected medical devices, which are less likely to be protected by information technology security safeguards such as end point detection and intrusion monitoring solutions. However, as noted, these devices can pose significant patient safety risks if they are infected with malware. The Cybersecurity Practices document describes the most impactful threats and provides general security information related to those threats; this document is then supported by Technical Volumes for Small [51] and Medium-to-Large [52] Healthcare Organizations that provide additional information regarding safeguards to prioritize.

Another contributing factor is the fact that often medical devices are built on off-the-shelf (OTS) operating systems that go out-of-support and present vulnerabilities that remain unpatched. It can be difficult to maintain patch currency; the device vendor will not release a patch until it has been tested against the proprietary device software to ensure that the patch does not impact the operation of the device; meanwhile the device remains vulnerable to security threats in the wild. The U.S. Food and Drug Administration (FDA) has emphasized that " . . . manufacturers [of medical devices that incorporate computing technology] should monitor, identify and address cybersecurity vulnerabilities and exploits as part of [the device's] postmarket management . . . " [53]. The use of OTS operating systems permits the manufacturer to focus on the application itself, without developing proprietary code for the operating system and other common functionality, but it prevents the manufacturer from exercising control over the entire software development life cycle [54]. The cadence of security updates, particularly those that relate to OTS, makes it difficult for medical device manufacturers to fully test and integrate OTS security updates into the medical device, and many device companies fear that such action would constitute a change requiring filing of a marketing update. The FDA has prescribed a risk-based approach to validation and implementation of cybersecurity patches, recognizing that responsibility for cybersecurity is shared, and that attention to the security of medical devices is required throughout the life of the device [53]. The FDA distinguishes between routine cybersecurity patches, which they define as "changes to a device to increase device security and/or remediate only those vulnerabilities associated with controlled risk of patient harm . . . " [53], and therefore do not trigger FDA reporting obligations, from remediation measures that are actions taken to manage an uncontrolled risk of patient harm caused by a cybersecurity vulnerability [53]. The FDA has stated clearly and repeatedly that most OTS security updates and patches are not considered changes to a medical device that require a report to the FDA under 21 CFR part 806 [53], and that typically such updates and patches do not constitute a change to the medical device that requires submission of a 510(k) [55].

It is not clear whether this interpretation remains reasonable. Since the issuance of the 2016 Postmarket Cybersecurity Guidance, ransomware attacks have increased to approximately 4000 per day. Hospitals have been forced to divert patients. There have been reports of patients impacted by the unavailability of resources to provide care, and a study has identified a statistically significant long-term adverse impact on mortality in patients with acute myocardial infarction [56]. In some cases, healthcare entities have permanently closed after refusing to pay the ransom resulting in destruction of all the entity's records, including backups which had been infected by the ransomware [57, 58]. These significant adverse outcomes suggest that ransomware that causes failures of medical devices and operational capacity might constitute an uncontrolled risk of patient harm.

8.5 Do No Harm

A more direct allegation of harm is reflected in the lawsuit filed against Springhill Medical Center, which suffered a ransomware attack in July, 2019 [59]. The lawsuit alleges that due to the ransomware attack, fetal heart monitors commonly used to monitor the baby's heart rate to identify distress during labor were not functional. As a result, indicators that the baby was suffering distress, which may have typically resulted in an emergency cesarean section, were missed.

Despite the threat that even a momentary disruption of healthcare technology services can pose, some cyber threat actors intentionally target healthcare. Some mistakenly believe that targeting healthcare will result in faster, more reliable payment of ransom. However, the attackers seem to not realize first, that any outage can result in damage; nor do they understand the complexity of the systems in question, which prevents an immediate recovery once operations are disrupted.

The impact is even greater when the disruption affects a hospital or health system that is already under stress, such as that experienced during the COVID-19 pandemic [60]. As hospitals moved to Crisis Standards of Care (CSC) to respond to the pandemic, patient flows were modified, in an attempt to maintain providing care to those in need. However, diversion of patients placed strain on the receiving facilities, which resulted in further diversion and, eventually, the inability to provide care to all in need. When a cyber incident is superimposed on this highly stressed system, it results in excess deaths—the difference between the expected number of deaths, and the observed number of deaths in a specified period [60]. This strain is not merely experienced during the acute phase of a ransomware attack but it continues to adversely impact the healthcare system for weeks or months after the attack [60].

8.6 Ransomware Across the World

On May 7, 2021, Colonial Pipeline, which is responsible for about 45% of the gasoline and petroleum products across the Eastern United States, announced that its information technology systems had been hacked. Relatively quickly, a hacker group called DarkSide was identified as responsible, and speculation began that a nation-state was behind the attack. DarkSide quickly responded to this allegation, stating that "...we are apolitical, we do not participate in politics, do not need to tie us with a defined government [sic]...our goal is to make money, and not create problems for society..." [61]. In fact, while this attack apparently did not affect Colonial Pipeline's operational technology, and Colonial successfully restored operations in about a week (reportedly after paying over $4 Million in ransom), this attack brought an intense spotlight on DarkSide. Rules related to transportation of petrochemicals in the United States were temporarily suspended [62] to decrease the impact although a run on gasoline still occurred, resulting in shortages. The FBI confirmed that they were working with the company and "government partners" on the investigation [63] confirming that the threat actor was DarkSide and issued a National Cyber Awareness System Traffic Light Protocol (TLP) Green Alert with Best Practices for preventing disruption [64].

The disruption caused by the DarkSide ransomware attack had far-reaching effects. DarkSide published on its blog site that it would "... introduce moderation and check each company that our partners want to encrypt to avoid social consequences in the future..." [65]. In less than a week, DarkSide's blog noted that it was going out of business, after its servers were seized by an unidentified country, and its funds were "... transferred to an unknown account..." [66]. In the same post, REvil representatives claimed that the REvil program was imposing restrictions on the types of entities that affiliates were permitted to hold for ransom, and that healthcare and educational institutions were off-limits [66]. Very few in healthcare cybersecurity felt reassured; a similar announcement had been made at the beginning of the COVID-19 pandemic but only a week after that announcement, another healthcare entity suffered a ransomware attack. Contrary to the claim of avoiding healthcare entities, some groups seem to target healthcare, knowing that access to data and devices is critical to restoring operations.

As another response to the Colonial Pipeline attack, the White House added the final touches to an executive order that was already in the works and released the Executive Order on Improving the Nation's Cybersecurity [67], setting forth significant actions intended to improve the cybersecurity posture of U.S. federal agencies. The Executive Order included actions intended to improve sharing of cybersecurity information by federal contractors; adopting zero-trust architecture as a federal computing system standard; improving software supply chain security; establishment of a Cybersecurity Safety Review Board, to conduct after-action review and reports related to cybersecurity events; creating standardized federal incident response playbooks and otherwise improving incident response and investigation capabilities; and improving detection of cybersecurity incidents on federal computer networks [67]. While the Executive Order focuses on federal computing systems, it will have a significant impact, as many of the mandates will "flow down" to U.S. government contractors that store or process data on behalf of the U.S. government.

News reports indicate that Colonial Pipeline recovered largely in spite of the payment of $4.4 million in ransom, not because of it. While in this case a decryption code was delivered, it worked very slowly [68] and much of the remediation was accomplished through traditional means by the Colonial Pipeline Information Technology (IT) team.

Barely a week later, the Irish health system, including both the Irish Department of Health and the ministry-level Health Service Executive (HSE), was hit by a ransomware attack by Conti, likely dropped by a cybercrime gang. The reported ransom demand was $20 million. After several days offline, and repeated statements by the HSE that no ransom would be paid, the threat actor announced that it was providing a decryptor without charge, to permit recovery of files critical to the operation of impacted health facilities. However, the threat of public disclosure of sensitive files, including identifiable health information, remained in place unless a ransom was paid. The HSE obtained from the Irish High Court an injunction prohibiting the sale, publication, sharing or making available of the stolen data, and further prohibiting the possession, transfer, or disclosure of information taken from HSE's computer network without consent from HSE [70]. While it is extremely unlikely that this will have any impact on the cyber criminals, it does put third parties that might unwittingly facilitate the crime, such as internet service providers, social media sites, and others, on notice that furthering the crime is not permissible.

On May 31, 2021, the criminal gang REvil reportedly hacked JBS SA, a multinational company headquartered in Brazil that is the world's largest meat packing company, deploying ransomware and halting operations in Australia and North America for several days [71]. Production lines were disrupted and there was concern regarding potential impacts on the supply chain. There were reports that meat processing operations decreased by 22% and wholesale prices for certain types of beef increased by 1% [72]. However, JBS reportedly had intact backup files, and recovery of operations was accomplished by June 3, 2021 [73]—just in time for Fujifilm to report that they had been attacked by ransomware. It was later reported that JBS paid a ransom of approximately $11 Million in Bitcoin to "avoid further disruption" [74]. Because there is no assurance of success, and because payment of the ransom or extortion demanded by the attacker often goes to fund further criminal behavior, law enforcement typically recommend against payment. There have been some who have proposed that it be made illegal to pay to recover from a ransomware attack. In one Op-Ed, the idea was postulated that payment of ransom should be made a federal crime, although the examples that the opinion opened with were municipalities that refused to pay, and ended up expending far more resources in rebuilding their systems [69]. Noting that the cost of ransom is often lower than the cost of rebuilding the system, the author stated that there is a moral imperative that municipalities, in particular, not support criminals by paying them for committing crime. An alternative approach is proposed, where the federal government provides support for recovery and prevention, including a focus on the "... need to have backups of critical data" [69]. While attractive at first blush, those who have actually dealt with ransomware in critical infrastructure quickly recognize that this approach is a bit too facile. While backups of critical data are indeed important, prohibiting the payment of ransom requires a more significant basis than simply an attempt to change an economic model of cybercrime.

8.7 Policy Action

This rash of attacks on major corporations garnered significant attention. The most senior levels have focused on the issue, including at the U.S. Department of Justice and the White House. A number of approaches have been proposed, including increased coordination of law enforcement, and communication through senior diplomatic channels to countries that harbor the hackers, demanding that action be taken to prosecute cyber criminals. The Department of Justice, via an internal memorandum, directed that all investigations involving ransomware be reported to the Cyber Task Force, to permit identification of connections between threat actors and improve the possibility of identifying points of disruption [75]. Calls to prohibit the payment of ransom have increased, claiming that ransomware and double-extortion will end if it ceases to be economically favorable.

A factor that is often missed in the discussions of whether payment of ransom is reasonable is the fact that the issue may not be related to recovery of data; it may be related to the need to recover operational capability, either as related to medical internet of things (IoT) devices, or operational technology such as elevators, HVAC systems, and lighting. While the proposals that seek to prohibit payment of ransom are well-meaning, the scenarios that are used in the underlying analysis address only the recovery of data. Rarely is the difference between loss of data and loss of technology distinguished. Analysts rarely, if ever, consider the role of ransom payments in the recovery of critical infrastructure operational technology. There is a fundamental difference in the cost-benefit calculus when considering the impact of remaining in an inoperable status when considering the functional technology of critical infrastructure. When critical infrastructure mission-critical devices are inoperable due to an attack, the speed of returning functionality may merit a much higher weight than the economic values that are typically cited in cost-benefit analyses.

On April 20, 2021, John Carlin, the Acting Deputy Attorney General for the U.S. Department of Justice (DOJ), issued an internal Memorandum advising of the creation of a Ransomware and Digital Extortion Task Force ("Task Force"). The goals of the Task Force are to sharpen and concentrate the resources of the DOJ to combat ransomware and digital extortion, through a number of mechanisms: improved training; improved coordination and leveraging of intelligence across the department; strengthening public–private partnerships and working with federal partners; and working in collaboration with international partners to share information and collaborate in preventing, responding to, and mitigating ransomware threats [76].

This was not the first action by the Department of Justice against ransomware. The Federal Bureau of Investigation (FBI) has been active in the investigation and support of ransomware victims for years. Three months earlier, the Department of Justice had participated in a "coordinated international law enforcement action . . ." against infrastructure components that were supporting the NetWalker ransomware [77]. In this case, one of the affiliates, a Canadian national, was indicted [78], $454,530.19 in cryptocurrency was seized, and a dark web portal taken down [79] in collaboration with European authorities. This was only days following the Emotet takedown, in which hundreds of servers that had been infected with Emotet were recovered and redirected [80].

Reflecting the sharply increased concern regarding ransomware, the Institute for Security and Technology (IST) convened a Ransomware Task Force (RTF), which issued a "Comprehensive Framework for Action: Key Recommendations from the Ransomware Task Force" [81] on April 29, 2021. The recommendations of the IST's

Ransomware Task Force, while US-centric, sought to emphasize the need for international cooperation and action, noting that ransomware is a global crime, which "... transcends business, government, academic, and geographic boundaries" [81]. Many of the suggestions involve the creation of additional governmental bodies, to take the lead on offensive strategies related to anti-ransomware campaigns, the exercise of governmental soft power to discourage nation-states from directly or indirectly supporting ransomware threat actors, and development of frameworks to prepare for, prevent, detect, respond to, and recover from ransomware attacks [81].

A common developing theme is the need for a holistic approach that disrupts the business model that supports ransomware as an economic activity. There have been a number of calls for criminalizing the payment of ransom to recover systems affected by ransomware. The basis for these calls range from an argument that payment simply encourages criminals to concerns that payment may constitute the provision of support to terrorist and other sanctioned organizations. On October 1, 2020, the U.S. Department of the Treasury issued an Advisory on Potential Sanctions Risks for Facilitating Ransomware Payments [82] (the "OFAC Advisory") in which the Office of Foreign Assets Control (OFAC) "... highlight[ed] the sanctions risks associated with ransomware payments related to malicious cyber-enabled activities ... " [82]. The OFAC Advisory stated that organizations that facilitated the payment of ransomware ransoms, including forensics and digital response firms and cyber insurance companies, might be at risk of violating OFAC regulations, if the recipient of the ransom is subject to sanctions.

8.7.1 Sanctions

The United States maintains several different sanctions programs, only some of which are administered by OFAC. The OFAC administered sanctions are intended to accomplish foreign policy and national security goals, and the bases for sanctions range from counterterrorism to countering narcotics trafficking. OFAC has specific authority for cyber-related sanctions, including the National Emergencies Act [83], the International Emergency Economic Powers Act [84], and the Information on Countering America's Adversaries Through Sanctions Act [85].

In understanding the intent and application of the sanctions rules, it is helpful to understand their history. In 2015, President Obama issued Executive Order 13694 [86], which authorizes the imposition of sanctions on individuals and entities that are determined to be responsible or complicit in malicious cyber-enabled activities that pose a threat to national security, economic health, or financial stability of the United States, and that results in harm, compromise, disruption of services, misappropriation of funds, trade secrets, or personal identifiers, or loss of availability of computers or networks of critical infrastructure, or that otherwise meet specified criteria. Executive Order 13757 was issued on January 3, 2017 [87], which amended Executive Order 13694 to cover misappropriation of information, and specifically identified certain individuals and entities based in Russia as subject to sanctions. Since the issuance of the Executive Orders, OFAC has added a number of individuals and entities to the Sanctions List that have been identified as responsible for significant malicious cyber activities and added to OFAC's Specially Designated Nationals and Blocked Persons List (SDN) [88]. Among the cyber threat actors that OFAC has sanctioned are Evgeniy Mikhailovich Bogachev, developer of CryptoLocker [89], Ali Khorashadizadeh and Mohammad Ghorbaniyan, who assisted with bitcoin exchange activities associated with SamSam ransomware attacks [90], North Korean hacking groups Lazarus Group, Bluenoroff, and Andariel [91], and Russian-based Evil Corp, including its leader Maksim Yakubets for development and distribution of Dridex malware [92]. In March, 2018, Russian cyber threat actors were sanctioned for election interference and malicious cyberattacks, including NotPetya [93] and in October 2020, sanctions were imposed against the State Research Center of the Russian Federation FGUP Central Scientific Research Institute of Chemistry and Mechanics (TsNIKhM), a Russian government-controlled research institution that developed the tools responsible for Triton malware, which attacked industrial control system (ICS) safety controls [94].

Despite the increased diligence due to the OFAC sanctioning process, nation-state hacking efforts continue to expand. In response, on April 15, 2021, President Biden issued the Executive Order on Blocking Property with Respect to Specified Harmful Foreign Activities of the Government of the Russian Federation [95]. This Executive Order authorized broad sanctions against Russian-based threat actors that engaged in any malicious cyber-based activities, including interference with elections and the SolarWinds breach. It further authorizes sanctions against any citizen or national of the Russian Federation, or an entity organized under the laws of the Russian Federation involved in " . . . cutting or disrupting gas or energy supplies to Europe, the Caucasus, or Asia . . . " [95]. A Fact Sheet, accompanying the Executive Order, specifically attributed the Solar Winds breach to a unit of the Russian Foreign Intelligence Service (SVR) " . . . also known as APT 29, Cozy Bear, and The Dukes . . . " [96]. The National Security Agency (NSA), CISA, and FBI also issued a *Joint Advisory on Russian SVR Targeting U.S. and Allied Networks*, with details regarding the five zero-day exploits used to compromise target networks [97, 98].

As a result of the April 15, 2021, Executive Order, several technology companies were added to OFAC sanctions lists for supporting Russian Intelligence Services: ERA Technopolis; Pasit, AO; Federal State Autonomous Scientific Establishment Scientific Research Institute Specialized Security Computing Devices and Automation (SVA); Neobit, OOO; Advanced Systems Technology, AO (AST); and Pozitiv Teknolodzhiz, AO (Positive Technologies). Neobit, AST, and Positive Technologies were also sanctioned under prior Executive Orders. Russian Intelligence Services, including the Federal Security Services (FSB), the Main Intelligence Directorate (GRU), and Foreign Intelligence Service (SVR) had been sanctioned previously, under prior Executive Orders. It is possible that the increased attention to the possibility of sanctions explains the immediate posting by DarkSide at the time of the Colonial Pipeline attack that they were only interested in money, and not motivated by geopolitical concerns.

As the list of sanctioned individuals and entities grows, the risk of violating OFAC sanctions laws when paying a ransom to recover devices locked by ransomware also grows. Generally, individuals and entities in the United States are prohibited under the International Emergency Economic Powers Act and the Trading with the Enemy Act [99] from engaging directly or indirectly in transactions with individuals or entities that are subject to sanctions under U.S. law. Civil penalties for violation of sanctions laws may be imposed on a strict liability basis; liability may exist even if the individual or entity did not know, and had no reason to know, that a payment constituted a prohibited transaction under the OFAC sanctions authority. OFAC has promulgated Enforcement Guidelines [100] which describe the factors that OFAC considers when determining the appropriate enforcement action, including possible assessment of a civil penalty. Among those factors are the existence of a risk-based compliance program, which is intended to mitigate exposure to sanctions violations.

The OFAC Advisory also notes that "...full and timely..." reporting of a ransomware attack will be considered a significant mitigating factor if ransom is paid, and if there is later determined to be a sanctions violation. The victim must self-initiate the report to law enforcement, and under OFAC's regulations, a report is considered self-initiated only if it is approved by senior management [100]. OFAC also encourages victims (and those assisting victims) to contact OFAC if "...they believe a request for a ransomware payment may involve a sanctions nexus" [82]. Theoretically, it is possible to receive a license from OFAC to overcome a transactions sanction; however, the OFAC Advisory notes that there is a "...presumption of denial" for license applications for permission to pay ransom related to malicious cyber activities [82]. Finally, OFAC cautions that some transactions related to payment of ransom may trigger regulatory obligations under Financial Crimes Enforcement Network (FinCEN) regulations [82].

The Department of the Treasury issued an Updated Advisory on Potential Sanctions Risks for Facilitating Ransomware Payments on September 21, 2021 (the "Updated Advisory"). In the Updated Advisory, OFAC noted that the demand for ransomware payments had increased during the COVID-19 pandemic and emphasized that the "...U.S. government strongly discourages all private companies and citizens from paying ransom or extortion demands..." [101]. Rather, the government encourages hardening computer environments and improving resilience to protect against ransomware attacks. OFAC emphasizes that sanctions violations are strict liability and notes that payments made to comprehensively sanctioned jurisdictions and to actors with a sanctions nexus merely perpetuate the ransomware problem and can fund other nefarious activities such as terrorism. However, under the OFAC Enforcement Guidelines, the "...existence, nature and adequacy of a sanctions compliance program..." may be considered by OFAC in determining the appropriate enforcement response to an apparent sanctions violation. A proactive development of a risk-based sanctions compliance program is an important measure to minimize the risk of sanctions violations; similarly, implementation of strong cybersecurity measures, including those in the CISA September 2020 Ransomware Guide [102], and immediate notification to and cooperation with law enforcement during a cyberattack, are all factors that may support a non-public response, such as a No-Action Letter, from OFAC. Because these rules impact the forensics vendors and cybersecurity insurers, significant due diligence is conducted prior to payment of the ransom in an attempt to minimize the risk that the payment is made to a sanctioned jurisdiction, individual, or entity. In the event, there is any reason to suspect a payment is made to a sanctioned party, notification to OFAC provides significant mitigation.

Taken together, the OFAC Advisory and the Updated Advisory provide a mixed message. The Treasury has made it clear that payment of ransom is against the policy of the United States and that a request for a license is likely going to be denied. However, the OFAC Advisory and Updated Advisory also seem to recognize that there may be times that payment is a reasonable decision. That flexibility will only be available to those entities that have taken steps to harden the environment and put appropriate controls in place, and that are willing to work with law enforcement. It will also require the conduct of due diligence in the midst of incident response to determine the likelihood that the ransomware threat actor is subject to OFAC sanctions. This introduces a wild card into the risk benefit analysis, particularly because the decision regarding payment of the ransom typically must be made early in the response effort, when there is limited information regarding attribution of the attack to the threat actor. There are some situations in which attribution is relatively clear; for example, in hacktivism situations, the threat actor is clearly identifiable through behavioral analysis or known indicators of compromise. In many cases, particularly given the prevalence of ransomware-as-a-service, it can be difficult to identify the threat actor with certainty early in the response. Even with the involvement and assistance of cyber law enforcement agents, there can be hesitancy to attribute the attack with certainty. While healthcare organizations tend to dismiss the possibility of sanctioned entities as the attacker, Chainalysis determined that 15% of all ransomware payments made in 2020 had a potential sanctions nexus [103]. Therefore, as a best practice, healthcare entities should consider adding to ransomware playbooks both consultation with law enforcement, querying of the OFAC SDN Sanctions List, and consultation with qualified legal counsel prior to payment of ransom.

8.7.2 Do Not Punish the Victim

The proposals regarding prohibition of the payment of ransom and imposition of strict liability on healthcare institutions and providers that pay ransom to recover critical health technology capabilities, however, should be carefully considered. In many ways, these proposals simply revictimize entities that are already victims. This is particularly true where the entity or institution has implemented reasonable technical, physical, and administrative safeguards, but is still subject to a successful ransomware attack. The fact that an attack is successful, or that a vulnerability remains, does not mean that the institution failed. Cybersecurity does not require that every possible vulnerability is addressed, and that no risk remains. To impose that standard ensures failure.

The principal theories of criminal justice in the United States on which criminal laws are based are restorative justice, retributive justice, and transformative justice. Classical criminal justice theory focuses on punishment—let the punishment fit the crime. Where an act has been declared to be illegal, retributive justice demands that any who commit that act must suffer a punishment, and the severity of the punishment must be proportionate to the harm caused by the crime. Retributive justice therefore focuses on deterrence—to prevent the crime, ensure that the punishment is both severe and repugnant, and demands accountability for the act that offends society. Restorative justice, in comparison, requires the offender to take responsibility, but permits those who are affected by the crime to help determine the punishment. The goal is to repair the harm caused by the crime. Transformative justice seeks to balance the inequality that is thought to underlie crime, encouraging social solutions to minimize criminal behavior.

Transformative justice and restorative justice theories are most commonly implemented in the context of interpersonal crimes, where social equities are identified as contributing to the criminal behavior. These approaches seem less apropos in the context of cybercrime, and particularly cyberattacks in which the threat actor is either a nation-state, a major criminal organization, or otherwise purely economically motivated. Therefore, the criminal justice theory that is most likely to apply is the retributive justice theory.

While attribution is always a challenge, to the extent a cyberattack can be attributed, retribution in the form of imprisonment for ransomware and extortion that sequesters and improperly discloses sensitive data is appropriate. Is it appropriate, however, to threaten retribution against an entity who seeks to recover that data by paying the criminal ransom? In that case, the organization is simply attempting to recover its property from the thief; it is seeking to protect the sensitive data of its patients, clients, or customers. Where the state imposes a punishment, it does so on the moral basis that the punished entity or individual acted to harm society. Thus, the question becomes whether payment to recover the functionality of critical infrastructure technology, or to protect sensitive data from exposure, is more protective of society, by returning the hospital to operation more quickly, by making healthcare services available to those in need with less delay, and by protecting private data; or is more damaging, by permitting a cyberattacker to operate another day.

To argue that payment of ransom is the greater societal harm assumes, first, that the ransomware was deployed for purposes of financial profit. While ransomware-as-a-service ("RaaS") has certainly grown into a significant economic activity, and there is a significant economic component to ransomware, not all ransomware is deployed for economic purposes. In fact, WannaCry, the ransomware that opened our discussion, has been attributed by some experts to Russian government-sponsored hackers [104]. The query remains whether the goal of the creators of

WannaCry was to collect ransom or to achieve other purposes. The same may be true of other ransomware variants.

It may be instructive to consider parallel criminal laws, such as criminal extortion. Under U.S. law, it is a crime to "... transmit[] in interstate or foreign commerce any communication containing any threat to injure the property or reputation ... " of the person or entity to whom the communication is addressed, or to another [105]. The "threatening nature of the communication ... " is the crux of what makes the communication illegal [106]. Further, under the Hobbs Act, it is illegal to interfere with interstate commerce, including by extortion, which is defined as "... the obtaining of property from another, with his consent, induced by wrongful use of actual or threatened force, violence or fear ... " [107]. The impact on interstate commerce need not be substantial to trigger the Hobbs Act; since the Supreme Court held that the market for illegal drugs meets standards for interstate commerce as a matter of law [108], without question, legitimate healthcare operations meet this standard. Further, the threat need not be of physical harm. In an unpublished opinion, the Ninth Circuit noted that the Hobbs Act followed the Travel Act; when not further limited, "extortion" included reputational threats [109].

8.7.3 Limiting the Impact

There is no question that cyber threat actors have every intention that the ransom notes that appear as ransomware is deployed, be viewed as threats; and, to ensure compliance, the threat actors carry out the threat to destroy or disclose sensitive data if the ransom is not paid in a timely manner. Further, it is clear that the reputation of healthcare organizations is damaged by ransomware threats and posting of sensitive and confidential information.

While the notification requirements decrease the protection from reputational damage that might be gained by paying the ransom, there might still be advantages in the time to recovery, if the decryption keys provided by the threat actor are effective, and the data is recovered in good condition. There is, however, a risk to data integrity that is associated with the encryption and decryption process that occurs with ransomware, and data integrity must be reviewed.

The question of whether it is appropriate to impose a penalty on entities that pay to recover their data and systems from cyber threat actors becomes even more complicated when one considers the fact that economic gain may not have been the motivation for the attack in the first place. There are two primary theories that support the proposal to prohibit payment of ransom, or extortion, to cyber threat actors. The first is that by removing the economic incentive for the attack, ransomware and extortion will decrease; in effect, crime will not pay. The second is that payments may be supporting terrorism or otherwise constitute payments in violation of sanctions and export laws. By penalizing the entity that pays the ransom or extortion payment, potential financial support to individuals and entities that have been identified by the government in question will be interdicted, thus furthering governmental policies.

These arguments are not without merit. Criminals do, indeed, go where there is profit; if there are no payments to be made, then there are those threat actors that will not engage in the crime. However, this view anticipates that the profit is made from the payment of the ransom or the initial extortion payment, and that there is no other financial benefit to the threat actor. This is a limited, and incorrect, perception. The crime has evolved. Originally, data was encrypted, and decryption was provided upon payment of the ransom. Then, when victims resisted payment, threat actors began exfiltrating data, and extorting payment by threatening to post the data. Now, threat actors are omitting the encryption; rather, there is simply the exfiltration of data and resulting extortion [110].

To penalize the victim by criminalizing one possible means of recovery fails to meet any of the goals of criminal justice philosophy. As noted by Europol, "[t]here is also the need to foster a culture of acceptance and transparency when organisations or individuals fall victim to cybercrime. Re-victimising victims after a cyberattack is counterproductive and a significant challenge, as law enforcement need companies and individuals who have been subject of a crime to come forward . . . ".[1] To identify, track, and prosecute cybercriminals, law enforcement needs the cooperation of the victim; the threat of prosecution for any action taken by the victim in response to a cyberattack will prevent the victim from engaging with law enforcement. In fact, for several years, healthcare entities were very resistant to communicating with law enforcement when they were attacked, due to fears that information learned by law enforcement would be used against the entity for enforcement actions. Through the diligent efforts of FBI and Secret Service cyber teams, the message that the entities are viewed as the victims has been clearly heard, and relationships have been developed that overcome this fear. To prohibit payment of ransom and threaten any type of enforcement action related to recovery from a cyberattack will destroy that relationship of trust and will slam the door on communication with law enforcement.

Neither is enforcement at the victim level the best approach to efficient enforcement. As is well demonstrated in Josephine Wolff's book *You'll see this message when it is too late*, enforcement action is most effectively taken at choke points— those steps in the process that provide single points, or limited points, of failure. Often, this is the point at which payment changes hands, as even with cryptocurrency there are limited means to transfer value. Through increased regulation of cryptocurrency, including extension of Know Your Customer (KYC) and Money Laundering regulations, the same goals of removing the economic incentives for the deployment of cryptocurrency can be accomplished much more efficiently.

---

[1] Internet Organised Crime Threat Assessment (IOCTA) Executive Summary.

8.7.4 Developing Protections and Resilience

There has been increasing focus on the threat that ransomware poses, and on the need for more effective responses to this threat. The recent Executive Order that focuses on improvements in cybersecurity for the federal government and its contractors, the creation of the Department of Justice Task Force and the report by the Institute for Security and Technology, the Department of Treasury's Advisory regarding the possible application of OFAC sanctions, and the imposition of sanctions on cyber threat actors, all demonstrate the increasing concern about the impact of ransomware on both critical infrastructure, and the international economy. The Department of Justice recently announced that it was establishing a Civil Cyber-Fraud Initiative to ensure that federal contractors who have responsibility for processing and safeguarding governmental data meet the required cybersecurity standards. Failure to comply with the regulatory and contractual standards applicable to federal contractors and grant recipients will be pursued as violations of the civil False Claims Act [111]. CISA, in collaboration with the FBI and the National Security Agency, continues to engage in information sharing to help identify threat actors and note trends to assist in defenses.

A multi-faceted, broad-based response to ransomware is critical, and that response must be coordinated internationally. However, recognizing the urgency of this reaction, further victimizing the victims is not the proper approach. Imposing sanctions on ransomware victims, either because payment of the ransom is the only way to recover devices that for some reason cannot be backed up or recovered, or because the time necessary for recovery puts critical infrastructure operations at unacceptable risk, is inadvisable. Attacking the problem at the narrowest point of failure, payment, is prudent, but it is critical to ensure that in doing so, we do not unduly tie the hands of those who seek to keep critical infrastructure operational.

A recurring theme is that of resilience. There have been many attempts to define resilience; in Presidential Policy Directive 21: Critical Infrastructure Protection and Resilience (PPD 21) [112] resilience is defined as "... the ability to prepare for and adapt to changing conditions and withstand and recover rapidly from disruptions." However, in today's world, resilience must mean more. According to NIST, cyber resiliency is "... the ability to anticipate, withstand, recover from, and adapt to adverse conditions, stresses, attacks, or compromises on systems that use or are enabled by cyber resources" [113]. Cyber resilient systems are able to withstand attacks and maintain operational functionality, and continuity of mission-critical operations, while ensuring that safety and security of information are preserved [113]. A key assumption is that the cyber resilient organization may be attacked by a skilled, tenacious adversary who is capable of establishing persistence in the network, living off the land and reacting to attempts to identify and eradicate the invader. To develop a cyber resilient system, not only is there an assumption of a successful attack; there is an assumption that the network has been compromised by an advanced persistent threat (APT), and that each move the defenders make will be countered; that the attackers can camouflage their responses to appear to be failures attributable to other sources—loss of power, structural failures, or simple human error [114]. Therefore, cyber resiliency contemplates more than simply defense in depth—it also contemplates defense in breadth; it requires the integration of planning and processes at all levels of the enterprise.

This requires a deeper level of integration between information security, biomedical engineering, and operations than has existed customarily. Without appropriate resilience and redundancy in hardware, software, and personnel, it is not possible to maintain operational capabilities in the face of an unrelenting attack. The benefits of an integrated approach to resiliency inure to the organization as a whole. Cyber threats do not present an isolated risk; the victimized organization suffers from reputational harm; patients may suffer from physical harm, which can lead to lawsuits; violation of regulatory standards may lead to imposition of fines and penalties.

The same techniques that provide resilience against adversarial attacks can also apply to other threats to the environment. For example, the development of a memorandum of understanding between hospitals, other health facilities, and emergency services in a local area which addresses the provision of support, similar to the memoranda of understanding currently used for natural disasters, could be developed to address potential consequences of a cyberattack. Disaster response laws should be updated to address cyberattacks, permitting the deployment of cyber response resources when the attack is significant. The development of regional depots of medical devices that could be quickly deployed and configured at a victim institution to replace affected devices might reduce the need to pay ransom gangs to restore operations. To allow any of these mitigation and remediation measures to work, however, victims must be protected against enforcement actions and other liability. The fact is that it is not possible, given the complexity of technology today, to have a completely secured network. As soon as a threat actor successfully penetrates and exploits a network, the vulnerability used becomes obvious—and it is easy to second-guess the IT staff for making the security decisions, given the outcome. There must be developed an objective standard which, once accomplished, protects the healthcare organization against enforcement actions and liability, as having demonstrated reasonable security.

8.8 International Cooperation

Internationally, the members of the North Atlantic Treaty Organization (NATO), in the Brussels Summit Communique on June 14, 2021 [115], recognized the critical threat posed by cybercrime and nation-state supported cyberattacks, and endorsed the NATO Comprehensive Cyber Defence Policy. NATO noted that cyberattacks are "... complex, destructive, coercive and becoming ever more frequent ... " [115] and pose a threat to the security of the members of NATO. Consistent with the role of NATO in defending the safety of its members and their citizens, NATO committed to "... employ the full range of capabilities at all time to actively deter, defend against, and counter the full spectrum of cyber threats, including those conducted as part of hybrid campaigns . . . " [115]. This commitment recognized that the " . . . impact of significant, cumulative, malicious . . . " cyberattacks could amount to an armed attack, which could trigger Article 5 of the NATO treaty, pursuant to which the NATO members commit to treating an attack against one member as an attack against all. While emphasizing defense and resilience, the Communique makes it clear that behavior that threatens the security of NATO members, whether in cyber or traditional domains, will be met with strength and determination.

This type of international cooperation is critical in the management of cyber threats. Traditional approaches to law enforcement fail in the cyber domain because the crime is committed across jurisdictional lines, and it is typically impossible to track and enforce without the cooperation of multiple jurisdictions. Where nations cooperate, investigations can be successful; for example, in June 2021, law enforcement authorities in the United States, Ukraine, and South Korea collaborated in arresting six suspected members of the Clop ransomware group [116].

Recognizing the international nature of cybersecurity and the complexity of response, the European Commission announced in June, 2021, the intent to establish a Joint Cyber Unit to respond to massive cyberattacks. The Joint Cyber Unit will have rapid reaction teams that provide operational and technical support to EU Member State entities [117]. The Joint Cyber Unit is one component of the EU Cybersecurity Strategy, which is intended to improve the resilience of the EU and Member States against cyber threats [118].

On July 1, 2021, a Joint Cybersecurity Advisory was released by the U.S. National Security Agency, the U.S. Cybersecurity and Infrastructure Agency, the FBI, and the UK National Cyber Security Centre regarding the use by the Russian General Staff Main Intelligence Directorate (GRU) 85th Main Special Service Center (GTsSS) of a Kubernetes cluster to conduct " . . . widespread, distributed and anonymized brute force attempts against hundreds of government and private sector targets worldwide" [119]. Through the brute force attack, GTsSS accessed confidential data, escalated privileges, moved laterally, and exploited vulnerabilities in target environments. The Joint Cybersecurity Advisory provided detailed information regarding the tactics, techniques, and procedures (TTPs) used by the GTsSS, as well as indicators of compromise and user agents. This coordinated notification provided both detection and mitigation information for an international audience and conveyed to Russia a unified front against nation-state supported hacking.

Almost simultaneously, an affiliate of the REvil group unleashed a ransomware attack against Kaseya, a provider of managed information technology services. Over the next several days, hundreds of companies internationally were impacted, with reported ransom demands of up to $5 million [120]. After about 4 days, REvil posted on its dark website an offer of a universal decryptor for all affected businesses for $70 million [120]. However, because the attack was timed to hit over the U.S. Fourth of July holiday, accurately determining the scope of affected entities was difficult. The scope of this attack demonstrates even more clearly the need for international cooperation in responding to cyberattacks.

8.9 Conclusion

The problem of ransomware is not a simple issue of technology. Ransomware is a complex political, economic, and public safety issue that will require a multi-faceted solution. It requires cooperation between the victim and law enforcement, as well as national-level exercise of soft power. It may, at some point, pose a sufficiently severe risk that NATO or another national or multinational power will determine merits the exercise of more direct intervention. Nation-states and private entities that knowingly provide infrastructure that supports ransomware should be held responsible, but interventions that punish victims should be avoided, to minimize the risk that victims further avoid seeking the assistance of law enforcement and limit information sharing. Through a common international commitment to information sharing and coordination of efforts, the threat posed by ransomware attacks against healthcare can be decreased.

References

1. The Comptroller and Auditor General. Investigation: WannaCry cyber attack and the NHS [hereinafter Comptroller's Report] https://www.nao.org.uk/wp-content/uploads/2017/10/Investigation-WannaCry-cyber-attack-and-the-NHS.pdf
2. Brewster T. 'Strong Links' Now Tie North Korea to WannaCry Ransomware Pandemic. FORBES (May. 23, 2017) https://www.forbes.com/sites/thomasbrewster/2017/05/23/north-korea-link-to-wannacry-ransomware-are-strong/?sh=56540c5451bc
3. Palmer D. Ransomware: Huge rise in attacks this year as cyber criminals hunt bigger pay days. ZDNET (Sept. 9, 2020) https://tinyurl.com/yy5vf5pm
4. CHECKPOINT. Global Surges in Ransomware Attacks https://blog.checkpoint.com/2020/10/06/study-global-rise-in-ransomware-attacks/ (last visited July 19, 2021)
5. U.S. GOVERNMENT INTERAGENCY. TECHNICAL GUIDANCE DOCUMENT. HOW TO PROTECT YOUR NETWORKS FROM RANSOMWARE (last visited July 19, 2021) https://www.justice.gov/criminal-ccips/file/872771/download
6. VERIZON. 2020 DATA BREACH INVESTIGATIONS REPORT 50 (2020), https://enterprise.verizon.com/content/verizonenterprise/us/en/index/resources/reports/2020-data-breach-investigations-report.pdf
7. HHS. FACT SHEET: RANSOMWARE AND HIPAA (last visited July 19, 2021) https://www.hhs.gov/sites/default/files/RansomwareFactSheet.pdf
8. Paquet-Clouston M, et al. Ransomware payments in the Bitcoin ecosystem, 5 J. of Cybersecurity, 1, 1 (2019), available at https://doi.org/10.1093/cybsec/tyz003 [hereinafter Journal of Cybersecurity]
9. Experian. https://www.experian.com/decision-analytics/synthetic-identity-fraud (last visited July 19, 2021)
10. DBIR. 2021 Data Breach Investigations Report (2021). https://www.verizon.com/business/resources/reports/dbir/
11. Cawthra J, et al. Data Integrity: Detecting and Responding to Ransomware and Other Destructive Events (December 2020) https://nvlpubs.nist.gov/nistpubs/SpecialPublications/NIST.SP.1800-26.pdf.
12. Crowdstrike. https://adversary.crowdstrike.com/ (last visited on July 19, 2021)

13. Crowdstrike. https://adversary.crowdstrike.com/adversary/twisted-spider/ (last visited July 19, 2021)
14. Toby L. The rise of ransomware, National Cyber Security Centre (Jan. 29, 2021) https://www.ncsc.gov.uk/blog-post/rise-of-ransomware
15. The White House Office of the Press Secretary, Presidential Policy Directive – Critical Infrastructure Security and Resilience (February 12, 2013) (on file with author) https://obamawhitehouse.archives.gov/the-press-office/2013/02/12/presidential-policy-directive-critical-infrastructure-security-and-resil
16. European Commission. Proposal for a DIRECTIVE OF THE EURO-PEAN PARLIAMENT AND OF THE COUNCIL on the resilience of critical entities (2020) https://ec.europa.eu/home-affairs/sites/default/files/pdf/15122020_proposal_directive_resilience_critical_entities_com-2020-829_en.pdf
17. ENISA. https://www.enisa.europa.eu/topics/critical-information-infrastructures-and-services/health (last visited July 19, 2021)
18. Nakamoto S. Bitcoin: A Peer-to-Peer Electronic Cash System (2008) https://bitcoin.org/bitcoin.pdf
19. Financial Action Task Force. Draft updated Guidance for a risk-based approach to virtual assets and vasps (2020) https://www.fatf-gafi.org/media/fatf/documents/recommendations/March%202021%20-%20VA%20Guidance%20update%20-%20Sixth%20draft%20-%20Public%20consultation.pdf
20. Chainalysis. https://www.chainalysis.com/ (last visited July 23, 2021)
21. Freedman L. Ransomware Attacks Predicted to Occur Every 11 Seconds in 2021 with a Cost of $20 Billion, Robinson & Cole (Feb. 13, 2020)
22. Paganini P. ClearEnergy ransomware aim to destroy process automation logics in critical infrastructure, SCADA and industrial control systems, Security Affairs (April 5, 2017), https://securityaffairs.co/wordpress/57731/malware/clearenergy-ransomware-scada.html
23. Kovacs E. Simulation Shows Threat of Ransomware Attacks on ICS, SecurityWeek (February 14, 2017) https://www.securityweek.com/simulation-shows-threat-ransomware-attacks-ics.
24. DHS, 2019 Public-Private Analytic Exchange Program. A Lifeline: Patient Safety & Cybersecurity (2019) https://www.dhs.gov/sites/default/files/publications/ia/ia_vulnerabilities-healthcare-it-systems.pdf
25. Lockheed Martin, Gaining the Advantage: Applying the Cyber Kill Chain Methodology to Network Defense 3 (last visited July 20, 2021) https://www.lockheedmartin.com/content/dam/lockheed-martin/rms/documents/cyber/Gaining_the_Advantage_Cyber_Kill_Chain.pdf
26. MITRE ATT&CK. attack.mitre.org (last visited July 20, 2021)
27. MITRE ATT&CK. https://medium.com/mitre-attack (last visited July 20, 2021)
28. Coley S, Chase P. Rubrics for Applying CVSS to Medical Devices (Oct. 27, 2020) https://www.mitre.org/sites/default/files/publications/pr-18-2208-rubric-for-applying-cvss-to-medical-devices.pdf
29. U.S. Food & Drug Administration. MDDT Summary of Evidence and Basis of Qualification, Rubric for Applying CVSS to Medical Devices (2017) https://www.fda.gov/media/143131/download
30. FDA, Medical Device Development Tools (MDDT). (Jun. 17, 2021). https://www.fda.gov/medical-devices/science-and-research-medical-devices/medical-device-development-tools-mddt
31. Mahn A. Identify, Protect, Detect, Respond and Recover: The NIST Cybersecurity Framework, nist (Oct. 23, 2018) https://www.nist.gov/blogs/taking-measure/identify-protect-detect-respond-and-recover-nist-cybersecurity-framework
32. Cybersecurity & Infrastructure Security Agency. https://www.cisa.gov/BadPractices (last visited July 20, 2021)
33. Goldstein E. Bad Practices, Cybersecurity & Infrastructure Security Agency (June 24, 2021) https://www.cisa.gov/blog/2021/06/24/bad-practices
34. Health Insurance Portability and Accountability Act of 1996, 42 U.S.C. § 1320d et seq.
35. American Recovery and Reinvestment Act of 2009, Pub. L. No. 111-5, Stat 13401 et seq.

36. Privacy of Individually Identifiable Health Information, 45 C.F.R. Subpart E § 164.
37. Standards for Safeguarding Customer Information, 15 C.F.R. § 314 and Interagency Guidance on Response Programs for Unauthorized Access to Customer Information and Customer Notice, 70 Fed. Reg. 15736 (3/29/2005)
38. Federal Trade Commission Act, 15 U.S.C. §§ 41-58 et seq.
39. Fair and Accurate Credit Transaction Act, 15 U.S.C. § 1681 et seq.
40. European Parliament and Council of the European Union 2016/679. art. 1-99, 2018 O.J. (L 100000) 1-88
41. UK Public General Acts (2018) (c.12). UK Data Protection Act 2018
42. CISA, ICS Advisory (ICSMA-19-164-01). https://us-cert.cisa.gov/ics/advisories/ICSMA-19-164-01, (Jun. 14, 2019)
43. Mayoral-Vilches V., et al. Industrial robot ransomware: Akerbeltz. arXiv:1912.07714v1 [cs.CR] 1, 2 (Dec. 16, 2019), https://arxiv.org/pdf/1912.07714.pdf
44. Applied Dexterity, History, https://applieddexterity.com/about/history/ (last visited July 20, 2021)
45. T. Bonaci T, et al., To Make a Robot Secure: An Experimental Analysis of Cyber Security Threats Against Teleoperated Surgical Robotics, arXiv:1504.04339v2 [cs.RO] 1, 1 (May. 12, 2015), https://arxiv.org/pdf/1504.04339.pdf
46. Alemzadeh H., et al. Targeted Attacks on Teleoperated Surgical Robots: Dynamic Model-based Detection and Mitigation, 46th Annual IEEE/IFIP International Conference on Dependable Systems and Networks, 395 (2016) https://faculty.virginia.edu/alemzadeh/papers/DSN_2016.pdf
47. Ralston W. The untold story of a cyberattack, a hospital and a dying woman, wired (Nov. 11, 2020), https://www.wired.co.uk/article/ransomware-hospital-death-germany
48. Sung Choi & M. Eric Johnson, Do Hospital Data Breaches Reduce Patient Care Quality, arXiv:1904.02058v1 [econ.GN] 1, 2 (Apr. 3, 2019), available at https://arxiv.org/pdf/1904.02058.pdf
49. Hargen E. Deputy Secretary of Health and Human Services, Health Industry Cybersecurity Practices: Managing Threats and Protecting Patients (last visited on July 20, 2021) (on file with the author) https://www.phe.gov/Preparedness/planning/405d/Documents/HICP-Main-508.pdf
50. Consolidated Appropriation Act, Pub. L. No. 114-113, Div. N.
51. Public Health Emergency, Technical Volume 1: Cybersecurity Practices for Small Health Care Organizations 3 (last visited July 20, 2021), https://www.phe.gov/Preparedness/planning/405d/Documents/tech-vol1-508.pdf
52. Public Health Emergency, Technical Volume 2: Cybersecurity Practices for Medium and Large Health Care Organizations 4 (last visited July 20, 2021), https://www.phe.gov/Preparedness/planning/405d/Documents/tech-vol2-508.pdf.
53. U.S. Food & Drug Administration. Postmarket Management of Cybersecurity in Medical Devices: Guidance for Industry and Food and Drug Administration Staff (2016) https://www.fda.gov/media/95862/download [hereinafter Postmarket Cybersecurity Guidance]
54. See U.S. Food & Drug Administration. Off-The-Shelf Software Use in Medical Devices: Guidance for Industry and Food and Drug Administration Staff (2019) https://www.fda.gov/media/71794/download#:~:text=Off%2Dthe%2DShelf%20Software%20(,software%20life%20cycle%20control
55. Establishment Registration and Device Listing for Manufactures And Initial Importers of Devices, 21 C.F.R. § 807.81 et seq. (2020)
56. Choi S, et al. Health Services Research, 54 Health Serv. Research 1 (Sept. 10, 2019)
57. Wood Ranch Medical, Wood Ranch Medical Notice to Patients. (Sept. 18, 2019) https://www.woodranchmedical.com/
58. Davis J, Michigan Practice to Shutter after Hackers Delete Patient Files. Health IT Security (Apr. 1, 2019) https://healthitsecurity.com/news/michigan-practice-to-shutter-after-hackers-delete-patient-files

59. Kiss v. Springhill Hospitals Inc., 02-CV-2020-900171, available at https://www.documentcloud.org/documents/21072978-kidd-amended-complaint
60. CISA Insight: Provide Medical Care Is In Critical Condition: Analysis and Stakeholder Decision Support to Minimize Further Harm, available at https://www.cisa.gov/sites/default/files/publications/Insights_MedicalCare_FINAL-v2_0.pdf
61. Krebs On Security. A Closer Look at the Darkside Ransomware Gang. (May 11, 2021) https://krebsonsecurity.com/2021/05/a-closer-look-at-the-darkside-ransomware-gang/
62. Regional Emergency Declaration 2021-002, 49 CFR § 390.23 (May 9, 2021) https://www.fmcsa.dot.gov/emergency/esc-ssc-wsc-regional-emergency-declaration-2021-002-05-09-2021
63. Federal Bureau of Investigation. FBI Statement on Compromise of Colonial Pipeline Networks (May 10, 2021) (on file with author) https://www.fbi.gov/news/pressrel/press-releases/fbi-statement-on-compromise-of-colonial-pipeline-networks.
64. CISA. Alert (AA21-131A) DarkSide Ransomware: Best Practices for Preventing Business Disruption from Ransomware Attacks, cisa (July. 8, 2021) https://us-cert.cisa.gov/ncas/alerts/aa21-131a
65. Brewster T. The Colonial Pipeline Hackers Are One Of The Savviest Criminal Startups In A $370 Million Ransomware Game, Forbes (May 12, 2021), https://www.forbes.com/sites/thomasbrewster/2021/05/12/the-colonial-pipeline-hackers-are-one-of-the-savviest-criminal-startups-in-a-370-million-ransomware-game/?sh=5e3e80ba7595
66. Krebs on Security, DarkSide Ransomware Gang Quits After Servers, Bitcoin Stash Seized. (May 14, 2021) https://krebsonsecurity.com/2021/05/darkside-ransomware-gang-quits-after-servers-bitcoin-stash-seized/ (quoting from screenshot)
67. The White House. Exec. Order No. 14028, 86 FR 26633 (2021) https://www.whitehouse.gov/briefing-room/presidential-actions/2021/05/12/executive-order-on-improving-the-nations-cybersecurity/
68. Turton W, et al. Colonial Pipeline Paid Hackers Nearly $5 Million in Ransom. Bloomberg (May 13, 2021) https://www.bloomberg.com/news/articles/2021-05-13/colonial-pipeline-paid-hackers-nearly-5-million-in-ransom
69. Washington Post. Opinion: Hackers are taking cities hostage. Here's a way around it (Jun, 23, 2019) https://www.washingtonpost.com/opinions/hackers-are-taking-cities-hostage-heres-a-way-around-it/2019/06/23/f08b79ea-9459-11e9-aadb-74e6b2b46f6a_story.html
70. Carolan M. HSE secures injunctions restraining sharing of hacked data. The Irish Times (May 20, 2021) https://www.irishtimes.com/news/crime-and-law/courts/high-court/hse-secures-injunctions-restraining-sharing-of-hacked-data-1.4570769
71. JBS Foods, (May. 31, 2021) (on file with author) https://jbsfoodsgroup.com/articles/jbs-usa-cyberattack-media-statement-may-31
72. CNBC, U.S. says ransomware attack on meatpacker JBS likely from Russia; cattle slaughter resuming, (June 2, 2021), https://www.cnbc.com/2021/06/01/big-north-american-meat-plants-halt-operations-after-jbs-cyberattack.html
73. JBS Foods, (June 3, 2021) (on file with author) https://jbsfoodsgroup.com/articles/jbs-usa-and-pilgrim-s-announce-resolution-of-cyberattack
74. Bunge J. JBS Paid $11 Million to Resolve Ransomware Attack, Wall Street Journal (June 9, 2021) https://www.wsj.com/articles/jbs-paid-11-million-to-resolve-ransomware-attack-11623280781
75. Bing C. Exclusive: U.S. to give ransomware hacks similar priority as terrorism, Reuters Online (June 3, 2021) https://www.reuters.com/technology/exclusive-us-give-ransomware-hacks-similar-priority-terrorism-official-says-2021-06-03/
76. Ferguson S. DOJ Launches Task Force to Battle Ransomware Threat, Bank Info Security (Apr. 22, 2021) https://www.bankinfosecurity.com/doj-launches-task-force-to-battle-ransomware-threat-a-16452, (citing Memorandum from John Carlin, Dep. Attorney Gen., U.S. Dep't of Justice, on Ransomware and Digital Extortion Task Force 1 (Apr. 20, 2021), https://dd80b675424c132b90b3-e48385e382d2e5d17821a5e1d8e4c86b.ssl.cf1.rackcdn.com/external/dojransomwarememo.pdf

77. Department of Justice. Department of Justice Launches Global Action Against NetWalker Ransomware (Jan. 27, 2021) (on file with author) https://www.justice.gov/opa/pr/department-justice-launches-global-action-against-netwalker-ransomware

78. Indictment, United States of America v. Sebastien Vachon-Desjardins, No. 8:20 (M.D. Fla. Dec. 02, 2020), https://embed.documentcloud.org/documents/20466053-492366128-u-s-v-sebastien-vachon-desjardins/?embed=1&title=1

79. Brown S. FBI Takes on Ransomware Giant NetWalker, OCCRP (Jan. 29, 2021), https://www.occrp.org/en/daily/13753-fbi-takes-on-ransomware-giant-netwalker; see also Akshaya Asokan, Another Takedown: Netwalker Ransomware Gang Disrupted, Bank Info Security (Jan. 28, 2021), https://www.bankinfosecurity.com/another-takedown-netwalker-ransomware-gang-disrupted-a-15875

80. Europol. World's Most Dangerous Malware Emotet Disrupted Through Global Action (Jan. 27, 2021) (on file with author) https://www.europol.europa.eu/newsroom/news/world%E2%80%99s-most-dangerous-malware-emotet-disrupted-through-global-action.

81. Institute for Security and Technology, Combatting Ransomware 1 (2021) https://securityandtechnology.org/ransomwaretaskforce/report/ [hereinafter RTF Report]

82. U.S Department of the Treasury. Advisory on Potential Sanctions Risks for Facilitating Ransomware Payments (Oct. 2020) https://home.treasury.gov/system/files/126/ofac_ransomware_advisory_10012020_1.pdf [hereinafter OFAC Advisory]

83. National Emergencies, 50 U.S.C. §§ 1601-1651 (1976)

84. International Emergency Powers, 50 U.S.C. §§ 1701-1706 (1998)

85. Countering America's Adversaries Through Sanctions Act, 22 U.S.C. § 9401 et seq. (2017)

86. Exec. Order No. 13694, 80 FR 18077 (2015)

87. Exec. Order No. 13757, 82 FR 1 (2016)

88. U.S Department of the Treasury. Office of Foreign Assets Control Sanctions List Search. https://sanctionssearch.ofac.treas.gov/ (last visited July 21, 2021)

89. U.S. Department of the Treasury. Treasury Sanctions Two Individuals for Malicious Cyber-Enabled Activities (Dec. 29, 2016) (on file with author) https://www.treasury.gov/press-center/press-releases/Pages/jl0693.aspx

90. U.S Department of the Treasury. Treasury Designates Iran-Based Financial Facilitators of Malicious Cyber Activity and for the First Time Identifies Associated Digital Currency Addresses (November 28, 2018) (on file with author) https://home.treasury.gov/news/press-releases/sm556

91. U.S Department of the Treasury. Treasury Sanctions North Korean State-Sponsored Malicious Cyber Groups (September 13, 2019) (on file with author) https://home.treasury.gov/news/press-releases/sm774

92. U.S. Department of the Treasury. Treasury Sanctions Evil Corp, the Russia-Based Cyber-criminal Group Behind Dridex Malware (Dec. 5, 2019) (on file with author), https://home.treasury.gov/news/press-releases/sm845

93. U.S. Dep't of the Treasury. Treasury Sanctions Russian Cyber Actors for Interference with 2016 U.S. Elections and Malicious Cyber-Attacks (March 15, 2018) (on file with author), https://home.treasury.gov/news/press-releases/sm0312

94. U.S. Department of the Treasury, Treasury Sanctions Russian Government Research Institution Connected to the Triton Malware (October 23, 2020) (on file with author), https://home.treasury.gov/news/press-releases/sm1162

95. Exec. Order No. 14024, 86 FR 20249 (April 15, 2021)

96. The White House. Fact Sheet: Imposing Costs for Harmful Foreign Activities by the Russian Government. (April 15, 2021) https://www.whitehouse.gov/briefing-room/statements-releases/2021/04/15/fact sheet imposing costs-for-harmful-foreign-activities-by-the-russian-government/

97. Joint Cybersecurity Advisory. Russian SVR Targets U.S. and Allied Networks (2021) https://media.defense.gov/2021/Apr/15/2002621240/-1/-1/0/CSA_SVR_TARGETS_US_ALLIES_UOO13234021.PDF/CSA_SVR_TARGETS_US_ALLIES_UOO13234021.PDF

98. Five Vulnerabilities SVR Is Exploiting Right Now 1 (last visited July 22, 2021) https://www.aha.org/system/files/media/file/2021/04/Infographic-five-vulnerabilities-svr-is-exploiting-right-now-and-how-to-stop-them.pdf
99. Trading with the Enemy Act, 50 U.S.C. § 4301 et seq.
100. Reporting, Procedures, and Penalties Regulations. 31 C.F.R. § 501 (referring to Appendix A to Part 501)
101. Updated Advisory on Potential Sanctions Risks for Facilitating Ransomware Payments. available at https://home.treasury.gov/system/files/126/ofac_ransomware_advisory.pdf
102. CISA MS-ISAC Ransomware Guide. September, 2020, available at https://www.cisa.gov/sites/default/files/publications/CISA_MS-ISAC_Ransomware%20Guide_S508C_.pdf
103. Chainalysis. The 2021 Crypto Crime Report 29 (February 16, 2021) www.chainalysis.com
104. Greenberg A. "Sandworm: A New Era of Cyberwar and the Hunt for the Kremlin's Most Dangerous Hackers" (Anchor Books, 2019)
105. Interstate communications, 18 U.S.C. 875(d)
106. Elonis v. U.S., 575 U.S. 723, 737-38 (2015)
107. Interference with commerce by threats or violence, 18 U.S.C. 1951 (a)(b)
108. Taylor v. U.S., 136 S.Ct. 2074 (2016)
109. U.S. v. Brank, No. 15-50467 (9th Cir. 2018) (citing to U.S. v. Nardello, 393 U.S. 286, 296 (1969))
110. Wellons MC, Javers E. The hacker group that went after one of Apple's suppliers found a new victim, cnbc (Jun. 14, 2021) https://www.cnbc.com/2021/06/11/revil-hacker-group-attacks-sol-oriens-with-ransomware.html
111. https://www.justice.gov/opa/pr/deputy-attorney-general-lisa-o-monaco-announces-new-civil-cyber-fraud-initiative
112. The White House. Presidential Policy Directive – Critical Infrastructure Security and Resilience (Feb. 12, 2013) (on file with author) https://obamawhitehouse.archives.gov/the-press-office/2013/02/12/presidential-policy-directive-critical-infrastructure-security-and-resil
113. NIST. Developing Cyber Resilient Systems: A Systems Security Engineering Approach Vol. 2 NIST SP 800-160 XIV (Nov. 2019) https://nvlpubs.nist.gov/nistpubs/SpecialPublications/NIST.SP.800-160v2.pdf
114. MITRE. Cyber Resiliency FAQ 4 (2017) https://www.mitre.org/sites/default/files/PR_17-1434.pdf
115. NATO, Brussels Summit Communique, Issued by the Heads of State and Government participating in the meeting of the North Atlantic Council in Brussels (Jun. 14 2021) (on file with author), https://www.nato.int/cps/en/natohq/news_185000.htm
116. Schwartz M. Ukraine Arrests 6 Clop Ransomware Operation Suspects, Data Breach Today. Data Breach Today (Jun. 16, 2021) https://www.databreachtoday.com/ukraine-arrests-6-clop-ransomware-operation-suspects-a-16885
117. European Commission, EU Cybersecurity: Commission proposes a Joint Cyber Unit to step up response to large-scale security incidents (Jun. 23, 2021) (on file with author), https://ec.europa.eu/commission/presscorner/detail/en/IP_21_3088
118. European Commission, New EU Cybersecurity Strategy and new rules to make physical and digital critical entities more resilient (Dec. 16, 2020) (on file with author), https://ec.europa.eu/commission/presscorner/detail/en/ip_20_2391
119. Cybersecurity Advisory, Russian GRU Conducting Global Brute Force Campaign to Compromise Enterprise and Cloud Environments 1 (2021), https://media.defense.gov/2021/Jul/01/2002753896/-1/-1/1/CSA_GRU_GLOBAL_BRUTE_FORCE_CAMPAIGN_UOO158036-21.PDF
120. The Associated Press, Scale, Details of Massive Kaseya Ransomware Attack Emerge, https://www.npr.org/2021/07/05/1013117515/scale-details-of-massive-kaseya-ransomware-attack-emerge

Chapter 9
TAP and Intelligent Technology for Connected Lifestyles: Trust, Accessibility, and Privacy

Katherine Grace August, Mathini Sellathurai, and Paula Muller

Contents

K. G. August (✉)
Stevens Institute of Technology, Matawan, NJ, USA

M. Sellathurai
Heriot Watt University, Edinburgh, UK

P. Muller
Sociavi, Keyport, NJ, USA
e-mail: paula@mullernj.us

© Springer Nature Switzerland AG 2022
F. D. Hudson (eds.), *Women Securing the Future with TIPPSS for Connected Healthcare*, Women in Engineering and Science,
https://doi.org/10.1007/978-3-030-93592-4_9

9.1 Background

In early 2020, the world was transformed by an unprecedented public health emergency—a global pandemic caused by Coronavirus and associated COVID-19—and a shattering cascade of consequences spreading most velociously through healthcare systems, the economy, education, government, transportation, justice, and virtually every aspect of life, both public and private, compromising resilience [1]. Technology, access to information, and technology disparity have emerged as pivotal in world affairs, and public policy, supply chain, and response to the emergency on a global scale has taken a higher priority in determination of systems requirements than ordinary goods and services, consumers, or product-driven markets [2]. It became clear that timely and comprehensive *access to intelligent technology and a connected lifestyle* should not be considered discretionary but compulsory for *every human being*.

The COVID-19 outbreak also made clear that fragmented, non-compatible, dispersive systems were unprepared, non-responsive, and in need of modernization; by global measures included in the Global Health Security Index, they serve neither present nor future needs [3]. Providing assistance (Accommodation), connection (Accessibility), safety and resources to people with differing abilities, for example, the elderly and those with hearing loss and other disabilities, underrepresented minorities, economically challenged, marginalized populations, and to frontline and essential workers, has become even more difficult and uncertain; without effective systems, each person must find their own solutions. There was a sudden awareness of shortages in preparedness and resources needed to address the emergency, such as personal protective equipment (PPE) and domestic manufacturing capabilities, respirators, treatments, systems, policies, technologies, and solutions, and then recognition of the profound lack of resilience of all systems [4]. Policy failed to include information needed, and society suffered from a crisis system's failure to plan [5].

While people with special needs are often served by separate or dedicated devices, formal or informal resources, and may be supported by alternative systems, their lack of availability and interoperability create major challenges. They have failed catastrophically during this pandemic, leading to excess harm and death, and in particular for those with special needs, which became obvious during the first few months of the COVID-19 pandemic [6]. These devices, systems, and processes serving people with special needs place undue burden on individuals and their particular support situation. They routinely leave many people vulnerable for a variety of reasons which cannot be easily mitigated. They fail for individuals every day; however, during the COVID-19 pandemic many individuals have been failed by the system because offices and services have been closed, overburdened, or unavailable. Therefore, the current systems are not sustainable, in the context of the United Nations Sustainable Development Goals (UN SDG) [7]. Inclusive and equitable systems providing accessibility and accommodation are necessary for sustainability and resilience. To improve trust requires a much higher level of commitment and must include protection of privacy.

The digital divide has amplified existing disparities, leading to great harm to many individuals, their families, and communities, with sickness and death, economic devastation, and tremendous suffering expected to impact families, communities, and nations for generations [8]. Health problems including underlying risk factors and pre-existing conditions are a burden to individuals, families, and communities. Without access to health, wellness, prevention and reliable healthcare, risks and health problems are attenuated and lead to catastrophe as people age, from any accident, in school and in the workplace, in congregant settings, and especially during any emergency. Sickness and/or death of a family member have significant consequences for everyone in the family. Some children will be left without a parent. Wage earners will become disabled and lose insurance. Many who survive COVID-19 will suffer long COVID with varying degrees of disability and healthcare needs. Early estimates of the global impact of COVID-19 on the UN Sustainable Development Goals to end poverty by 2030 indicate that poverty could increase for the first time since 1990, representing a reversal of a decade of the world's progress [9].

Previous forecasts about Internet of Things (IoT) connected lifestyles, with predictions of tremendous increases, nevertheless did not anticipate the present unprecedented needs of the society as a whole, affecting every one of its constituents. There is a great expansion of IoT connected healthcare where Trust, Accessibility, and Privacy (TAP) are even more relevant and integrally linked with intelligent technology and connected lifestyles. There is an urgent, immediate, ubiquitous, and increasing demand for connected healthcare solutions and connected lifestyles from stakeholders of every type, including traditional consumer systems, and also those required for resilience, while there is a widening diversity of users. Improving trust of individuals and stakeholders, which is multifactorial, can improve participation; there is influence of general trust, as well as trust involving issues specific to a given topic, for example, COVID-19. Through trust, health outcomes, and well-being may be improved, for example, by increasing COVID-19 protective behaviors [10]. Intelligent technology and connected lifestyles in this context will improve not only safety and security, but will also support resilience and allow the best fit for essential interactions with the world. The envisioned world of IoT-connected healthcare, intelligent technology, and connected lifestyles will be possible under a system of Trust, Accessibility, and Privacy (TAP).

There is a great expansion of IoT-connected healthcare where Trust, Accessibility, and Privacy are even more relevant and integrally linked with intelligent technology and connected lifestyles. There is an urgent, immediate, ubiquitous, and increasing demand for connected healthcare solutions and connected lifestyles from stakeholders of every type, including the traditional consumer system, as well as those required for resilience, with a widening diversity of users.

9.2 TAP: Trust, Accessibility, and Privacy Defined

9.2.1 Trust

We strive to trust, to believe, to have confidence in the reliability, truth, and ability of the systems we use; in addition, we trust in someone, we trust in a system, when we turn over something of value to another person or to a system. In this context, trust is afforded to systems when the experience reflects the expectations of the user. Trust allows everyone to participate willingly.

Coronavirus and the associated COVID-19 pandemic catapulted many aspects of trust to the forefront, from small villages to the global economy, in the blink of an eye. This was because many more users were in need of connected systems, and the number and variety of stakeholders widened, each with their own requirements for which the systems were not originally designed. Transparency was questioned by the new stakeholders. The pandemic raised suspicions and distrust of many organizations, governments, policy makers, and individuals, widened the divide, and as a result, challenged trust and transparency in decisions and systems for many. While the United States received the top score of 195 countries assessed and was ranked number one in the Global Health Security Index in 2020, they scored a zero in the public confidence category, indicating a low level of confidence among the public (less than 25%) [3]. Solving these issues is an ambitious undertaking where governments, vendors, and standards bodies should participate to develop appropriate methods to regain confidence and ensure trust for a connected lifestyle.

9.2.2 Accessibility

Accessibility is the capability of an object, system, or environment to admit and accommodate abilities, needs, and preferences of any and each individual, class, and group, in any context, time, and place. Accessibility can be described from several aspects, such as: (1) accessibility to use or operate the capabilities of the systems, what could be referred to as User Interaction and Experience (UIX), ensuring the UIX is adequate for every individual independent of their abilities through accommodations; (2) accessibility to infrastructure such as adequate connectivity to network communications, internet, and devices; and, (3) accessibility and interoperability among systems, for example, medical devices, and electronic records such as medical, financial, and others. COVID-19 challenged all aspects of accessibility.

Many people with disabling conditions rely on others for information, live in groups, and suffer economic inequities. Technology can theoretically enable access to all people in all contexts. However, often and especially during COVID-19, individuals had to deal with many situations without adequate accessibility support or solutions. Early in the pandemic, people with disabling conditions suffered, became sick, and died at a higher rate due to exacerbation of existing vulnerabilities. Many shocking news stories and statistics reflect this ongoing disparity [6].

One can see that people find themselves in a wide range of situations where their abilities or access to systems and information may be influenced by a set of factors, which might be both internal and external, resulting in a level of personal resilience as a function of the fitness of the solution. For example, an individual's resources to afford, understand, gain access to, and implement the solution, and the ability of available solutions to map to the needs of the individual, impact the personal resilience and vulnerability of the family and the community.

Conditions, abilities, and contextual needs are variable and may even be unique to the individual. They may be influenced by, or representative of, the family or social group. There may be cultural influences, religious traditions, linguistic identity, or varied levels of literacy, subject matter expertise, etc. All of these variables may be subject to influence during interactions with a specific solution such as a human interpreter, prosthetic, software, or other technology. There may be external elements outside the sphere of influence of the individual, family, or group, such as legislated processes and/or solutions, or infrastructure such as fitness and availability of special parking, proximity to accessible doors, suitability of ramps, and examination tables in a clinic. There are processes, for example, to be fitted for, order, and obtain needed equipment or solutions which can constrain a person and delay or prevent them from receiving appropriate solutions. Another consideration is compatibility and usefulness of enhanced communication systems which might require advance preparation, reservations which may be subject to being able to find the reservation system, finding help to access the reservation system, availability of human interpreters or communication equipment, transparency of use, fitness and resources available within the reservation system at each institution, public place, venue or event, and more. Then there must be compatibility of equipment, effectiveness and specificity of the solution for the person in the context, such as an augmented hearing support system for a person on jury duty during a trial, or a family member attending the trial, and more. Various conditions complicate the scene leading to dysfunctional inclusion, access, and interoperability. Most of these so-called accommodation systems failed during COVID-19. Interpreters, both formal and informal, were not permitted due to lockdown and precautions including medical, education, workplace, public transportation, etc. Some employers accommodate people at the office but not at home leaving some unable to work remotely. Legislation such as the U.S. Americans with Disabilities Act (ADA) is clearly not sufficient for a sustainable solution [11].

Even though there has been significant progress in accessibility and usability, there are "continued gaps" as mentioned in a 2020 Biennial Report to Congress [12]. While network coverage has expanded through the years, there are still many people who have no access to the internet or to mobile phones. After many promises of interoperability, systems still do not fully integrate with each other, causing inefficiencies and limiting access to crucial information with consequences. In healthcare, for example, not obtaining timely, comprehensive access to one's private medical data may lead to dreadful health outcomes.

Even when technology systems are available, there may be disparities that attenuate access, such as income, physical or cognitive abilities. We have to understand that *people are not disabled but they are experiencing disabling conditions* because there is a mismatch between their abilities and the systems that they try to use. People would benefit from inclusive design that provides all fairness in technology solutions, so that they are available to everyone who may need them, independent of their abilities. Furthermore, individuals can more easily engage with these systems when there is a suitable fit and the person recognizes that he or she is included.

Another situation arising from limited accessibility is that technology solutions may be available at very high and sophisticated levels, but since neither access nor inclusion is universal the results are disparity in outcomes. Comprehensiveness and timeliness of accessibility and inclusion is, at present, inadequate. For example, our medical system includes high-tech medical wearables and implants such as pacemakers, but not all environments around the world support these devices to enable the best cardiac care. Other products are available through the discretion of those who can afford them. Therefore, solutions are obtainable for few people, and comprehensive solutions for far fewer. For those with little or no access to connectivity, consequences are extreme, resulting in functional disability. We aim for a future with the highest level of accessibility and inclusion with systems, methods, and solutions that reduce disparity and accommodate a wide range of abilities. Since COVID-19, it is even more apparent how urgent it is for all to be included with effective care. It is urgent for individuals and society. People are vulnerable not only to the infectious condition of COVID-19, but also to comorbidities and other conditions, especially when the medical infrastructure is engaged and overwhelmed by the pandemic.

9.2.3 Privacy

Privacy is a fundamental human right. It underpins human dignity and other values such as freedom of association and freedom of speech. It has become one of the most important human rights of the modern age [13].

Privacy can be preserved in a trustworthy environment where access to information relevant to an individual is limited to trusted entities that are authorized, and their trusted intermediaries. These trusted entities are expected to have no malicious intent. It is expected that they will avoid known predatory practices, man-in-the-middle eavesdropping, and acquisition without specific authorization or privileges, either on purpose, through neglect or apathy, or by accident.

Having a system that provides comprehensive and ready accessibility is critical for appropriate delivery of care, safety, and for preservation of the very welfare and well-being of all constituents of our society. Promoting trust and protecting privacy makes possible effective connected lifestyles that will not only address goals of business and consumer services, but also address public health, safety, and resilience issues rising in importance worldwide.

9.3 Virtual Spaces Framework

Living through COVID-19 has made it evident that the boundaries between physical and virtual spaces have blurred, and the world will most likely continue to evolve in this way, shifting, for example, virtual surgery transitions from "touch to talk" for building trust between patient and healthcare practitioner in a new model [14].

Virtual spaces employ technology to create entirely new environments. Virtual spaces can replace and overlap physical spaces. As we move in and out of virtual spaces, the principles of TAP (Trust, Accessibility, Privacy), and security are crucial. From telehealth consultations to remote learning and virtual gathering, we are building a new ecosystem anywhere a person is located.

Lack of access to connectivity in the time of the COVID-19 pandemic created shocking disparities, adding to existing inequities for underrepresented minorities, those with disabling conditions, elders, and those with pre-existing health conditions. These individuals became vulnerable to catastrophic outcomes including economic devastation, sickness, and death. Such impact is long lasting, consumes families and communities, and will cross generations. As we redefined our daily interactions, migrating to virtual spaces for work, school, healthcare, shopping, social gatherings, entertainment, telemedicine, accommodation of disabling conditions, and for many other purposes, many of us were able to adapt, while others found these situations much more difficult. Whereas previously there was more access to human assistance, for example, for sign language interpreters, hospital volunteers, and family members, at the time of this writing these resources are greatly reduced. Experiencing connected lifestyles is the way we will evolve, and ensuring TAP in this realm is crucial and recognizes each human with dignity and respect. TAP is needed for systems to be more easily and equitably configured, managed, and operated in this more frequently adopted, automatic and remote conduct of operation. Even after the current restrictions of human contact, movement and travel are lifted, these systems and processes will remain. Incorporating TAP will inspire more people, professionals, and communities to accept and actually embrace connected healthcare and connected lifestyles.

Inequalities and disparities at many levels have become apparent during these times. In order to reduce them, it is essential to move away from the historically separate, siloed, expensive accommodation systems, and transition to systems that enable users to be untethered from bulky, costly dedicated-purpose devices and solutions. Our inclusive and accessible vision of the future through cloud connectivity provides smooth transitions among virtual spaces and physical spaces without custom development. In this embodiment, there are context-specific features which may be enabled through artificial intelligence (AI) virtual agents and robots on a mainstream network of networks, connected to service providers and databases. Virtual agents provide features which allow them to learn to adapt to differing abilities and provide personalization for individual preferences. These virtual agents use their experiences to build a library of features and recommendations, enabling diverse and inclusive accessibility. They connect to useful devices, sensors and

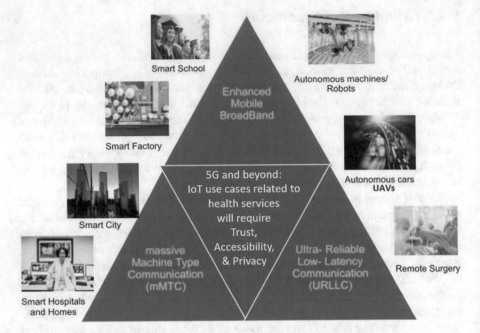

Fig. 9.1 IoT use cases related to health will require Trust, Accessibility, and Privacy

actuators, manage transactions and connections among people and resources, and address power management. They also provide means for analysis, accounting for those on the network and those not, with robust levels of security, while understanding context, with learning and intelligence. Awareness about these solutions is increasing. A selection of IoT use cases related to health which will require Trust, Accessibility, and Privacy (TAP) are illustrated in Fig. 9.1.

9.3.1 Scenarios

Our user scenarios highlight how assumptions and cyber engagements will change over the next few years, when heretofore postulations have been altered by a global pandemic, adding an entirely new vocabulary to every aspect of societal life. Even with regard to how people perceive Trust, Accessibility, Privacy, and security in connected lifestyles, what people expect as a result of the COVID-19 pandemic is likely to be markedly different from anything anticipated by forecasts, models, or forward-looking scenarios from before the COVID-19 pandemic. Influencers of the future are likely to include different considerations, stakeholders, and policy makers. There may be an increased willingness to rapidly share private information with others to achieve safety and well-being. Applications unfamiliar before the pandemic will be key including health status, track, and trace, and at the time of this writing, vaccination status [16].

9.3.2   Pivot Point in Connected Healthcare: United States in a Pandemic

There are a variety of medical delivery models around the globe. One that was barely used at the beginning of 2020 was telehealth as shown by several reports and surveys. In the United States, in February 2020 prior to the COVID-19 Public Health Emergency (PHE), less than 1% (0.1%) of Medicare primary care visits was telehealth. By April 2020, following the announcement of the COVID-19 PHE which was accompanied by warnings of severe illness increasing with age and stay at home orders, 43.5% of Medicare primary care visits were telehealth. It is likely to be some time before effects of COVID-19 will entirely disappear, yet in May 2020, Medicare opened up again to in-person primary care. Still, there is a continued demand for telehealth from patients, also confirmed by a survey of approximately 300 oncologists, specialists, and primary care healthcare providers. According to the survey, prior to the COVID-19 PHE, only about 9% of appointments were telehealth, but they increased to 51%. A report from the U.S. Department of Health and Human Services (HHS) noticed that people are now more willing to embrace telehealth including providers, policy makers, and patients, forecasting 21% of all patient–provider interactions will remain telehealth in the future, and shifting infrastructure needs from centralized points to a highly distributed model. A distributed model would require a significant investment in connectivity, effective collaborative models, associated systems and services [15, 17, 18].

Telemedicine has replaced in-person visits for a significant amount of healthcare; leveraging key wearables or specialty devices such as cardiac implant monitors provides an excellent opportunity to substantially improve healthcare, accessibility, and outcomes for patients.

9.3.3   Accessibility Facts

As communicated with the United Nations Sustainable Development Goals (SDGs) related to the COVID-19 pandemic, "The pandemic provides a watershed moment for health emergency preparedness and for investment in critical 21st century public services" [7]. Action is needed in order to achieve SDG Goal 3, Good Health and Well-Being, which is vital to avoid further catastrophe during the COVID-19 pandemic and beyond. People have been facing challenges to good health and well-being as individuals, families, marginalized, disabled, underrepresented minorities, culturally or linguistically diverse, uninsured, aging, and economically challenged, for many reasons. There is undue burden placed upon individuals to survive any emergency with their own resources. If an individual cannot afford routine healthcare, prevention, interpreters, housing, or access to a computer or broadband for telehealth, they are vulnerable not only because they cannot see a healthcare professional, but also because they cannot receive important public health information. They cannot remain safe. If the person is living in a congregant setting, or if they require an interpreter, or mobility assistance, they are relying on others to provide safe and vital care. During the COVID-19 pandemic, we have seen the most vulnerable suffer the greatest impact. Lack of effective systems and support, together with ongoing healthcare needs, takes a great toll upon those who are vulnerable. Preparedness for each individual, and communities, globally, particularly for the most vulnerable, is essential to the UN SDGs including Good Health and Well-being.

As noted by the United Nations Development Program (UNDP), "While every society is vulnerable to crises, their abilities to respond differs significantly around the world. For example, the most developed countries—those in the very high human development category—have on average 55 hospital beds, over 30 physicians, and 81 nurses per 10,000 people, compared to 7 hospital beds, 2.5 physicians, and 6 nurses per 10,000 people in a least developed country. And with widespread lockdowns, the digital divide has become more significant than ever. Around the globe, 6.5 billion people—representing 85.5% of the global population—still don't have access to reliable broadband internet, which limits their ability to work and continue their education" [19]. These facts provide insight into the scope and scale of the situation and challenges present during ordinary times and also in times of crisis.

As previously mentioned, in the United States, Medicare expanded telemedicine benefits during the COVID-19 pandemic through emergency rulemaking adding 135 services, increasing types of practitioners, locations for services, and eliminating video requirements allowing people to connect by voice only, resulting in an increase in patient participation from 14,000 to over 10.1 million patients in 5 months. At the same time, the Health Insurance Portability and Accountability Act (HIPAA) penalties will not be imposed for violations in connection with "good faith delivery of telehealth using non-public facing technologies." Questions remain about whether these changes will become long term or permanent [15, 20, 21].

Telehealth offers many opportunities to modernize healthcare and improve outcomes. Yet a large segment of the population remains underserved for a number of reasons, inspiring our efforts to reduce disparities. The pandemic provides a unique opportunity to study the healthcare system, with an eye towards transforming overall healthcare, to reach more people, with equitable healthcare, with wearables and expanded connected healthcare as key enabling elements, and influences such as public health accountability. It also provides an opportunity to uncover even more inadequacies of systems, policies, and practices [22].

Another aspect of the impact of limited accessibility is demonstrated by the fact that technology disparity has arisen as a differentiator in mortality and morbidity in all geographic locations, in all nations, around the globe. For example, people without access to broadband could not protect their health by working or shopping from home, or by keeping up with the latest coronavirus recommendations and information. Many could not participate in education or telemedicine for themselves or their children or for elders in their care. Neither society nor infrastructure was prepared. Already before the pandemic, there were measurable disparities in life expectancy, causes of death, participation in treatment, preventive health, and poor statistics on time-to-treatment for chronic and acute conditions, associated with rural versus urban life even in rather wealthy economies such as the United States. Although the COVID-19 pandemic began in the United States in March 2020, even early effects of mortality rates for the first half of 2020 indicate reduced life expectancy. Male life expectancy at birth fell 1.2 years, from 76.3 years in 2019 to 75.1. Female life expectancy dropped 0.9 years, from 81.4 years to 80.5. The gap between male and female life expectancy increased from 5.1 years in 2019 to 5.4 in 2020. Racial statistics indicate the expectancy gap between non-Hispanic white and Black people widened from 4.1 years in 2019 to 6 years in the first half of 2020, the largest since 1998 [23, 24].

Approximately 25% of the US population lives in rural areas, where they are experiencing additional barriers to healthcare. These barriers include living great distances from medical and trauma centers, lack of prevention, screening, and treatment, longer waits, and fewer specialists. This has widened the healthcare gap between rural and urban dwellers. The U.S. Department of Health and Human Services regions organize the geographic and population diverse healthcare system into regions which are illustrated in Fig. 9.2. Within each region, there are issues

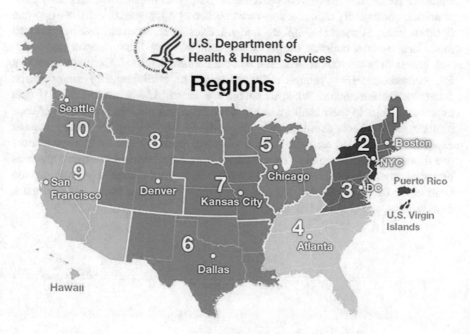

Fig. 9.2 Regional Offices of the Office of Intergovernmental and External Affairs [30]

related to resources, distances, and the nature of healthcare needs, and impact of the capacity and capabilities of the systems available within the region. It is important for agencies to understand these variabilities and resources in order to plan, coordinate, and provide healthcare and meet the needs of people in the regions.

In some regions, there are counties without hospitals or primary physicians, for example. In some regions, there is a lack of healthcare transportation such as ambulances or the capability of dealing with rescues. In some regions, people must travel from rural areas to the major urban areas, even in emergencies, to receive appropriate levels of care. The nature of health emergencies might be different between regions, for example, population composition, age of the population, burden of disabling conditions, nature of work in the region, cold weather regions which experience different health emergencies from hot weather regions. Even smoking and alcohol habits vary which affect health risks and need for healthcare. Some regions have a high burden of recreational emergencies such as outdoor sports, or higher roadway speed limits which affect health and injury risk in motor vehicle accidents. The distance and time involved in a rescue and also traveling to an appropriate level of care increases the risk of a poor outcome which is reflected in regional statistics and in urban versus rural burden of disease. Important examples include head injury from motor vehicle accidents, and stroke or cardiac emergencies. In 2014, even though the death rate in the United States reached a historically low number, the rural mortality rates (830.5 per 100,000 population) decreased less than the urban mortality rates (704.3 per 100,000 population) from the five most common causes of death, and many were preventable [25]. This translates to mortality rates which are consistently higher in non-metropolitan or rural areas than in metropolitan or urban areas, as shown in Figs. 9.3 and 9.4. Even in urban areas, underrepresented minorities, women, children, the uninsured, economically disadvantaged, and others lack access to in-person medical care and the communication infrastructure needed for telemedicine. Even though resources might be available, they might not be accessible to individuals. When resources are unavailable or inaccessible, people experience risks to their health that are immediate and also accumulate over their lifetime. This affects families and communities. Modernization should include expanding the needed technology infrastructure, methods, and systems to address healthcare within the regions. Telemedicine may help improve the mortality rates by increasing access to healthcare, to supplement but not entirely replace in-person healthcare, for example, for prenatal care, high risk pregnancies, preeclampsia, emergencies, and birthing [26–29].

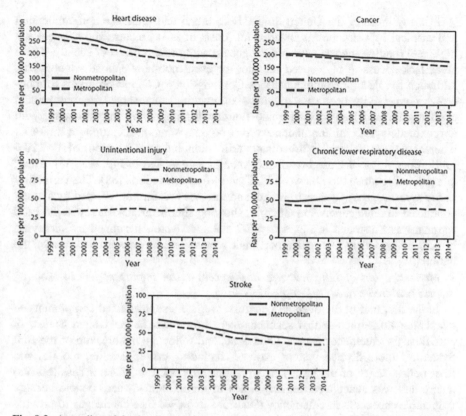

Fig. 9.3 Age-adjusted death rate among persons of all ages for five leading causes of death [31]

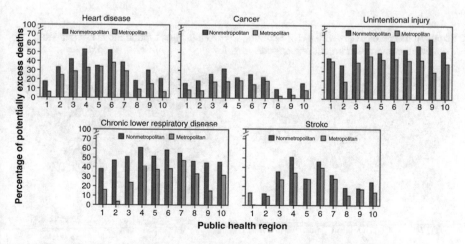

Fig. 9.4 Percentage of potentially excess deaths among persons aged <80 years [32]

In many areas of the United States, both urban and rural, the communication and medical infrastructure is insufficient, costs of infrastructure and services are high, and funding models have not caught up with present needs of society. These areas lack access to high-speed internet, or even mobile telephone connectivity. Although the Federal Communications Commission (FCC) has programs to modernize connectivity or access, methods of tracking underserved regions remain controversial and lead to inadequate funding for improving infrastructure, with approximately 14.5 million underserved people in America according to the FCC, whereas Microsoft reports broadband utilization indicates approximately 120.4 million people do not use broadband internet as depicted in Fig. 9.5 [33]. There is a gap in broadband use between FCC and Microsoft reports [33]. The variability in the reporting about access to broadband internet was further revealed by a study conducted in three counties in Georgia, showing significant inaccuracy in the FCC estimates as illustrated in Fig. 9.6. FCC statistics were determined by surveying broadband providers who self-report their service in each census block across the nation [34].

Modernization of infrastructure and access is an important key to meeting diverse healthcare needs of people globally.

In the first half of the twentieth century, we had a sophisticated comprehensive telephonic infrastructure that reached every household in the United States, in particular for emergency access. Over time, and following the breakup of the Bell System, a more diverse system evolved, including cable, satellite, mobile, and fiber optics. Much of the legacy network that supported universal access fell into disuse and was abandoned, leaving holes in service areas where people became vulnerable especially in emergency situations. Now we face challenges to provide universal services to people all across the country, and around the globe. Even

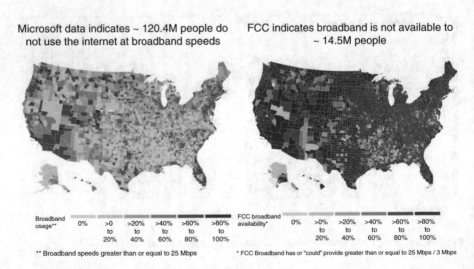

Fig. 9.5 FCC and Microsoft Broadband Maps [33]

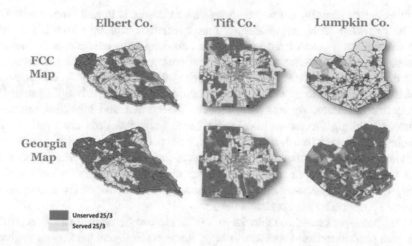

Fig. 9.6 Georgia rural broadband situation worse than FCC maps showed, new mapping underway. (Emma Hurt, Sep 13, 2019 [34])

though programs exist to make communications services more affordable for low-income consumers, like the FCC Lifeline program that provides discounts on the monthly fees, these services may not be sufficient to address the need, particularly when the infrastructure fails to reach every household. Even when family members wish to help their parents at a distance, there are locations where internet and mobile services limit their ability to connect monitoring and health applications for their loved ones. Connected healthcare represents an urgent need to drive policy makers and technology innovators to shift resources towards the important goal of reducing the characteristic and widening gap of death and poor outcomes among rural populations, uninsured, underrepresented minorities, and other underserved people. For further reading about legacy systems, see the report about the Breakup of AT&T, information about lifeline services and universal access [35, 36].

9.4 Improvements and Infrastructure

Improvements in accessibility and inclusion will be led by innovations in communication technologies, standards, and policies. Over the past decade, the internet has transformed into the cloud backbone connecting a variety of "smart" systems and devices for the ever-demanding connected lifestyle, including health monitoring and network connected actuators. These improvements enable novel service and also emergency models that can rapidly increase system capacity, reach, timeliness, and geographic diversity. For example, unmanned aerial vehicles (UAVs) can be deployed to a crash scene or natural disaster, enabling quick response so that the scene can be assessed. These approaches can expand limited local resources and enable effective planning for first responders and hospitals in real time. Assistance can be provided from anywhere, so that specialists can be identified at any time without delays associated with remote and dangerous conditions. Advancing connected systems taps into sophisticated network resources and AI/ML solutions that can be brought more effectively into each situation which would otherwise be limited to time consuming and physical methods of problem solving. Connecting to network resources, for example, reduces the burden and logistical problems of humans calling around to find where needed hospital beds are available for a stroke, heart attack, crash trauma patient, or a pediatric emergency. Networked solutions can also bring remote care to the scene more effectively reducing need for quick transportation to the nearest hospital or medical center. Traffic and logistics management in the network can also be used to find a better fit for a hospital or resource appropriate to the patient's need.

Many bottlenecks and roadblocks to healthcare can be addressed by improved inclusion, accommodation, and accessibility through intelligent networked systems. For example, people who travel to appointments from a distance are sometimes late or must wait upon arrival. Networked services can be used to provide more flexible appointments, directions and information for travelers, using the Global Positioning System (GPS), plus weather, traffic and other information to arrange a more flexible and accommodating schedule. This can improve accommodation and accessibility for many needed services such as preventive care, screening, drug and alcohol substance programs, psychological therapy, prenatal care and more, to reduce risk factors and improve wellness for everyone. Such intelligent networked systems can also be employed to find medical resources available for immediate need for a visit to a hospital or clinic, to reduce the number of people who must resort to utilizing more expensive resources such as emergency rooms where certain services might not even be available.

In particular, the advent of the Internet of Things (IoT) has been a major driver for the evolution of novel and diverse applications such as smart homes, smart cities, health monitoring, remote surgery, long-term monitoring of water quality, marine life, oil and gas, connected cars, navigation, and remote and autonomous vehicles of various types, as illustrated in Fig. 9.1. Critical challenges and constraints associated with large volumes of IoT and next-generation wireless networks include providing consistent low latency, highly reliable network communications, signal processing, as well as information extraction of big data, supporting automated decision-making, with energy efficiency. Many of these devices are also expected to be low cost, low complexity, and battery-operated user equipment (UE). These challenges and constraints necessitate novel, fast-convergent, energy-efficient solutions. Moreover, a number of problems in these fields are computationally complex to the extent that they are referred to as technically "NP-hard" (non-deterministic polynomial-time hard) and therefore motivates the incorporation of machine learning and artificial intelligence as the underlying novel framework [37]. The IoT scenario presents a variety of applications, whose demands and value can be contrasted to that of conventional human-to-human (H2H) communication. While the IoT was a small consumer marketplace at one point, the combined experience of COVID-

19 telemedicine and multiple possible scenarios will lead to many innovations for a connected lifestyle that far exceed even our most ambitious vision of the IoT-enabled future.

We envision telemedicine will soon evolve beyond a one-to-one H2H connection between the patient and the doctor or nurse for one appointment, one measurement, or one transaction. Telemedicine enabled by wearable and implanted devices will become part of a comprehensive medical model, part of a connected lifestyle with humans and machines in the loop. An IoT wearable device involving a simple thermometer has greater significance in a cloud-connected healthcare and connected lifestyle scenario, which can be leveraged in telemedicine scenarios. People everywhere will be served on a secure set of resources and functions enabled by an interconnected public network served by multiple levels of security and privacy, with service providers delivering value to individuals and groups. Together with demographics, medical history of the individual, health status, stage of life, and more identity-related information, including knowledge of the context or location, awareness of time and day, and body temperature tracked by a wearable device, there is a robust amount of data which may be accessed and interpreted by various network agents. These network agents/robots such as the ones that analyze the weather and room temperature, air flow, and humidity and adjust the thermostat, will incorporate sensor-measured body temperature, health status and age of individuals in the environment, understanding if they are athletic or frail, for example [38–40]. Incorporating information and models, knowledge and learning, the network agent/robot will provide features adding up to more than the sum of the parts, which will be shared, with the ability to improve meaningful function for individuals and populations. This vision provides a model for designers and developers to leverage in serving widely diverse knowledge domains and populations, even while processing multivariate features. This vision breaks down barriers for those with disabling conditions providing best-fit solutions, reduces the burden upon individuals and, at the same time, benefits society. Over the years, projects have explored and filled in this vision of a comprehensive, cloud-enabled connected lifestyle.

9.4.1 For Aging Adults, Accommodation, Chronic Conditions

We envision a scenario where individuals are connected with their loved ones using a secure and trusted platform, which provides accessibility for virtual spaces including telemedicine and social interaction, trusted remote operation of features, and more. Privately, objective measures are gathered using wearable devices and the cloud connected system processes.

In this scenario, an aging adult living at home, or at a senior living setting such as a skilled nursing facility, an assisted living facility, or a memory care facility, depends on several caregivers and care providers. Many aging adults have multiple chronic conditions and need the attention of several care providers. The caregiving responsibilities may be shared by several siblings or family members. Other individuals like financial advisors, elder law attorneys, money managers, government insurers like Medicare in the United States, private insurers, and others have access to personal and private information of this aging adult individual. Having immediate access to the relevant information to make adequate decisions for the care and well-being of this aging adult is critical, but it is crucial that this access is trustworthy and ensures the privacy of the aging adult.

As seen in this scenario, Trust, Accessibility, and Privacy (TAP) of connected lives is critical to provide adequate care and to guarantee the well-being of the aging population.

Another embodiment of this scenario relates to the body temperature of the individual living alone who is elderly or suffers a debilitating condition. They might need a human to assist with activities of daily living including monitoring body temperature and adjusting room temperature. A connected healthcare application as described can provide accommodation for that person, improving independence without the need for a human intervention [39].

The system can be further extended to monitor the temperature of other persons in the physical environment that are processed by the telemedicine system to infer the health status of each individual, and use that learning to offer features to others through the cloud. Temperature measurement has been used as one part of the assessment for COVID-19. However, traditionally considered fever temperature ranges may not apply to the elderly, and therefore such a prognostication system has to adapt to the conditions of the individual to minimize the risk of infection and disease. Such a system should also consider the potential history of exposure, incorporating the identity of the individual and those with whom they may have come into contact [40].

It is of importance to understand the health of others in the environment of the individual and to be able to infer the implications for them. The scenario which has emerged since COVID-19 is an excellent illustration of the dynamics and the timely need for information across a population in order to improve outcomes in a connected lifestyle, and connected health of an individual and society. One can now appreciate the value across many additional use cases, in particular, to improve resilience to unexpected permutations and new problems not represented in IoT consumer models.

The vision of connected healthcare includes transparency, reliability, and resilience; our vision involves curating and updating models, algorithms, data, performance, and confidence measures to improve trust. The vision endorses inclusive connected healthcare access, with culturally and linguistically adaptive systems, that reflect the individuals, the latest features, as well as knowledge, information, and learning shared across the cloud. In light of COVID-19, one can easily recognize that knowledge of properties, characteristics, and features of individual patients, their symptoms, treatment, and outcomes can improve performance of a knowledge-based connected healthcare system. For example, knowing that specific patients with a specific pre-existing condition and/or taking a specific medication had a poor outcome on a specific treatment for COVID-19 could improve performance of an AI/ML system being used by healthcare providers. However, previous knowledge used to design algorithms, and databases used to train algorithms, might not apply as well to the COVID-19 situation. Timely and ongoing system and application performance checks will be required to improve curation of algorithms, data, and more. Even appreciating symptoms of patients such as body temperature of aging persons whose screening test was positive for COVID-19 might pose challenges in decision-making. An AI/ML system which may advantageously use knowledge about the population and body temperature measures to improve performance of a system, while updating the training data with real patient cases with as many variables as possible, would be ideal. Then ongoing verification of system performance can detect changes in a variety of aspects of the ecosystem, for example, the presence of variants, vectors, risks to particular populations, effect of vaccine, and effect of treatment. [41].

It is most important to recognize that individuals and people with pre-existing health risks or conditions might have physiological characteristics and experiences to consider during monitoring, diagnosis, and care. For example, people with impaired immune systems might have an inability to fight an infection, and they might not be aware of their status which can result in an inability to fight an infection and/or mount a temperature. They might neither recognize risks nor symptoms. Also as people age, they develop changes of clinical importance. Elderly patients are often not capable of mounting a strong inflammatory response, for example, to infection and disease. During COVID-19 surveillance, this is of great significance because elderly and other persons might fail to register a temperature traditionally considered to be a fever. Not only is a fever used as a diagnostic indicator, it is also a prognostic indicator. These are important considerations and together with history, evidence must be included in systems and methods when screening, diagnosing, and treating individuals, for example, by lowering temperature ranges when examining elderly persons [39, 40].

Addressing these issues, connecting the unconnected, inclusion, accommodation, improving healthcare, is consistent with the United Nations Sustainable Development Goals (UN SDGs), in particular, Goal 3 Good Health and Well-being, part of the 17 UN SDGs illustrated in Fig. 9.7 [7].

During a pandemic, many traditional accessibility accommodations pose unforeseen challenges. At the time of this writing, a variety of measures have been implemented to avoid spread of the COVID-19 virus. Many of the measures confuse people and change frequently. We have social distancing and face masks. Travel, indoor venues, and social activities are limited. Schools once opened have closed again, shifted to hybrid, and at times change again on a moment's notice. Worldwide, many people have been quarantined to reduce risk of infection. Individuals are isolated away from family and friends, many in senior communities. Effective quarantine is a complex concept. Those known to be exposed to COVID-19 are expected to quarantine to avoid spreading it, or certain other infectious diseases. Many other people are forced to risk themselves and the health of their families going out to work, school, raising children, and living in multigenerational homes. With a vaccination, various people will not necessarily have symptoms making the process even more complex. People are denied cognitive, hearing and speech, or language interpreters or companions during health visits, as well as at school, work, court, the bank, etc. Systems reliant upon the Americans with Disabilities Act (ADA) procedures are unavailable during lockdown, and even after facilities reopened, making ADA unsustainable. Technologies can provide important solutions, but many are not connected. Non-essential procedures, including hearing-related and other surgeries, are suspended in order to reduce endangerment, preserve hospital and medical system resources, and reduce demand on personal protective equipment (PPE) [42]. Face masks impair lip reading and reduce audibility of the voice and intelligibility of speech or other sounds. Altogether life has become even more challenging, while increasing loneliness and despair.

TAP for these populations, no longer provided in human assistance, compromised by transitioning from physical to virtual spaces or to new locations, requires attention. Accessibility will rely more on virtual agents and virtual robots in virtual spaces.

Virtual spaces and physical spaces rely on accurate identity, identification of individuals, as well as the associated information conveyed through ordinary interactions in physical spaces, to establish meaningful and secure virtual and physical transactions, and provide access to needed data. Visits to the doctor and waiting in the waiting room convey a great deal of information about the healthcare provider, staff, and also the individual patient and their support system. A physical space conveys multivariate information including a sense of permanence, identity, education, certification, and other qualifications of the provider. This information is conveyed through diplomas on the wall, other employees in the space, quality of the furnishings, coffee or informative materials, others waiting to see the provider, etc. Patients and their companions can be identified with photo identification, and others in the waiting room convey a sense of endorsement. Changes of aging and other

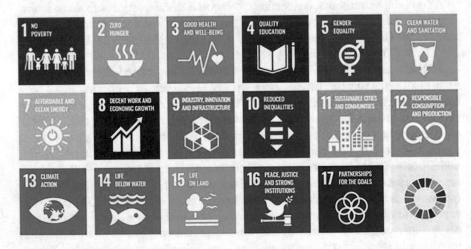

Fig. 9.7 United Nations Sustainable Development Goals [7]

conditions might not be obvious through telemedicine encounters. During COVID-19, a long interval has passed when people rely on remote care. Providers and services have changed. Many of the implicit information and assurances associated with traditional interactions will need to be addressed in order to provide trust, and appropriate levels of care.

Incorporating accessibility into IoT peripheral and wearable devices supported by cloud connections on a mainstream communication infrastructure using the latest techniques transforms what was once impossible and expensive into a practical enabling technology. Such an approach is necessary as we can see from COVID-19 experiences. Improving such interactions will improve the reach of connected healthcare to a greater percentage of the population who can transition among virtual spaces and will lay the groundwork for the future of TAP and connected lifestyles.

Our imperative is to address the urgent and universal need for accessibility. We are concerned with advancing technology for humanity, to reduce suffering and disparity, including healthcare disparity, and improve quality of life consistent with the United Nations Sustainable Development Goals [7]. This presents a complex and multidimensional challenge. People have abilities along a continuum experiencing disabling conditions only under certain circumstances, or during certain phases of life. Accessibility and accommodation may vary by time of day, situation, and environment. Populations have been living with disparities of many types for a long time and the pandemic is revealing the dramatic, and truly tragic negative risks and outcomes of long-time disparities. For example, for those not connected, for those who are disabled, underrepresented, minorities, indigenous peoples, the elderly, the marginalized, and those with pre-existing conditions. The systems designed and developed to support the mainstream consumer market often overlook those with little to no access to technology and/or differing abilities; we seek to provide accessibility on mainstream networks and to reach as many as possible with features and services that can provide smooth transitions for all.

9.4.1.1   Accommodation

The global pandemic has raised awareness of the needs for accommodation for those with disabling conditions in order to reduce disparities. Even in the best of times, accommodation often fails to meet the needs of individuals and populations. Accessibility assists those with needs for hearing, vision, mobility, cognition, abilities, protection, aging, or more, and others with invisible disabilities and those who do not identify as disabled which has become a greater challenge during the pandemic. Social distancing and other pandemic measures leave many people without human assistance, making them vulnerable. The digital divide further exacerbates disparities, especially for people who are unable to conduct their many needs online such as working at home, shopping online, telemedicine, educating themselves or their families, and the like. There is a catastrophic impact on individuals, families, groups, and everyone in society. Solutions for access and accommodation are high cost, sometimes custom, cumbersome, and not interoperable. Many accommodation solutions suffer proprietary interfaces, are often complex, and follow siloed approaches. These solutions are not available or affordable to many; therefore, they fail to help the very people who need them most. Accommodation systems are often not effective in the new pandemic reality. Examples of accommodations for accessibility include expensive hearing aids or specialist sign language interpreters, and captioning for those with hearing loss; screen readers, canes, or guide dogs for those with vision loss; wheelchairs, walkers, canes, and dogs for mobility loss.

We envision mainstream systems infrastructure on interoperable networks of networks provided by collaborative service providers, incorporating accessibility. For example, IoT integrated into communication systems that include accommodation for those with hearing loss or other communications issues, supported by standards, including open source solutions. This would include the most effective technologies, on cloud-connected slim mainstream devices and the lowest cost configurable platforms, balancing needs of society, and with smooth transitions across virtual spaces, to achieve connected lifestyles.

9.4.2 Failure of Inclusion Equals Failure of Resilience

Failure of inclusion represents failure of resilience. Multiple systems failed during the COVID-19 pandemic. For example, communication methods failed for those with hearing loss.

9.4.2.1 Hearing Loss

People with hearing loss experience inequities in their lives including social, educational, healthcare, business, employment, income, justice, etc. and miss out on many popular experiences. One-third of people over age 65 have hearing loss; 5% of the population of the world, 466 million children and adults worldwide, have disabling hearing loss, according to the World Health Organization (WHO). Only about 17% of those who would benefit from hearing aids actually use them. The impact of unaddressed hearing loss costs an estimated 750 billion US dollars annually worldwide and can interfere with many aspects of life [43].

Hearing loss affects functional, social, emotional, economic, and all aspects of life. Partnerships to introduce innovative strategies and disruptive solutions, for standards, prevention, hearing loss identification, and treatment, such as affordable hearing aids, cochlear implants, and evidence-based services worldwide, can reduce disparity and improve quality of life in the near term and into the future [44, 45]. Many people who would benefit from hearing aids do not have them; researchers have identified a number of reasons including but not limited to cost, access to insurance, geographic location, or cultural influences [46].

However, even in countries where hearing aids are available, people choose not to use them, perhaps because they do not fulfill their needs. For example, in the UK 11 million people have hearing loss making it the second leading disabling condition. Whereas 6.7 million could benefit, only about two million use hearing aids. For the 4.4 million people with hearing loss who are of working age, the employment rate is 65% compared to 79% for those without long-term health issues or disability. On average, people with hearing loss are paid £2000 less per year than the general population; this amounts to £4 billion per year in lost income across the UK [47]. These issues are particularly urgent. The stakes are very high during a pandemic as disparity amplifies impact on humans all around the globe.

There are limitations to the usefulness of hearing aids, and in our vision, cloud-connected hearing assistance can advance the ability for people with varying degrees of hearing loss to engage more fully in life. Even people with mild hearing loss are challenged to understand speech. In the pandemic, people wearing masks reduces the volume of voices by an estimated 10 dB. Masks may obscure visibility of the face, so even more people are experiencing difficulty understanding speech [48]. Understanding communication is now a matter of life and death, health and information, learning and work, loneliness and comfort. The most important thing we can do is to work as a team, including every stakeholder, policy makers, and industry, to promote equitable access for all using mainstream cloud-connected IoT. Those with hearing, vision, mobility, or cognitive issues, or any other situation leading to disparity in jurisdictions all over the world should be included in this equitable distribution of technology enabling assistance.

Identity is a key to providing security, trust, and privacy. Whereas pre-pandemic interactions in physical spaces enabled individuals to recognize the faces and/or voices of other individuals, many transactions are now being conducted in virtual spaces.

9.4.2.2 Use Case: Hearing Assistance to Authenticate Identity

One of the most essential methods of security is to recognize a person, by face or voice. A person's hearing must be relatively good in order to recognize the voice of an individual to confirm identity, to communicate, recognize environmental threats including fire alarms, sirens, wind, thunder, hear a sink dripping, and more. Some people with hearing loss lose their ability to recognize voices. Elders or a differently abled person may be unaccustomed to telemedicine, they may be unfamiliar with a person, or for another reason, they may be unable to recognize voices. Inability to recognize voices of family members, friends, teachers, healthcare providers, or others leaves them vulnerable to identity spoofing in a physical or virtual space. An unscrupulous person can take advantage of the individual by telling them they are a trustworthy individual.

Trust, Accessibility, Privacy, and security through cloud connectivity can provide a means to first provision biometric measures for voice identity databases, then to authenticate people by biometrics of voice using virtual spaces for connected lifestyles.

When an individual goes into the physical medical center or doctor's office, the staff recognizes the individual, whether with a picture, through person-to-person human recognition, or by a biometric technology, such as facial, voice, or hand vein recognition. In a physical space, or even in a video interaction, a human or facial recognition application could be used for security. However, some algorithms have been performing poorly, attracting negative attention. More importantly, facial recognition is not always possible during the pandemic. A first line of prevention for coronavirus is to wear a mask, and socially distance. Wearing masks reduces the practical usefulness of facial recognition technology and causes problems for those with hearing loss when speaking through the mask which lowers acoustic transmission, the volume of speech, and prevents lip reading [48].

We look to our experience in a wide range of communications-related topics, including innovating, designing, developing, regulatory issues, standards, human factors, and large-scale services on public and private infrastructures. We bring to TAP over 40 years of experience participating in the communications evolution, providing connectivity, services, security, emergency systems, and more that represents the gold standard in the industry. Claude Shannon introduced Information Theory, which provides insight into many aspects pertaining to providing high quality reliable technology, connectivity, security, and services that are interoperable, scalable, and can reach everyone, everywhere [49, 50]. The present environment includes networks of networks, with a variety of equipment and service providers, in a combination of regulated spaces. Where security, trust, and privacy might previously have relied upon location and physical properties of a transaction, we see the emerging scene of virtual spaces, virtual transactions, blended experiences, and an urgent need to provide smooth transitions among physical and virtual spaces. The needs of society have evolved beyond standalone use cases. We must seamlessly bridge individual use cases, physical spaces, virtual spaces, virtual transactions, and accessibility for a connected lifestyle experience.

It is crucial to provide accessibility and to include as many people as possible to reduce disparity and improve quality of life and safety for everyone. Previously limited by consumer uptake of products and services, with the pandemic, we have reached and quickly passed a tipping point of value to stakeholders, regulators, and for the benefit of public health everywhere. Connected healthcare is a fact of our society. With smooth transitions across virtual spaces, connected healthcare enables today's connected lifestyle for diverse populations under one mainstream network of networks, in a cloud-connected communication model. Planning TAP for connected lifestyles now is key to integrity and success.

Failure of inclusion led to failure of resilience for people with disabling conditions during the COVID-19 pandemic due to complex mechanisms, leaving many people vulnerable. Disabling conditions have been identified as a differentiator in COVID-19 impacts and deaths. In a report from the UK examining COVID-19 deaths, disabled people made up 6 in 10 (60%) of all deaths involving the coronavirus (COVID-19). For comparison, disabled people made up 17% of the study

COVID-19 Cases, Hospitalizations, and Deaths, by Race/Ethnicity				
Rate ratios compared to White, Non-Hispanic persons	American Indian or Alaska Native, Non-Hispanic persons	Asian, Non-Hispanic persons	Black or African American, Non-Hispanic persons	Hispanic or Latino persons
Cases[1]	1.8x	0.6x	1.4x	1.7x
Hospitalization[2]	4.0x	1.2x	3.7x	4.1x
Death[3]	2.6x	1.1x	2.8x	2.8x

Race and ethnicity are risk markers for other underlying conditions that affect health, including socioeconomic status, access to health care, and exposure to the virus related to occupation, e.g., among frontline, essential, and critical infrastructure workers.

Fig. 9.8 COVID-19 cases, hospitalizations, and death, by race/ethnicity [52]

population, therefore suggesting that disabled people have been disproportionately impacted by the COVID-19 pandemic.[51].

In addition to disabling conditions, race and ethnicity are risk markers for other underlying conditions. These conditions affect health in complex ways including socioeconomic status and access to healthcare. In addition, there is varied exposure to the virus related to occupation, for example, frontline, essential, and critical infrastructure workers. For more information about COVID-19 cases, hospitalizations, and deaths, by race/ethnicity, see Fig. 9.8 [52].

Perhaps the most shocking statistics in the United States reported in November 2020 are that 40% of the COVID-19 deaths have been in long-term care facilities. In three states, long-term care COVID-19 deaths accounted for over 70% (New Hampshire, Rhodes Island, and Connecticut). In 18 states, these deaths account for at least half of all deaths due to the pandemic (three mentioned above plus Minnesota, Kentucky, Pennsylvania, Massachusetts, Nebraska, Maine, North Dakota, Ohio, Delaware, Washington, Oregon, Indiana, Vermont, Maryland, North Carolina) [53].

With connected lifestyles and connected healthcare, we can transform the model of care. We can reach people where they are instead of gathering them in long-term care facilities or isolating them, which makes people dependent, uninformed, vulnerable to infectious diseases, loneliness, depression, domestic abuse, and other complications.

Accessibility and inclusion examples include implanted cardiac devices. How can we use a device like an implanted cardiac device as an IoT device for the delivery of care and how can we ensure privacy and accessibility for every stakeholder involved in the delivery of care?

Devices such as pacemakers and implanted cardiac defibrillators are connected with a wireless inductive coupler to a patient monitor, which is connected to a communications network. A service provider receives periodically transmitted data and creates a report for the physician, who assesses the performance of the device as a prescribed aid for the health of the patient. The patient receives a report with medical provider notes. During an in-person check-up, data is reviewed and patient healthcare is provided.

During the pandemic, patients remain at home, and they are not seen for elective surgeries, battery changes, and other important procedures. Recommendations from the American Heart Association and others include conducting frequent transfers of cardiac device data as well as extensive analysis of data. We envision opportunities to expand accessibility and inclusion for the patient, during this difficult time and continuing into the future. Through virtual spaces, aware of the patient implant and virtual agents that perform more sophisticated analysis, the world can be transformed.

Among all the pre-existing conditions, heart conditions pose specific risks. Some of these risks are well understood. Others, for those individuals having cardiac implants, are related to the function of the device itself. For example, electromagnetic fields (EMF) in the environment, even in healthcare settings, include a risk that might be hidden from both the patient and other people, such as magnetic resonance imaging (MRI) systems, or another incompatible environment [54]. In such a case, the smart building and virtual space, sensing the presence of the implanted device, perhaps through a mobile phone app, near-field communication (NFC), or another method, can engage a virtual agent or virtual robot for continual surveillance, assistance, and notifications. In our view, this accessible and inclusive system recognizes the context and the specific need of the human. The human does not have to self-identify when they walk into a building or when the Emergency Medical Services (EMS) people show up for an emergency. The H2H model fails to help in such situations. An inclusive system would be prepared to accommodate, transforming the experience so the person is no longer "disabled" when challenged by incompatible EMFs or episodes with EMS in a given virtual space. Trust, a person's expectation of being safe from cardiac health risks associated with the cardiac condition, can be improved by avoiding emergency events such as accidental exposure to MRI, EMFs, and other perilous situations. If there is an emergency in the smart building, a virtual agent or virtual robot can inform the EMS that the person with a cardiac condition is present in the physical space. People with implanted devices are encouraged to live a normal lifestyle; with inclusive connected healthcare and connected lifestyles, accommodation can in fact be achieved through virtual agents and virtual robots in virtual spaces, incorporating temporary conditions, augmented reality, and physical spaces.

The accurate test of trust in connected healthcare, as part of a connected lifestyle, is not simply what takes place in the physician's office or with home monitoring, but what happens in a virtual space when the patient steps into the real world—into their normal life.

9.5 Innovating for the Extraordinary Needs of Connected Lifestyles

Extraordinary demand for practical IoT, connected healthcare, and connected lifestyles has arrived. It is essential to the very survival of humans and the success of society everywhere. Meanwhile, the unprecedented growth of wireless communications and services in recent years has led to highly congested radio spectrum in the useful frequency range, leaving no further scope for future applications and consequently resulting in the looming spectrum crunch. With currently available wireless technologies, it is becoming increasingly difficult to facilitate more data and users into the congested spectrum. Fueled by the need to support the explosive growth of mobile data traffic, the quest for next-generation mobile networks has already begun through a range of research activities internationally. The primary targets of the next-generation mobile networks are to deliver 10–100× today's data rate, 1000× capacity per unit area, 10–100× the number of connected devices, <1 ms roundtrip latency, 10× spectrum and energy efficiencies, and support for IoT and other emerging applications. In other words, the next-generation mobile networks need to be significantly faster, resilient, cost and energy-efficient, and accommodate an extraordinarily large number of connected devices that can communicate very fast and reliably without any noticeable lags or delays. In particular, the IoT evolution demands the support of an enormous number of devices and machine-to-machine communications with varying capabilities and is expected to revolutionize the way we live and the applications we use on a daily basis. This brings the new generation of wireless technologies, the fifth-generation (5G) wireless communication technologies, to life.

The fifth-generation (5G) wireless communication technologies have three main operating categories—(1) enhanced mobile broadband (eMBB), (2) massive machine type communication (mMTC), and (3) ultra-reliable low-latency communication (URLLC). While the focus of eMBB is to provide a very high data rate and improved coverage, the mMTC and URLLC are tailored towards the Internet of Things (IoT) scenarios. Currently, most of the research and development in the telecommunications industry are targeting the needs of the people and industries in the urban areas. However, the International Telecommunication Union (ITU) estimates that 3G (third-generation wireless mobile telecommunications technology) covers 69% of the world's population which means that almost two billion people have no coverage. This will hardly change since the telecom operators and the people who live in such areas are not able to financially afford the installation of the expensive infrastructure that is needed. Recently, companies like Google and Facebook are aiming to tackle this technological inequality, the digital divide. However, providing coverage to these areas requires a massive momentum in research and development towards providing low-cost and low-power solutions for the rural and underdeveloped areas. Moreover, these solutions would easily be classified under eMBB/mMTC/URLLC for 5G rural operation. The deployment of unmanned aerial vehicles (UAVs) to enhance the coverage area is promising, and at the same time a challenging approach. The main advantage of using UAVs is that they are able to travel to remote areas and their density can vary according to the requirements at a particular region.

For eMBB applications, it is desired that the link can exchange a high amount of data related to all the uses in the designated cells. At the same time, it should not interfere with the transmission of the users. An ideal candidate for such scenarios can be millimeter wave communication as it enables high data rate exchange in the line-of-sight scenarios (suitable for the UAV type applications). In millimeter wave scenarios, a large number of antennas can be fit into a small area, and it is possible to achieve the benefits of massive multi-input multi-output (MIMO). Equipping each antenna element with a dedicated power-hungry and expensive radio frequency chain prohibits the use of digital signal processing techniques to design the beamformer. Hence, analog and hybrid beamformers are known to be the alternative solution. For delay-tolerant IoT applications, there is potential to use the backhaul satellite link itself for communication between the drones. The number of devices requesting service might be large. The use cases include applications where multiple smart meters are requesting and reporting data (smart-grid scenario), multiple vehicles carrying industrial assets need to be tracked simultaneously, and data of multiple patients needs to be monitored (eHealth).

When the focus is on extending the support for IoT, with both mMTC and URLLC being investigated, mMTC aims to serve many devices hosting delay-tolerant applications such as health monitoring, and URLLC mainly deals with the communication aspects of delay-sensitive, critical IoT applications like remote surgery. Also, new technologies like massive multi-input multi-output (MIMO) [55, 56] and non-orthogonal multiple access (NOMA) are being considered to further improve the 5G IoT performance [57]. In massive MIMO, the base station employs many antennas to serve the devices. The increased number of antennas provides an additional dimension domain, which can be utilized for beamforming (to improve coverage and transmit directed messages to the devices), improved channel estimation, and enhanced detection of user signals. In traditional 4G technologies, each user is allocated a separate set of orthogonal resources, which limits the number of simultaneously served users. In order to support the IoT scenarios with a large number of users, new access methods like NOMA are being evaluated, where two or more users share the same set of orthogonal resources, but are either separated in the power domain or the code domain. These technologies have rekindled the interests of academics and industry researchers towards developing novel mechanisms for efficiently supporting the IoT evolution through the 5G network.

IoT can be broadly categorized into four domains—(a) communications, (b) data handling, (c) security, and (d) energy efficiency. In the following, we outline a methodology in each of these domains.

Health monitoring IoT communications scenarios are characterized by a large number of health devices with a significant portion of these devices requiring low-data rate communication (very low-data rate to communicate health data). To this end, efficient mechanisms for small packet transmission need to be developed. The performance metrics considered to evaluate these mechanisms incorporate the network throughput, probability of outage, and latency aspects of the IoT devices. These small packet transmission methods have to be accompanied by a reliable method of network access. Many IoT plans consider only the monitoring, whereas actuating and controlling devices is integral to healthcare as well. Connected healthcare promises to go well beyond monitoring. Connected healthcare promises to deliver a comprehensive healthy lifestyle.

In addition, it is important to recognize the global level of network access. At present, many people in the United States and elsewhere do not have sufficient minimum download speed for broadband internet, for example, in March 2020 (according to M-Lab) only 62% of counties across the United States have it [58]. Healthcare applications must be able to deal with variable levels of connectivity gracefully, and a comprehensive plan to address the digital divide is essential to the safety and security of humans everywhere.

For health data handling, the presence of a massive number of IoT devices, each having its own data stream, would lead to a "big-data" phenomenon [59]. The IoT big data is not only large in volume, but also diverse (due to the variety of IoT applications) with a variable arrival rate (depending on the frequency of reporting/collection of the underlying IoT application). This demands novel mechanisms for data handling in terms of (1) recognizing similar data and exploiting data correlation to minimize storage requirements, (2) developing methods for faster data processing, and (3) designing networks that adapt to the data dynamics. The underlying complexity in developing these mechanisms is very large (often NP-hard). Therefore, we propose the need to explore and develop machine learning-based solutions to address these problems. Steps towards addressing these problems include (but are not limited to)—(1) developing novel device grouping mechanisms using data correlation-based k-means clustering and self-organizing maps, along with novel methods for data caching in IoT, (2) using compressive sensing and reinforcement learning for fast-convergent data processing, and (3) developing Q-learning and deep learning-based algorithms for self-organizing networks (SONs) to efficiently host the IoT. Moreover, with a considerable amount of IoT data involving sensors with human interaction, we would also recommend exploring the incorporation of social and behavioral learning for the relevant IoT applications.

Now let's turn to security. Securing data is a major issue in IoT since it has to co-exist with low-complexity data communications and should handle large data volumes. From the physical layer perspective, the presence of a large number of devices provides an increased number of dimensions for eavesdropping [60]. To this end, we would recommend developing artificial noise and compressive sensing-based physical layer security solutions having low complexity. From a network security point of view, we would recommend design methodologies to address security against distributed denial of service (DDoS) attacks through a form of secure transmission over the air. One approach would be to develop a mechanism for superposition of different user signals that reduces the transmission time. This prevents the attacker from having a long enough signal to find temporal correlation patterns to launch a DDoS attack. From a signal processing perspective, multiuser detection is required to superpose user signals. The data set of possible users is large, but the number of active users is small. This enables the evaluation of compressive sensing-based signal detection on a big data set. NOMA, with its associated multiuser detection strategies, is a good candidate to be explored in this regard. Again, machine learning algorithms can be explored for these purposes.

Energy efficiency is critical for health IoTs. The use of low-complexity and low-data rate operations also demands extended lifetime of the IoT devices. Therefore, constraints on energy consumption should be imposed while addressing the issues. While the communication mechanisms can be energy efficient by the introduction of enhanced sleep mode and power saving modes [61], other approaches towards addressing the energy consumption include wireless energy harvesting and ambient backscattering.

There is a need to develop novel techniques based on multiple antenna transmission and beamforming to further enhance the performance of wireless energy harvesting and ambient backscattering.

9.6 Looking Towards a More Evolved Environment for Humanity

Our vision is to define methods for a more resilient and evolved future in a connected lifestyle, utilizing sophisticated infrastructure resources and intelligence enabled through the cloud to create virtual spaces that are interoperable. In our vision, a connected lifestyle provides access and accommodates humans to reduce disparity and improve quality of life for everyone. Connected lifestyles will provide a future with the best fit for individuals where adaptive accessible systems respond to people's needs and where they don't need to self-identify or explain themselves. People will not be differentiated or categorized unnecessarily. People will be recognized where they belong, and where they choose to engage, and systems will provide for their needs. In the future, identity and privacy can function well in systems to meet the needs of individuals improving trust, safety, and more.

Local and global awareness of the important relationship of healthcare with lifestyle has been greatly elevated since the COVID-19 emergency, and the ongoing, expanding, and all-encompassing situation has transformed our society for the foreseeable future. Our vision of a connected lifestyle and integral connected healthcare reduces suffering, improves independence, enables people to reach their potential, and improves quality of life for everyone; it is established upon a firm foundation of Trust, Accessibility, and Privacy.

Our vision incorporates an enabling concept such as virtual agents that will manage the real and virtual experience and will manage and improve the smooth transition among our necessary connections, our resources, and our real environment, continually reviewing, learning, and recommending. An enabling concept such as our virtual space combines real and synthetic objects, slim and complex edge devices such as wearables, implanted devices, robots of a variety of types, and more innovations of devices and solutions as they become available in the environment.

Whereas we once focused on a narrow set of user needs, we find the reality of the COVID-19 global pandemic emergency has greatly expanded awareness of the need to eliminate the digital divide for the well-being and survival of humanity, and to rapidly facilitate the IoT layer to its greatest potential.

The digital divide and associated disparity have already impacted many humans around the globe, and continue to impact every aspect of life including healthcare, telehealth, education, work at home, opportunities for work, social connections and in their absence, loneliness, and depression, and so much more. As time goes on, this becomes a more significant influence. The impact of the COVID-19 global pandemic upon individuals, families, communities, and society will be extensive and disparities will be felt for many years and many generations to come. Directly, sickness and death associated with COVID-19, and indirectly associated reluctance to seek healthcare and lack of healthcare resources available for routine wellness, early diagnosis of serious illness, treatment, and care will have noticeable effects. In addition, growing unemployment and economic distress will lead to fewer people with access to health insurance and means to seek healthcare.

Traditional methods of care have proven ineffective, and in some cases they have proven deadly. For example, although only 1.3 million individuals of the US population resided in long-term care facilities as of 4 March 2021, 34% of those who died from COVID-19 were residents of these settings [62]. New models of connected healthcare including early data analysis, identification of simple measures to reduce spread of infectious disease, access to and sharing information, and providing access to healthcare through alternative methods such as hospital at home might reduce such risk. Distributed networks of care, rather than brick and mortar centers, might serve society more effectively, now and into the future.

Millions have been impacted by COVID-19, and there is no end yet in sight. Economic impact alone will affect education and earning opportunities for many, leading to multi-generational disparity.

We have come to a more global awareness of connected healthcare as an essential element of a connected lifestyle, and the vital need to provide infrastructure, access, and accommodation to all humans everywhere. Infrastructure, standards, methods, regulatory updates, and new funding models are needed. Such problems are no longer an issue for consumer business alone. Public health and welfare are now elevated in importance which includes public policy, government, and expanded technology innovations.

The systems and objects in connected healthcare provide features for people who have a wide range of medical needs from casual exercise monitoring to complex chronic health conditions. Those systems may include hospital at home, enabling interoperable individualized intelligent and accessibility features, negotiating transactions, protecting identity and privacy. Many people with complex chronic health conditions rely on others as caregivers to assist in their care, and exemplify the varied requirements for privacy in connected healthcare. Systems will be needed across geographic locations instead of in centralized medical care facilities alone. Multiple providers will share information about a patient, and communicate with more individuals routinely, including patients and patient representatives. For example, a parent might be sharing information about the patient who is a child, or a spouse or legal representative might be in control of a patient's information making privacy quite complex. During the COVID-19 emergency, many of these communications with their associated privacy issues are urgent and time sensitive.

Public health matters such as COVID-19 have greatly expanded complexities and awareness of requirements surrounding Trust, Accessibility–Accommodation, and Privacy (TAP). This was particularly exposed because of regulatory matters and Centers for Disease Control (CDC) safety restrictions, and also because the workforce is overwhelmed at healthcare facilities and through the entire workflow of healthcare, and because many caregivers cannot even be present when healthcare decisions are being made [63]. While during the COVID-19 emergency several significant and swift changes were made in infrastructure, we encourage local and national governments, regulators, organizations, and companies to move swiftly to improve infrastructure that will continue to improve reliable connectivity and sustain the new models to benefit all. Innovations in government policies and regulations must continue, even following the emergency. Such policy changes will help to address the big issues, direct resources to the situation, and reduce digital and healthcare disparity.

We advocate for connected healthcare enhanced through access to a resource-rich infrastructure, through cloud connections, bringing together a variety of relevant locations into one virtual space perspective, so that multiple consistent features and devices can be supported. At present, the COVID-19 emergency has enabled connected healthcare across state lines in the United States and enables Medicare and Medicaid insurance payments. In addition, regulations were changed to allow voice-only calls for certain specialties which is not ordinarily allowed by regulation. We advocate a continuation of these enabling regulatory models to improve access to centers of excellence, expand professional services, reduce distress, reduce time to appointments, increase compliance and treatment potentials, and more. We advocate for infrastructure efforts and new models to provide broadband to rural, urban, and suburban areas which are not currently covered by broadband and/or mobile services or support for individuals currently without access. With new programs to modernize infrastructure, more people should have access in a future connected healthcare system. There are people today who do not have broadband and or mobile phones and are limited in their ability to connect to telemedicine, and all the associated lifestyle measures that reduce risk and improve success in life. Communication infrastructure is now essential to healthcare in the way the Centers for Medicare and Medicaid Services (CMS) has provided for the nation's healthcare infrastructure through a network of hospitals and facilities [63]. We advocate government and policy planning, expanding communication infrastructure to provide for connected healthcare in a more comprehensive manner into the future to complement the brick-and-mortar centers of the CMS system.

Access to databases and technologies including AI/ML that exist for commercial or other purposes can be very helpful for connected lifestyles and connected healthcare. This increases independence for people, solves problems, improves recommendations, accommodating many more needs of users as individuals and as groups, and not bound to one healthcare or service provider. This supports better privacy and identity over all interrelated elements brought together into a virtual space. Over time, more features can be accessed through network connectivity, more sophisticated features can be pushed into the network, and edge devices can become even more intelligent and slim, simplifying upgrades, flexibility, and enriching capabilities at all levels. By virtue of connectivity, standards, networking and learning, improvements can be identified and supported in every layer and every aspect of connected lifestyles, improving outcomes.

We promote accommodation through specialized resources and interfaces that are planned and integrated into all systems and products from the very beginning, for example, for those with mobility, cognitive, vision, or hearing loss. Influencers and standards are needed to achieve this goal. Leadership is needed for the planning of global standards for products including IoT that incorporate interfaces for those with vision and or hearing loss, and feedback to others who interact with them to manage expectations. Screen readers with text to speech and captioning are examples of accommodation for products and IoT systems. At present, people must invest in accessories, devices, and systems from other vendors to provide accommodation after products are built. For each situation, compatible software or hardware must be purchased and integrated at great expense for individuals, companies, and groups. If standards supported transferring data to appropriate applications to process and or display information to those who need alternative interface design, then interoperability will be achieved and complexity reduced. At the moment, although the Americans with Disabilities Act (ADA) [11] requires accommodation, reasonable cost is a consideration and can be used as an excuse to hesitate on such development. We advocate building in accommodation to new products and IoT at the beginning, in the planning stages, making sure they interconnect effectively with screen readers and captioning, for example. We believe having these accommodations built-in rather than retrofitting them will have a greater impact and will lead to inclusion and more effective connected lifestyles, and connected healthcare, including in these difficult times of the public health emergency of COVID-19. This will enable people to more effectively participate in their own healthcare, education, workplace, etc. and advocate for themselves. We advocate for planning and development that engages people with all abilities. We also believe built-in accommodation and accessibility will be impactful for businesses for many reasons including that the products will be informed by inclusion, leveraging experience with the wider community, and enabling economic opportunities in the wider community to reduce disparities and benefit everyone. Products will reach more people, and they will expand the community, and enable more people to participate in the economy.

By meeting expectations for accessibility and inclusion on a continuum, connected lifestyles must fit and serve the people who need them, enabling everyone to be part of the connected village and global community. There are variability and evolving properties in the data associated with healthcare. Systems should not further attenuate inequalities and disparities, or propagate bias. Systems should fit the individual needs of each person, over time, and throughout life. Overall, systems should move away from episodic models and disease models focusing instead upon human-centered life and well-being models. Connected lifestyles should fit people regardless of health and ability. They should fit the athlete and the frail, those with acute or chronic conditions. Consider the athletic person who might have a watch or other device to help achieve training goals in one dimension, one who might have been a typical connected healthcare client before the COVID-19 emergency.

Consider the diabetic person who must manage several aspects of their health and lifestyle such as diet and exercise as another model in the connected healthcare model. Further, consider people who are frail or who have an acute illness. In a connected healthcare system, data from these populations may differ dramatically and bias can result from the way and the nature of the data used to train the systems, as is demonstrated by bias in pulse oximeter devices [64]. Systems must also fit those with disabling conditions without requiring new and extra development, or re-engineering. We can see there are many aspects of health that must be considered over a lifetime. Future systems must be able to update, evolve, and accommodate all of these and many more circumstances of human health and life.

Systems that use cloud connectivity, virtual spaces/agents, artificial intelligence (AI), and machine learning (ML) will provide a more adaptive and flexible model capable of working well with highly variable characteristics, needs, and resources. Systems can learn about changes involving age and hearing, vision, balance, and mobility in an individual and across populations, and with a variety of conditions. Systems can learn how to best adapt the environment to fit the need. For example, as we age or if we have reduced vision, we might require additional light to walk safely to the bathroom in the middle of the night. At the same time, systems can learn about individuals and their needs, finding others with similar needs as in social networks, to learn solutions, consolidate the learning across many solutions, and share optimized as well as personalized recommendations. For example, some users prefer hearing aid algorithms to allow them to hear high frequencies but other users do not. One high-tech solution for a given situation might not make every user happy. Maintaining capabilities not only to recommend solutions but also to enable personal choices would be ideal.

In this way, we can reach a baseline for systems where people don't have to look at a situation and get a message that "this is not for me." Instead, there will be less need to ask for special accommodations, and no need to label the people. People will see accommodation strategies in use all around. People will be able to find what fits—and recommenders will share what fits—because the accommodations and adaptive principles are already incorporated into the system, and the system learns and adapts. Systems should provide at least enough information in useful reconfigurable formats to support decision-making by a range of users including but not limited to patients, caregivers, healthcare professionals, stakeholders, policy makers, etc.

AI/ML testing and standards will be critical to support more widespread deployment of effective, trustworthy systems. Data used to train systems should be robust enough to serve the community and applications. There should be transparency about how the systems are trained. Performance of these algorithms should be measured and reliable. Thresholds of performance of systems, especially in terms of data used for training, must be transparent. AI/ML algorithms should function with reasonable levels of confidence and report results generated at those performance levels. Over time those system needs might change. Reliable test data should be maintained and publicly available. Disaggregated data are essential to meet the needs of diverse populations and improve well-being for individuals.

Systems should have a default mode, even a manual mode, to adapt when AI/ML is not performing adequately, or when communication is not robust enough to support the desired function. Systems should be poised to certify, change, track, report, and update training data to more effectively answer the questions posed over time. For example, if systems are trained on data from one population of people such as men, but then the system will later be used by women, the system might not perform with a high degree of confidence or accuracy. Training data should be supporting equitable systems, and updated to include the target populations, features, conditions, etc. Confidence levels reported by the system should reflect an identified goal of the application. Systems should improve outcomes in a quantifiable way, for example, through precision, reliability, reduced errors, improved throughput, and availability or frequency of process. The system should improve healthcare by some identified characteristics of the application, task, skill, logistics, or process. Results should represent an improvement in fact, or in access, such as to important surveillance or tests when experts or hospitals are not available. Systems must be more reliable than healthcare would be without the system, for example, by improving performance of healthcare professionals, by providing timely data, by improved personalized processing of data, through targeted recommendations, or through process improvement for experts and the like. Such a personalized approach will rely on privacy to improve trustworthiness and confidence in systems. If system performance is only addressed after errors are noticed by the public and reported in the media, consequences can be severe and long lasting.

Connected lifestyle systems must be trustworthy by meeting expectations for accessibility and inclusion; they must serve the people who need them, enabling them to be part of the village and global community, and not further attenuate inequalities and disparities, but to foster independence.

9.7 Conclusions and Discussion

Connected healthcare presents an urgent need to drive policy makers and technology innovators to shift resources towards the important goal of reducing the characteristic and widening gap of poor outcomes and deaths among rural populations, uninsured, underrepresented, minorities, and other underserved people.

The already existing technology divide afflicting people everywhere of all backgrounds became even more evident with the pandemic of COVID-19. These unprecedented times made apparent the need for re-engineering our systems to be more equitable, accessible, accommodating, trustworthy, and inclusive. The suffering experienced by people with disabling conditions, the elderly, underrepresented, minorities, economically challenged, and marginalized populations during this pandemic because of lack of support and isolation is inexcusable. It impacts every aspect of life and impacts dignity and well-being of individuals and communities locally and globally.

Technology and, for the most part, connected lifestyles and connected healthcare were previously perceived to be a luxury. Many of the connected healthcare apps were available as a premium service or as an accessory for expensive implanted devices. Before COVID-19, Medicare did not cover telemedicine. However, because of the emergency of COVID-19, at one point 80% of medical appointments were by telemedicine and covered by Medicare. In actuality, the old model created technology disparity, healthcare disparity, and in a pandemic, threatened not only the individual but also the family, community, and population. The old model of resilience was shattered under COVID-19.

The COVID-19 pandemic also raised awareness of disparity, bias, and social inequities of healthcare. The impact has been across the globe. We have yet to fully see the effect of the hardships of disparity. They very quickly result in suffering, sickness, and/or death. Many members of our families and society are vulnerable immediately and cannot avoid risks. We are learning of many more impacts of disparities upon individuals, families, communities, and societies. These impacts will be passed along to future generations.

We have an opportunity to build a vision, to share and engage with others, and to reinvent connected healthcare as an accessible, accommodating, and inclusive part of the connected lifestyle for all of humanity. We envision a modern infrastructure that shifts focus away from brick and mortar centralized physical places, such as hospitals in cities, doctors, and other healthcare providers in distant places, inflexible schedules and models, and standalone factories and schools. Our vision incorporates more planning and investment in connected lifestyles, for example, communications including broadband and mobile, culturally and linguistically appropriate systems, and adaptive systems that can reach every person.

We recognize the need for a new conceptualization of infrastructure because we realize interactions with the world are more fluid. Needs are more fluid. Our interactions continue to transition from physical to virtual spaces for every aspect of life: health delivery systems, work, education, entertainment, and social interactions. All places and all hours, individual well-being is crucial. We expect these fundamental needs for connectivity and healthcare will continue even after the COVID-19 pandemic is over.

The impact of the COVID-19 event will change how we view things we do in our ordinary life. Unless we do our best to capture this opportunity to understand the nature of inequities and needs, and to translate them into works of action, we will continue to see impact upon many people well into the future.

The great expansion of IoT extended to connected healthcare with its requirements for trust and privacy, is all now integrally linked with connected lifestyles. As a result, there is an urgent, immediate, ubiquitous, and increasing demand from stakeholders of every type, and a widening diversity of users. Intelligent technology and connected lifestyles in this context will improve not only safety and security, but it will allow our best fit essential interactions with the world. The envisioned world of IoT-connected healthcare, intelligent technology, and connected lifestyles will be only possible under a system of Trust, Accessibility, and Privacy (TAP).

We propose the vision of augmenting our systems to accommodate and/or compensate for human variabilities, disabilities, and other conditions to engage everyone—all of humanity, where all individuals are included, protected, and cared for and to truly support an egalitarian society. Thus, we need to address our infrastructure, standards, and applications. It is not possible to engage society when only 62% of the counties in the United States have broadband access, for example [58]. The situation is unfair to everyone. Our applications, systems and processes must incorporate inclusive design principles, and effectively integrate personalization. Therefore, we must create processes and standards for interoperability, security, and protection of privacy that allow users to trust the systems we build and operate. These requirements must be planned up front during system and product design because retrofitting is not as effective. ADA and other legislated methods have proven unsustainable, in particular during lockdowns associated with COVID-19 when human interpreters, for example, were not permitted in hospitals to assist those with hearing loss or language needs. Such methods have been demonstrated to be an obvious failure.

Retrofitting disproportionally places burden and expense on individuals, another form of disparity. New methods such as connected healthcare standards should include interoperability or plug and play with systems or devices used by those with vision or hearing loss, cognitive, or mobility needs rather than placing the burden on the person with needs having to advocate for special development efforts to support them. Technology solutions informed through standards have great potential to improve well-being.

The proposed solution will rely on two technological developments: (1) IoT and (2) virtual agents, all connected to a highly interconnected network and supported by continuous AI and machine learning.

For this vision to become a reality, the principles of TAP and security as foundational pillars must apply, upon a bedrock of interoperable, accessible, and accommodating infrastructure, in order to achieve our future of connected lifestyles.

Systems today rely more upon artificial intelligence, deep learning, machine learning, and the like. Great advances can come from excellent, transparent use of these technologies. However, because of the very nature of these technologies, they can jeopardize trust and privacy if misused or wrongly used. For example, mislabeling an individual belonging to a particular demographic for identity verification has caused a backlash of bias in systems causing mistrust of facial recognition technology and resulting in potential banning of its use.

In addition, even when intelligent systems are used in today's environment, there are often medical specialists present to supervise, detect, and correct issues that might arise in systems. Over time, however, more systems might be combined with others, and they might be used by different users without expert skills. It will be more difficult to detect if and where errors might be introduced. It will become more evident that stronger formal controls might be necessary.

It is also important to recognize there will be greater need for experts who understand the requirements and risks associated with the medical and healthcare environment as well as all the many layered issues associated with the connected healthcare systems, which represents a lot of technology expertise and experience. The risks impact human life.

We have to create the mechanisms for transparency and quality processes surrounding how the technology is implemented. To begin we would like to suggest collaborative community efforts including transparent access and ongoing updates to quality verifiable data training sets, making sure that the data is not biased one way or another but is proven in performance metrics to cover all the space of the problems in question with statistical evidence, and that is stated clearly, and updated on an ongoing basis. It is important to provide transparency and demonstrate how effectively the algorithm performs, to explain the performance, and to indicate variables that change recommendations. In particular in cases unique to medicine and wellness, the data should include all types of patient populations, and over time, more options for recommendations and treatments. There must also be a way to enforce transparency and appropriateness of one recommendation over another, and potentially indicate the scope of alternatives considered. These recommendations will require iterative development because systems will grow organically. Not all healthcare solutions, providers, or modalities will be available on connected healthcare at once. Effects of the scope, scale, and data content might not be obvious to users. The system must help in decision-making while indicating context and limitations.

As standards are being penned, we can craft guidance to improve connected healthcare. Use of technology must be appropriate and transparent. It is important for us to find appropriate ways to improve trust and privacy in the use of AI and associated technologies. At present, artificial intelligence is used with palm vein recognition to identify patients, for example. One way to improve trust and privacy might be for product developers to provide access to the data used to train the application, enable members of the community to participate in building and curating the databases and algorithms, and conduct ongoing verification of performance. In these ways, inclusive diverse systems can become possible, trust can be fostered, and privacy can be maintained.

Clarifying our vision for TAP and intelligent technology for connected lifestyles—Trust, Accessibility, and Privacy (TAP) is empowering particularly at this time in history. Everyone, everywhere, on the entire planet, is turning to science and technology to ensure the very survival of humanity, for health, education, work, communication, and society. Scheduling and tracking COVID-19 vaccinations for the entire population is a major undertaking with delays and difficulties in communication. Previous experience with healthcare, along with current confusing communication and information, can result in loss of trust. Many topics presented to the public are new, for example, COVID-19 testing. Individuals are hired to conduct contact tracing, but other individuals resist. Analysis and understanding of what it all means must be timely, and conditions can change yet again. Translating all the data into effective, understandable actions requires new notions and implementations to improve resilience. We have new concepts of COVID-19 symptom tracking, diagnosis, treatment, and ongoing care for people with COVID-19, especially and importantly for those who have what has become known as long-haul COVID. These issues are new to society and they are not simply a matter of discretion; they are essential to humanity. All of this is on top of the fact that people are still suffering from all the rest of the healthcare issues as usual. Many will suffer consequences of preventable negative outcomes because of overstressed healthcare systems and fear of exposure to COVID-19. This is no time to leave anyone behind. In particular, this is no time to leave out those at risk to poor outcomes from preventable health problems.

We call for a collective vision of the future— to rise to the moment with all our best skills, our voice and actions to inspire others through that vision. We encourage researchers, stakeholders, standards bodies, influencers, policy makers, students and the community, both locally and globally, to inspire change where each contribution is vital, significant, and meaningful. Now is the time to establish a vision and to create a resilient future that is inclusive, greater, and transformative for the dignity and benefit of all.

We can seize this moment together to make our mark—to leave our signature— on that vision of the future.

References

1. Bryce C, Ring P, Ashby S, Wardman, JK. (2020). Resilience in the face of uncertainty: early lessons from the COVID-19 pandemic, Journal of Risk Research, 23:7-8, 880-887, DOI: https://doi.org/10.1080/13669877.2020.1756379 To link to this article: https://doi.org/10.1080/13669877.2020.1756379

2. Yin Y, Gao J, Jones BF, Wang D. (2021). Coevolution of policy and science during the pandemic Science 371 (6525), 128-130. DOI: https://doi.org/10.1126/science.abe3084 8 JANUARY 2021

3. Global Health Security Index. The U.S. and COVID-19: leading the world by GHS Index score, not by response [Internet]. Washington (DC): GHS Index; 2020 Apr 27 [cited 2020 Dec 3]. Available from: https://www.ghsindex.org/news/the-us-and-covid-19-leading-the-world-by-ghs-index-score-not-by-response/ [Accessed 19 Sept 2021].

4. Daszak P, Keusch GT, Phelan AL, Johnson CK, Osterholm MT. (2021). Infectious Disease Threats: A Rebound To Resilience doi: https://doi.org/10.1377/hlthaff.2020.01544 Health Affairs 40, NO. 2 (2021): 204–211 This open access article is distributed in accordance with the terms of the Creative Commons Attribution (CC BY-NC-ND 4.0) license, https://www.healthaffairs.org/doi/pdf/10.1377/hlthaff.2020.01544 [Accessed 19 Sept 2021].

5. National Academies of Sciences, Engineering, and Medicine. (2021). Crisis standards of care: Ten years of successes and challenges: Proceedings of a workshop. Washington, DC: The National Academies Press. https://doi.org/10.17226/25767. https://www.nap.edu/catalog/25767/crisis-standards-of-care-ten-years-of-successes-and-challenges [Accessed 19 Sept 2021].

6. Rotarou ES, Sakellariou D, Kakoullis EJ, Warren N. (2021). Disabled people in the time of COVID-19: identifying needs, promoting inclusivity. J Glob Health 2021;11:03007. https://www.ncbi.nlm.nih.gov/pmc/articles/PMC7897447/ [Accessed 19 Sept 2021].

7. United Nations Sustainable Development Goals https://www.un.org/sustainabledevelopment/health/ [Accessed 19 Sept 2021].
8. Buheji M, da Costa Cunha K, Beka G, Mavrić B, do Carmo de Souza YL, Souza da Costa Silva S, Hanafi M, Yein TC, (2020). The Extent of COVID-19 Pandemic Socio-Economic Impact on Global Poverty. A Global Integrative Multidisciplinary Review. American Journal of Economics 2020, 10(4): 213-224 DOI: https://doi.org/10.5923/j.economics.20201004.02http://article.sapub.org/10.5923.j.economics.20201004.02.html [Accessed 19 Sept 2021].
9. Sumner A, Hoy C, Ortiz-Juarez E. (2020). Estimates of the impact of COVID-19 on global poverty, WIDER Working Paper, No. 2020/43, ISBN 978-92-9256-800-9, The United Nations University World Institute for Development Economics Research (UNU-WIDER), Helsinki, https://doi.org/10.35188/UNU-WIDER/2020/800-9. This Version is available http://hdl.handle.net/10419/229267 [Accessed 19 Sept 2021].
10. Smith AC, Woerner J, Perera R, Haeny AM, Cox JM. (2021). An Investigation of Associations Between Race, Ethnicity, and Past Experiences of Discrimination with Medical Mistrust and COVID-19 Protective Strategies. J. Racial and Ethnic Health Disparities (2021). https://doi.org/10.1007/s40615-021-01080-x [Accessed 19 Sept 2021].
11. U.S. Department of Labor Americans with Disabilities Act (ADA) https://www.dol.gov/general/topic/disability/ada [Accessed 19 Sept 2021].
12. 2020 Biennial Report To Congress As Required By The Twenty-First Century Communications and Video Accessibility Act of 2010 Report01_18_19-Sharing-Data-Saving-Lives_FINAL.pdf https://www.fcc.gov/document/2020-cvaa-biennial-report-congress [Accessed 19 Sept 2021].
13. Rotenberg M. (2000). Protecting Human Dignity in the Digital Age. In: Proceedings of the Third National Educational, Scientific and Cultural Organization Congress on Ethical, Legal and Societal Challenges of Cyberspace (UNESCO 2000). http://webworld.unesco.org/infoethics2000/report_151100.html [Accessed 19 Sept 2021].
14. Rosen, C.B., Joffe, S.; Kelz, R.R. (2020). COVID-19 Moves Medicine into a Virtual Space, *Annals of Surgery*: August 2020 - Volume 272 - Issue 2 - p e159-e160 doi: https://doi.org/10.1097/SLA.0000000000004098
15. HHS Press Office. HHS Issues New Report Highlighting Dramatic Trends in Medicare Beneficiary Telehealth Utilization amid COVID-19. U.S. Department of Health & Human Services. July 28, 2020. https://www.hhs.gov/about/news/2020/07/28/hhs-issues-new-report-highlighting-dramatic-trends-in-medicare-beneficiary-telehealth-utilization-amid-covid-19.html [Accessed 14 March 2021].
16. Kapelke C. (2020). The Post-Pandemic Future of Cybersecurity. CLCT Bulletin Center for Long-Term Cybersecurity at US Berkeley. August 24, 2020. https://medium.com/cltc-bulletin/the-post-pandemic-future-of-cybersecurity-7956c6c1292f [Accessed 19 Sept 2021].
17. HRS COVID-19 Task Force Update April 15, 2020. https://www.hrsonline.org/COVID19-Challenges-Solutions/hrs-covid-19-task-force-update-april-15-2020 [Accessed 19 Sept 2021].
18. Dobkowski D. (2020). Arrhythmia management during COVID-19 incorporates remote monitoring, virtual visits.Healio.com News August 14, 2020. https://www.healio.com/news/cardiology/20200814/arrhythmia-management-during-covid19-incorporates-remote-monitoring-virtual-visits [Accessed 19 Sept 2021].
19. UNDP COVID-19: New UNDP data dashboards reveal huge disparities among countries in ability to cope and recover (2020). April 29, 2020. https://www.undp.org/content/undp/en/home/news-centre/news/2020/COVID19_UNDP_data_dashboards_reveal_disparities_among_countries_to_cope_and__recover.html [Accessed 19 Sept 2021].
20. Lakkireddy DR, Chung MK, and Russo AM, et al. (2020). Guidance for rebooting electrophysiology through the COVID-19 pandemic from the Heart Rhythm Society and the American Heart Association Electrocardiography and Arrhythmias Committee of the Council on Clinical Cardiology. Endorsed by the American College of Cardiology. The Heart Rhythm Society, the American Heart Association, Inc., and the American College of Cardiology Foundation. Published by Elsevier Inc. on behalf of

Heart Rhythm Society. https://doi.org/10.1016/j.hrthm.2020.06.012https://www.hrsonline.org/COVID19-Challenges-Solutions/hrs-covid-19-task-force-update-april-15-2020 [Accessed 19 Sept 2021].

21. Guidance for Cardiac Electrophysiology During the Coronavirus (COVID-19) Pandemic From the Heart Rhythm Society COVID-19 Task Force; Electrophysiology Section of the American College of Cardiology; and the Electrocardiography and Arrhythmias Committee of the Council on Clinical Cardiology, American Heart Association. *Circulation* 2020;Mar 31:[Epub ahead of print]. https://www.acc.org/latest-in-cardiology/ten-points-to-remember/2020/03/30/12/17/guidance-for-cardiac-electrophysiology-covid [Accessed 19 Sept 2021].

22. floe The Inclusive Learning Design Handbook. https://handbook.floeproject.org/UnderstandingAccessibilityandInclusivity.html [Accessed 19 Sept 2021].

23. CDC: Life expectancy declines by 1.5 years in 2020 (2021). Jul 20, 2021. https://www.aha.org/news/headline/2021-07-22-cdc-life-expectancy-declines-15-years-2020 [Accessed 19 Sept 2021].

24. Arias E, Tejada-Vera B, Ahmad F, Kochanek KD. (2021). Provisional life expectancy estimates for 2020. Vital Statistics Rapid Release; no 15. Hyattsville, MD: National Center for Health Statistics. July 2021. DOI: https://doi.org/10.15620/cdc:107201. [Accessed 19 Sept 2021].

25. Garcia MC, Faul M, Massetti G, et al. (2017). Reducing Potentially Excess Deaths from the Five Leading Causes of Death in the Rural United States. MMWR Surveill Summ 2017;66(No. SS-2):1–7. https://doi.org/10.15585/mmwr.ss6602a1externalicon. [Accessed 19 Sept 2021].

26. Harrison E, Megibow E, (2020). Three Ways COVID-19 is Further Jeopardizing Black Maternal Health, July, 30, 2020. https://www.urban.org/urban-wire/three-ways-covid-19-further-jeopardizing-black-maternal-health [Accessed 19 Sept 2021].

27. Howell E A. (2018). Reducing Disparities in Severe Maternal Morbidity and Mortality. Clinical obstetrics and gynecology, 2018 June; 61(2), 387–399.

28. Bosworth A, Ruhter J, Samson LW, Sheingold S, Taplin C, Tarazi W, and Zuckerman R. (2020). Medicare Beneficiary Use of Telehealth Visits: Early Data from the Start of COVID-19 Pandemic. Washington, DC: Office of the Assistant Secretary for Planning and Evaluation, U.S. Department of Health and Human Services. July 28, 2020. https://www.aspe.hhs.gov/pdf-report/medicare-beneficiary-use-telehealth [Accessed 19 Sept 2021].

29. CMS Fast Facts, February 2020, https://www.cms.gov/Research-Statistics-Data-and-Systems/Statistics-Trends-and-Reports/CMS-Fast-Facts [Accessed 19 Sept 2021].

30. U.S. Department of Health & Human Services, Regional Offices, Figure 9.2. Source: https://www.hhs.gov/about/agencies/iea/regional-offices/index.html [Accessed 19 Sept 2021].

31. Figure 9.3. Source: Moy E, García MG, Bastian B, et al. Leading causes of death in nonmetropolitan and metropolitan areas—United States, 1999–2014. MMWR Surveill Summ 2017;66(No. SS-1) https://doi.org/10.15585/mmwr.ss6601a1 [Accessed 19 Sept 2021].

32. Figure 9.4: Percentage of potentially excess deaths among persons aged <80 years for five leading causes of death in nonmetropolitan and metropolitan areas, by year and public health region—National Vital Statistics System, United States, 2014. MMWR Surveill Summ 2017;66(No. SS-1) https://doi.org/10.15585/mmwr.ss6601a1 [Accessed 19 Sept 2021].

33. Source Figure 9.5: Kahan J., Lavista Ferres J. (2020). United States Broadband Usage Percentages Dataset. John Kahan Vice President, Chief Data Analytics Officer, Juan Lavista Ferres Chief Scientist, Microsoft AI for Good Research Lab. Please contact for questions. https://github.com/microsoft/USBroadbandUsagePercentages [Accessed 10 October 2021].

34. Hurt E. (2021). Georgia Rural Broadband Situation Worse Than FCC Maps Showed, New Mapping Underway Emma Hurt • Sep 13, 2019 https://www.wabe.org/georgia-rural-broadband-situation-worse-than-fcc-maps-showed-new-mapping-underway/ [Accessed 19 Sept 2021].

35. Federal Communications Commission Report on Lifeline Access https://docs.fcc.gov/public/attachments/DA-20-820A1_Rcd.pdf [Accessed 19 Sept 2021].

36. Federal Communications Commission Report on the Breakup of AT&T https://www.everycrsreport.com/files/19840810_IP0257A_38f13e13d3220c8f7c56fd39ad97d87f5fe325ed.pdf [Accessed 19 Sept 2021].

37. Ericsson, (2017). "Tracking IoT complexity with machine intelligence," Available [Online] https://www.ericsson.com/en/publications/ericsson-technology-review/archive/2017/tackling-iot-complexity-with-machine-intelligence (2020) [Accessed 19 Sept 2021].
38. Qi Zhao Q, Quo Y, Ye T, et al. (2021). Global, regional, and national burden of mortality associated with non-optimal ambient temperatures from 2000 to 2019: a three-stage modelling study. The Lancet Planetary Health Volume 5, ISSUE 7, e415-e425, July 01, 2021 Open Access Published: July, 2021 DOI: https://doi.org/10.1016/S2542-5196(21)00081-4 [Accessed 19 Sept 2021].
39. Geneva II, Cuzzo B, Fazili T, & Javaid W. (2019). Normal Body Temperature: A Systematic Review. Open forum infectious diseases, 6(4), ofz032. https://doi.org/10.1093/ofid/ofz032
40. Norman DC. (2000). Fever in the Elderly, (2000) Clinical Infectious Diseases, Volume 31, Issue 1, July 2000, Pages 148–151, https://doi.org/10.1086/313896
41. Planas D, Veyer, D, Baidaliuk A, et al. (2021). Reduced sensitivity of SARS-CoV-2 variant Delta to antibody neutralization. Nature 596, 276–280 (2021). https://doi.org/10.1038/s41586-021-03777-9
42. Welkoborsky HJ, Dietz A, Deitmer T. (2020). Laryngo-Rhino-Otologie. 2020 May 8; 99(6): 370-373 British Society of Otology; 2020. Guidance for undertaking otological procedures during COVID-19 pandemic. http://www.yoifos.com/sites/default/files/ent_uk_guidance_for_covid-19_for_otology_procedures._25-mar-2020.pdf
43. World Health Organization Deafness and Hearing Loss. https://www.who.int/news-room/fact-sheets/detail/deafness-and-hearing-loss [Accessed 19 Sept 2021].
44. The Lancet Commission on Hearing Loss https://globalhearinglosscommission.com/ [Accessed 19 Sept 2021].
45. World Health Organization Safe Listening Devices and Systems: A WHO-ITU Standard. https://apps.who.int/iris/bitstream/handle/10665/280085/9789241515276-eng.pdf [Accessed 19 Sept 2021].
46. Arnold ML, Hyer K, Small BJ, et al. (2019). Hearing Aid Prevalence and Factors Related to Use Among Older Adults From the Hispanic Community Health Study/Study of Latinos. JAMA Otolaryngol Head Neck Surg. 2019;145(6):501–508. doi:https://doi.org/10.1001/jamaoto.2019.0433 [Accessed 19 Sept 2021].
47. Hearing Link Facts about deafness & hearing loss. Hearing loss statistics in the U.K. https://www.hearinglink.org/your-hearing/about-hearing/facts-about-deafness-hearing-loss/ [Accessed 19 Sept 2019].
48. Brooks L. (2020). CNN; April 2, 2020. For the deaf or hard of hearing, face masks pose new challenges. https://edition.cnn.com/2020/04/02/opinions/deaf-hard-of-hearing-face-masks-brooks/index.html [Accessed 19 Sept 2021].
49. Shannon CE. (1948). A Mathematical Theory of Communication - The Bell System Technical Journal, 1948.
50. Gappmair W. (1999). IEEE Communications Magazine (Volume: 37, Issue: 4, April 1999) Page(s): 102 – 105 Date of Publication: April 1999 ISSN Information: INSPEC Accession Number: 6223109 DOI: https://doi.org/10.1109/35.755458
51. Updated estimates of coronavirus (COVID-19) related deaths by disability status, England: 24 January to 20 November 2020. https://www.ons.gov.uk/peoplepopulationandcommunity/birthsdeathsandmarriages/deaths/articles/coronaviruscovid19relateddeathsbydisabilitystatusenglandandwales/24januaryto20november2020 [Accessed 19 Sept 2021].
52. Centers for Disease Control and Prevention Risk for COVID-19 Infection, Hospitalization, and Death by Race/Ethnicity. https://www.cdc.gov/coronavirus/2019-ncov/covid-data/investigations-discovery/hospitalization-death-by-race-ethnicity.html [Accessed 19 Sept 2021].

53. Chidambaram P, Garfield R. (2020). KFF COVID-19 Has Claimed the Lives of 100,000 Long-Term Care Residents and Staff. *KFF*. Nov 25, 2020. Rachel Garfield Follow @RachelLGarfield on Twitter, and Tricia Neuman Follow @tricia newman on Twitter. https://www.kff.org/policy-watch/covid-19-has-claimed-the-lives-of-100000-long-term-care-residents-and-staff/ [Accessed 2 Oct 2021].
54. American Heart Association Devices that May Interfere with ICDs and Pacemakers. (2021). https://www.heart.org/en/health-topics/arrhythmia/prevention%2D%2Dtreatment-of-arrhythmia/devices-that-may-interfere-with-icds-and-pacemakers [Accessed 2 Oct 2021].
55. Masouros C, Sellathurai M, and Ratnarajah T. (2014). "Maximizing Energy-Efficiency in the Vector Precoded MU-MISO Downlink by Selective Perturbation," IEEE Trans. on Wireless Communications, pp. 4974-4984, Vol. 13, No. 9, Sep. 2014.
56. Payami S, Ghoraishi M, Dianati M, Sellathurai M. (2018). Hybrid Beamforming With a Reduced Number of Phase Shifters for Massive MIMO Systems, IEEE Transactions on Vehicular Technology, Year: 2018, Volume: 67, Issue: 6 Pages: 4843 - 4851.
57. Xue J, Biswas S, Cirik A, Du H, Yang Y, Ratnarajah T, and Sellathurai M. (2018). Transceiver design of optimum wirelessly powered full-duplex MIMO IOT devices, IEEE Transactions on Communications. 66, 5, p. 1955-1969 15 p. May 2018.
58. Measurement Lab (M-Lab) is led by teams based at Code for Science & Society, Google, Inc; and supported by partners around the world. M-Lab is an open source project with contributors from civil society organizations, educational institutions, and private sector companies, and is a fiscally sponsored project of Code for Science & Society. https://www.measurementlab.net/who/ [Accessed 10 October 2021].
59. Min C, Mao S, and Liu Y. (2014). "Big data: A survey." Mobile Networks and Applications 19, no. 2 (2014): 171-209.
60. Mukherjee A. (2015). "Physical-layer security in the internet of things: Sensing and communication confidentiality under resource constraints." *Proceedings of the IEEE* 103, no. 10 (2015): 1747-1761.
61. Mysore Balasubramanya N, Sellathurai M, Lampe L, and Vos G. (2018). "Overview of wireless communication technologies for the Internet of things (IoT).," Submitted to World Forum on Advances in Science, Engineering and Technology (Cambridge Summit 2018), Cambridge, U.K., 2017.
62. March 2021: About 8% of people who live in US long-term-care facilities have died of COVID-19—nearly 1 in 12. For nursing homes alone, the figure is nearly 1 in 10. https://covidtracking.com/analysis-updates/category/long-term-care [Accessed 2 Oct 2021].
63. Centers for Medicare & Medicaid Services. https://www.cms.gov/ [Accessed 2 Oct 2021].
64. Sjoding MW, Dickson RP, Iwashyna TJ, Gay SE, and Valley TS. (2020). Racial Bias in Pulse Oximetry Measurement. (2020). December 17, 2020 N Engl J Med 2020; 383:2477-2478. DOI: https://doi.org/10.1056/NEJMc2029240. [Accessed 2 Oct 2021].

Chapter 10
The Rise of IoMT: Leveraging a Polycentric Approach to Network-Connected Medical Device Management

Cory Brennan and Emily Dillon

Contents

10.1 Introduction

Every day, all around the world, physicians rely on advanced medical technology to assist in diagnosing patients' life-threatening conditions. In many instances, time is critical in such diagnoses. For example, if a patient's visual symptoms include slurred speech, numbness or weakness in limbs, and facial weakness, then the initial diagnosis may be a stroke. However, strokes can be caused by either internal bleeding or a blood clot in the brain. This means that the wrong treatment (e.g., blood thinning medication) is very risky and can result in a long-term disability or even death of the patient. Consider now, that without advanced medical technology to diagnose what is not outwardly visible, the consequences could be disastrous and deadly.

Clearly, medical devices have become critical components to the delivery of healthcare services, and with each passing breath these devices become more

C. Brennan (✉)
Hall Render, Indianapolis, IN, USA
e-mail: cbrennan@hallrender.com

E. Dillon
Indiana Health Information Exchange, Indianapolis, IN, USA

© Springer Nature Switzerland AG 2022
F. D. Hudson (eds.), *Women Securing the Future with TIPPSS for Connected Healthcare*, Women in Engineering and Science,
https://doi.org/10.1007/978-3-030-93592-4_10

technologically advanced. Now, most medical devices are part of what is called the Internet of Medical Things (IoMT), referring to an amalgamation of medical devices and applications that can connect to healthcare information technology systems using networking technologies. While this amalgamation makes our medical systems more sophisticated and the delivery of healthcare more technically capable, it also creates a threat to the essential availability of these devices we depend upon.

10.2   The Rise of IoMT

In 2019, there were an estimated 14.2 billion connected medical devices used in hospitals and healthcare provider offices across the United States [1]. This includes a vast amount of legacy medical equipment which typically requires frequent operational updates and presents a greater vulnerability to security threats. Even with an increasing number of IoMT, many health systems are woefully operating without a coordinated medical device security management plan, creating compliance and security gaps as devices go missing or become overdue for security patches and preventative maintenance.

Similarly, there has been a significant increase in the number of cyber attacks in the United States focused on IoMT. In August of 2019, 82% of healthcare organizations, IoMT manufacturers, and other organizations that use IoMT devices had faced a cyberattack focused on IoMT within the past year. The trend is disturbing because just 18% of healthcare providers reported an attack on their medical devices in October 2018 [2].

Cyberattacks targeting network-connected medical devices have an impact even more significant than a typical computer system. The potential impact of these types of attacks includes a remarkably heightened risk to patient safety, clinical outcomes, service disruptions, and loss of patient data leading to consequential compliance problems. In order to adequately counter a threat such as this, healthcare providers have been forced to increase the resources available to address these adverse impacts. Typically, these resources should include the people, processes, and tools required to manage a program focused solely on protecting the organization's IoMT and reducing the sublime risk to clinical operations.

10.3   Managing IoMT Security and Compliance

Unfortunately, there are many challenges involved with acquiring and developing adequate resources to manage IoMT security and compliance. Initially, the human aspect of the resources required is one of the greatest challenges. There is an underwhelming number of individuals with an understanding of the cybersecurity needs surrounding medical devices. Alas, due to the distinctive clinical nature of most medical devices, it is extremely challenging to manage them to typical cybersecurity best practices. Because of the sophisticated and complex clinical nature of the equipment, medical devices are typically managed by a clinical engineering professional. According to the American College of Clinical Engineering (ACCE), a Clinical Engineer is a professional who supports and advances patient care by applying engineering and managerial skills to healthcare technology.

The role of a Clinical Engineer has increasingly become the bridge between modern medicine and equally modern engineering. However, medical devices were originally designed as appliances that simply required general upkeep and preventative maintenance; thus, the clinical engineering practicum does not ordinarily include information technology and systems security requirements. This allows for an expertise gap in the area tottering between typical clinical engineering management of medical devices and an emphasis on cybersecurity protocols that is required to maintain IoMT in a secure manner.

Hence, decades of treating medical devices as physical assets rather than sophisticated equipment with software and computer components has created a process of management that underestimates the technological advancements of these devices. This is primarily where concern around the adequate "processes" component of the resources required to manage IoMT security and compliance becomes highly prevalent. Due to disparate and antiquated processes, it is very common to see network-connected medical devices in service for more than 15 years, especially considering the high dollar investment in certain IoMT systems.

10.4   Software as an Angle of Attack

The long life cycle of IoMT devices means that the underlying software operating system was likely "new" between 15 and 20 years ago. When these medical devices are examined, they are found to be running Microsoft Windows 98, 2000, or 2003—all of which are past the end of their lifetime and are no longer supported by the software vendor. Devices designed 15–20 years ago were generally not designed to be upgraded or patched and have limited memory or onboard storage. Cyberattackers are aware of this situation, which exposes legacy devices, while many of these vulnerabilities were corrected years ago with newer operating systems.

For example, healthcare organizations that still operate medical devices acquired in 2006 may find that those devices rely on legacy systems and insecure Wired Equivalent Privacy (WEP), a security protocol used in wireless networks, which requires the use of a single shared "key" to connect. In order to keep those devices operational, the organization must manage a separate WEP wireless network, resulting in a very high risk that a cyberattacker could compromise the network and, ultimately, the entire organization. Once a legacy medical device is compromised, those vulnerabilities allow medical devices to be susceptible to a variety of malware that may infiltrate and be present on an organization's network. Other information technology systems may not be vulnerable to such malware; however, medical devices could be and may also serve as the conduit or index device that would continually re-infect other vulnerable systems as they are brought onto the network.

Similarly, with over 10,000 medical device manufacturers, healthcare organizations find themselves struggling to develop and maintain an accurate IoMT inventory, and, more importantly, acknowledging which operating system each device is running and what vulnerabilities exist. As Dr. Christian Dameff, a cybersecurity researcher and informatics fellow at the University of California San Diego Health, stated, "When [the] WannaCry [ransomware attack] hit, hospitals were scrambling to figure out which medical devices were impacted. These devices are often black boxes to hospitals" [3].

However, when it comes to the tools available to a healthcare organization to leverage in support of a holistic IoMT security and compliance program, there is nearly an endless supply. Unfortunately, without the people and processes to manage and reinforce such tools, it is likely to be a futile use of resources to implement a tool that will not be appropriately utilized. For instance, typical information security teams are at a distinct disadvantage as an organization's customary network and end-point vulnerability scanning tool cannot be used to perform a scan on a medical device the way it is done for traditional IT systems. A medical device may not require access to the organization's network except when it is being utilized for direct patient care, and active vulnerability scans present the risk of causing a device to malfunction and cause patient harm.

Simply put, medical devices are an entirely different animal than traditional IT systems on the network. It is nearly impossible to preemptively discover an attack or the presence of malware on the device until the device has begun to lose critical functionality. And, when a medical device has lost critical functionality, the effect on hospital operations can become immediately apparent. If a piece of critical life-support equipment loses its functionality, the impact to patient care is remarkably unmistakable.

Similar to cybersecurity issues in any industry, the scope of impending threats and the diversity of the resources involved in protecting against those threats creates an environment that has become increasingly difficult to navigate and almost impossible to successfully regulate. A multi-level, multi-purpose, and multi-functional model of governance must be considered.

10.5   A Polycentric Approach

The idea of polycentricity is a fundamental concept in common scholarship that suggests a form of governance with multiple centers of semi-autonomous decision-making. If the decision-making centers take each other into account in competitive and comparative relationships, and have recourse to conflict resolution mechanisms, they may be regarded as a polycentric governance system.

The government is only one of many actors in a polycentric system. It is the "desire to address a common concern that ties together the various state and non-state actors in a system of polycentric governance" [4]. As history has shown, a single governmental entity is often incapable of managing something as malleable and intangible as cybersecurity. A polycentric approach recognizes that diverse organizations working at multiple levels can create different types of policies that can increase levels of cooperation and compliance [5].

A polycentric approach to governing cybersecurity has been championed by scholars as it challenges orthodoxy by demonstrating the benefits of self-organization, networking regulations "at multiple scales," and examining the extent to which national and private control can in some cases coexist with communal management [6]. A system of governance is fully polycentric if it facilitates creative problem-solving at all levels [7].

A common theme is the clear need for collaboration amongst the many different groups attempting to manage network-connected devices. This includes more than just the technical support groups within each individual hospital, but also the medical device equipment manufacturers, local and federal governments, and the international regulatory bodies concerned with this same issue. These communities must have a defined stake in the outcome to effectuate good governance, which can be accomplished by codifying and enforcing best practices.

Older medical equipment was also never intended to use anti-virus software. Standard end-point protection software, something ubiquitous to every workstation, can't be used to protect medical devices. Although encryption is used to protect workstations and is the foundation of a "safe harbor" defense, medical devices that contain patient data cannot benefit from the same technology. Hospitals that experience lost or stolen devices containing patient data must presume they have experienced a breach of patient confidentiality. Only recently have we seen medical device manufacturers include encryption as an option, but even then, safe harbor cannot be proven if generic user IDs and access controls are used.

In the past, the healthcare industry focused on medical device quality and safety risks predominantly as standalone devices rather than interoperable devices. Even with an increasing number of network-connected medical devices, many hospitals are still operating without a coordinated medical device security management plan, creating compliance and security gaps as devices go without essential patches and upgrades. These devices are essential for patient care delivery; however, due to their high susceptibility to technical exploits combined with a disjointed security management plan, hospital operations, and patient safety are at an increasingly high level of risk and noncompliance.

10.6   Guidance and Standards

In an attempt to assist Health Delivery Organizations (HDOs) with implementing a medical device security program and including network-connected medical devices into a health system's current security practices, prominent industry leaders have issued guidance and standards documents illustrating best practices. However, the majority of the recommendations in these guidance and/or standards, as listed in Table 10.1, are not enforceable by any active regulating or auditing bodies but are meant to encourage those responsible to bring medical device security to fruition.

Table 10.1 Guidance and standards

Date issued	Guidance/standard	Description
December 2000	Health Insurance Portability and Accountability Act (HIPAA) Privacy Rule—Final Rule	The Rule requires appropriate safeguards to protect the privacy of personal health information and sets limits and conditions on the uses and disclosures that may be made of such information without patient authorization.
January 2005	FDA Guidance: Cybersecurity for Networked Medical Devices Containing Off-the-Shelf (OTS) Software	A growing number of medical devices are designed to be connected to computer networks. Many of these networked medical devices incorporate off-the-shelf software that is vulnerable to cybersecurity threats such as viruses and worms. These vulnerabilities may represent a risk to the safe and effective operation of networked medical devices and typically require an ongoing maintenance effort throughout the product life cycle to assure an adequate degree of protection. The FDA issued this guidance to clarify how existing regulations, including the Quality System (QS) Regulation, apply to such cybersecurity maintenance activities.
July 2010	21 CFR part 11; Electronic Records, Electronic Signatures	Established to ensure that electronic records and electronic signatures can be trusted as much as paper records and ink signatures.
April 2012	21 CFR 820.30 Design Controls	Drafted to establish and maintain procedures to control the design of the device in order to ensure that specified design requirements are met.
July 2012	ISO/TR 80001-2-2-2012—Application of risk management for IT-networks incorporating medical devices—Part 2-2: Guidance for the disclosure and communication of medical device security needs, risks, and controls	A technical report that creates a framework for the disclosure of security-related capabilities and risks necessary for managing the risk in connecting medical devices to IT-networks and for the security dialog that surrounds the IEC 80001-1 risk management of IT-network connection.

(continued)

Table 10.1 (continued)

Date issued	Guidance/standard	Description
February 2014	NIST Cybersecurity Framework Version 1.0	The Framework is voluntary guidance, based on existing standards, guidelines, and practices for organizations to better manage and reduce cybersecurity risk. In addition to helping organizations manage and reduce risks, it was designed to foster risk and cybersecurity management communications amongst both internal and external organizational stakeholders.
October 2014	FDA Final Guidance: Content of Premarket Submissions for Management of Cybersecurity in Medical Devices	In addition to the specific recommendations contained in this FDA guidance, manufacturers are encouraged to address cybersecurity throughout the product life cycle, including during the design, development, production, distribution, deployment, and maintenance of the device.
October 2014	Center for Internet Security (CIS) and Medical Device Innovation, Safety and Security Consortium (MDISS)—The Security Benchmark Mapping Guidance	Configuration guidelines covering a multitude of different technologies developed in collaboration with healthcare providers, manufacturers, cybersecurity experts, and government entities for system hardening best practices.
June 2015	IEC 62304:2006—Medical device software life cycle processes	Focuses on software risk management, configuration management, and problem resolution. Accompanies ISO 14971 and ISO 13485 or 21 CFR Part 820.
December 2016	FDA Final Guidance: Postmarket Management of Cybersecurity in Medical Devices	This FDA guidance provides recommendations to industry for structured and comprehensive management of postmarket cybersecurity vulnerabilities for marketed and distributed medical devices throughout the product life cycle.
September 2017	UL2900-2-1 Safety Software Cybersecurity for Network Connectable Products	A cybersecurity testing standard for connected medical devices for structured penetration testing, evaluation of product source code, and analysis of software bill of materials.

(continued)

Table 10.1 (continued)

Date issued	Guidance/standard	Description
April 2018	FDA Medical Device Safety Action Plan	The Plan aims to improve patient safety, explore regulatory solutions, and advance medical device cybersecurity nationwide with five key areas of focus.
October 2018	FDA Draft Guidance: Content of Premarket Submissions for Management of Cybersecurity in Medical Devices	Provides recommendations to industry regarding cybersecurity device design, labeling, and documentation to be included in premarket submissions for devices with cybersecurity risk.
January 2019	HPH HSCC Medical Device and Health IT Joint Security Plan (JSP)	A set of recommendations for cybersecurity best practices for health providers. Experts identified the five most prevalent cyber threats and the ten best practices to deal with them which should lead to measurable risk reduction.
September 2019	AAMI TIR97:2019 Principles for medical device security: Postmarket risk management	A technical information report that provides guidance on how medical device manufacturers should manage security risk throughout the entire life cycle of a medical device.
September 2019	AAMI TIR57:2019—Principles for medical device security—Risk management	A report that provides guidance on specific methods manufacturers can use to perform information security management in the context of ISO 14971:2019. It is intended to be a companion to TIR97.
December 2019	MDCG 2019-16 Guidance on Cybersecurity for medical devices	This guidance aligns with the IMDRF guidance and explains both the premarket and postmarket requirements to help companies ensure an adequate balance between the benefits and risks during all of a device's possible operation modes.
March 2020	IMDRF WG/N60: Principles and practices for medical device cybersecurity	This document strives to harmonize medical device cybersecurity principles and best practices internationally. It's the first IMDRF document to focus on the topic, and it goes well beyond recommendations for manufacturers by also including advice on reducing cybersecurity risks to healthcare providers, regulatory, and users.

10.7   A Holistic Approach

Security experts have been advocating for a more holistic approach when it comes to properly managing connected medical devices [7]. This includes aligning organizational resources needed to address the problem. Security officers, privacy officers, Chief Information Officers (CIOs), procurement, clinicians, physical security, and clinical engineering cannot unilaterally implement solutions, but all have a critical role in management processes. While an all-inclusive style is ideal, the array of overlapping standards and regulations makes the selection process difficult for these typically siloed groups. Clinical engineering departments and Information Security teams tend to take a different approach to security practices which is reflected within the frameworks and guidance documents issued for medical device security.

For example, the National Institute of Standards and Technology (NIST) cybersecurity framework was issued in 2014 as a way to "focus on using business drivers to guide cybersecurity activities and considering cybersecurity risks as part of the organization's risk management processes." The NIST Framework will help an organization to align and prioritize its cybersecurity activities with its business/mission requirements, risk tolerances, and resources. However, this approach was established with more traditional IT assets in mind and wasn't fully translated over medical device assets until more recent years, thus leading to a lack of understanding from a clinical engineering perspective. When taking the clinical engineering perspective into account, there is a whole other set of regulations and standards to consider when it comes to safely managing medical devices. Outside of federal and state regulation requirements for properly maintaining medical devices for safe use, many hospitals and health systems must follow strict guidelines from accrediting bodies, the most popular being that of The Joint Commission. Although The Joint Commission does not have specifics in place for addressing network-connected medical devices from a security standpoint, which does illustrate an overall gap in how Clinical Engineering departments approach safely maintaining a medical device throughout the device life cycle, they do have standards in place that facilitate security best practices.

The Joint Commission standards include maintaining an up-to-date medical device asset inventory, which includes documenting medical devices that are considered Cannot Locate (CNL) and responding to product notices and recalls [9]. Although inventory standards are not cybersecurity focused, they support the bigger picture by allowing Information Security teams to quickly and appropriately respond to an incident by having an accurate inventory which should include items like network capability, operating system version, MAC address, IP address, etc. Additionally, having a process established to ensure that hazard and recall information is received, communicated to the necessary personnel, and required action is taken as well as documented, is another way the standards aid in network security and patient safety. The FDA's Medical Device Reporting regulation is "a mechanism for FDA and manufacturers to identify and monitor significant adverse events involving medical devices" (Center for Devices and Radiological Health). Traditionally, hazards and recalls were related to break/fix malfunctions; however, these alerts also include cybersecurity related incidents and vulnerabilities.

Having an established medical device inventory also assists from a compliance standpoint. This is due to the fact that medical devices that may contain sensitive information or protected health information, but cannot be found within the health systems during scheduled maintenance intervals, may require escalation steps in accordance with the HIPAA Security Rule.

10.8 The Future

The Internet of Medical Things (IoMT) is growing every day, as is the related cybersecurity risk. We need a holistic polycentric approach to have the most effective network-connected medical device management. Leaders in the industry including federal agencies, such as the FDA, DHS, and NIST, are providing effective guidance and frameworks to support this effort. We have the responsibility to deliver on the promise of safe and secure connected healthcare, and this approach will enable that to be our future reality.

References

1. https://www.forbes.com/sites/forbestechcouncil/2019/03/01/prognosis-for-health-care-iot-six-predictions-for-2019/?sh=694d440efddd
2. Hewitt C, Blacketer C (2020) Compliance-driven risk reduction strategies for medical devices. Compliance Today - January 2020. https://compliancecosmos.org/compliance-driven-risk-reduction-strategies-medical-devices#footnotes
3. Wetsman N. (2010) Health Care's Huge Cybersecurity Problem. Cyberattacks Aren't Just Going After Your Data. The Verge. Apr 4, 2019. https://www.theverge.com/2019/4/4/18293817/cybersecurity-hospitals-health-care-scan-simulation
4. Ostrom, Elinor (2010) Beyond Markets and States: Polycentric Governance of Complex Economic Systems. American Economic Review, 100(3):641-72. https://www.aeaweb.org/articles/pdf/doi/10.1257/aer.100.3.641
5. Keohane R, Victor D. (2011). The Regime Complex for Climate Change. Perspectives on Politics, 9(1), 7-23. doi:https://doi.org/10.1017/S1537592710004068
6. Shackelford S. (2016) Protecting Intellectual Property And Privacy In The Digital Age: The Use Of National Cybersecurity Strategies To Mitigate Cyber Risk. Chapman Law Review. https://dlc.dlib.indiana.edu/dlc/bitstream/handle/10535/10251/SSRN-id2635035.pdf?sequence=1&isAllowed=y
7. McGinnis M. (2011) Costs and Challenges of Polycentric Governance. Workshop in Political Theory and Policy Analysis and Department of Political Science, Indiana University, Revised February 16, 2011. https://mcginnis.pages.iu.edu/core.pdf

8. Zhang M, Raghunathan A, Jha N. (2013) MedMon: Securing Medical Devices Through Wireless Monitoring and Anomaly Detection. IEEE Transactions On Biomedical Circuits And Systems, Vol. 7, No. 6, December 2013. https://web.archive.org/web/20160508141752id_/http://www.utdallas.edu:80/~gxm112130/CE7V80SP16/medmon.pdf
9. The Joint Commission. (2020) What equipment is required to be included in a medical equipment inventory and how is high-risk equipment and maintenance strategies determined? The Joint Commission. Reference EC.02.04.01. Last updated on June 01, 2020 https://www.jointcommission.org/standards/standard-faqs/critical-access-hospital/environment-of-care-ec/000001244/

Index

Printed in the United States
by Baker & Taylor Publisher Services